A. G. Brown

Nerve Cells and Nervous Systems

An Introduction to Neuroscience

With 212 Figures

Springer-Verlag
London Berlin Heidelberg New York
Paris Tokyo Hong Kong

A. G. Brown, BSc, MB ChB, PhD, FIBiol, FRSE
Professor of Veterinary Physiology, University of Edinburgh,
Summerhall, Edinburgh EH9 1QH, UK

ISBN 3-540-19637-4 Springer-Verlag Berlin Heidelberg New York
ISBN 0-387-19637-4 Springer-Verlag New York Berlin Heidelberg

British Library Cataloguing in Publication Data
Brown, Alan G. *1940–*
Nerve cells and nervous systems.
1. Mammals. Nervous system
I. Title
599.0188
ISBN 3-540-19637-4

Library of Congress Cataloging-in-Publication Data
Brown, A. G. (Alan Geoffrey)
Nerve cells and nervous systems: an introduction to neuroscience/A. G. Brown.
p. cm. Includes bibliographical references and index.
ISBN 0-387-19637-4 (alk. paper). – ISBN 3-540-19637-4 (alk. paper)
1. Neurophysiology. I. Title.
[DNLM: 1. Neurons. 2. Nervous System. WL 102.5 B877n]
QP355.2.B76 1991 591.1'88—dc20
DNLM/DLC
For Library of Congress   90-10412
                                                                CIP

Typeset by Best-set Typesetter Ltd., Hong Kong
Printed by The Bath Press, UK
2128/3830-543210   Printed on acid-free papger

Preface

For the past 15 years I have given a set of Introductory Lectures to a Master of Science course. Initially the course led towards an MSc in Neurophysiology, but later the course title was changed to an MSc in Neuroscience, to reflect more accurately the content of the course as it had changed over the years. This textbook has its origins in my notes for those Introductory Lectures.

Students arriving to start the MSc were from a wide background. Some had received a professional training, in Veterinary Medicine or Nursing, others had come from the biological sciences, with degrees in Physiology, Biochemistry, Psychology, Zoology etc., and a few came from the physical sciences. Because of these different backgrounds, the individual students varied widely in their knowledge of the nervous system: some knew quite a lot of neuroanatomy and/or neurophysiology, others were weak in these areas but had a broader knowledge of animal biology or a detailed knowledge of biochemistry etc. A few students knew very little biology at all. The aim of my Introductory Lectures was to present the students with some general principles of the organization and function of the nervous system.

The aim of presenting general principles is also the aim of this textbook. I have attempted to present these principles in the context of experimental neuroscience. Neuroscience is essentially an experimental science, and our current understanding is based on the interpretation of experimental observations. Wherever possible I have included indications of how this understanding has been derived from experiments and have also illustrated the text with figures from original papers. In my opinion, the sooner students come to terms with the original literature the better, and I hope that by including such illustrations the reader will be encouraged to investigate that literature. Furthermore, in these times when it is often considered unfashionable to read anything that is more than 5 years old, I have unashamedly included material that can be considered classical, in the sense that the experiments were not only excellent in design and execution but have had important repercussions. For those readers who wish to know a little more, often more about experimental techniques, a series of "Boxes", amplifying certain material, is included.

In an introductory text of this sort a lot of selection of material is inevitable. Some of the selection reflects my personal interests and biases. I have deliberately avoided, as far as possible, a "systems" approach. There is, for example, no pedagogic presentation of the anatomy and physiology of the various sensory pathways in mammals or of the control of posture and locomotion, as is found in the standard medical texts. Rather, I have developed the material from the single neuron level, through the interactions between two neurons, to small groups of neurons, and then considered particular functional attributes of nervous systems. This approach, I believe, fills a gap in the available introductory texts, although there are undoubtedly some excellent books available, such as *From Neuron to*

Brain by Kuffler, Nichols and Martin and *Neurobiology* by Shepherd, as well as the much larger *Principles of Neural Science* by Kandel and Schwartz.

I hope that this book will be useful to anyone starting a study of the nervous system, at both the undergraduate and immediate postgraduate levels. But, more than anything, I hope that this introductory text will encourage readers to pursue further the fascinating subject of neuroscience.

Acknowledgements

I should like to thank Heather Anderson, Debbie Hall and Colin Warwick for preparing the large number of illustrations and Michael Jackson and his colleagues at Springer-Verlag for encouragement and advice. Finally, I thank my past students for their interest, difficult questions and many discussions, which have really been the inspiration responsible for this book.

A. G. Brown
Edinburgh, 1990

Contents

1 Introduction to Nerve Cells and Nervous Systems

The essence of nervous system function is control by means of communication. Unicellular (acellular) organisms, such as amoeba or paramecium, can perform every function necessary to sustain their lives. They can take in nutrients from their external environment, organize their metabolic reactions, excrete waste products into their external environment and move towards or away from entities in their environment, that is, they can perform simple behavioural adjustments to that environment. In multicellullar organisms the constitutent cells have become specialized into organs and tissues for carrying out specific functions, such as digestion and assimilation of foodstuffs, respiration, circulation of the blood to carry oxygen, metabolites and hormones etc. to the tissues, reproduction and so on. The nervous system and the endocrine system together carry out the functions of control and communication, between the various organs and tissues of the body and between the organism and its external environment. In this book we shall consider the structure and function of the nervous system, with special emphasis on vertebrate animals. But invertebrates will be discussed, especially where they illustrate a particularly important principle of neuroscience or where the experimental evidence is compelling. The endocrine system will also be mentioned where appropriate, since there is the closest relationship between nervous and endocrine mechanisms. Some nerve cells function as endocrine cells, and some endocrine cells are modified nerve cells. The main difference in action between nervous and endocrine systems relates to the directness of control.

The Nervous System and Control

The nervous system, along with the endocrine system, controls the organism's internal environment. In fact, for the most part, the nervous system also controls the endocrine system. Changes in the internal environment are monitored by sensory receptors. Control over the internal environment is achieved by control of the various effector cells of the body: the smooth muscle of the viscera, the cardiac muscle and the various gland cells. Furthermore, the nervous system also monitors the external environment by means of sensory receptors (sense organs) and, at the simplest level, reacts to those changes so as to maintain the internal environment within physiological bounds (e.g. in the dog by panting in response to increased external temperature that causes the body temperature to rise).

Interaction with the external environment can lead to complex behaviour. The nervous system controls the organism's skeletal (striated) muscle and therefore controls the movement of its body in space, for example away from potential harm, or towards potential gain such as a meal or a member of the opposite sex.

In the more complex organisms this interaction with the external environment is further developed. The animal does not just react to the environment passively, but actively explores it. Such exploration is well-developed in mammals and probably most highly developed in primate species. Young mammals spend a considerable time playing, which is really an active exploration of the environment. Human beings may spend most of their lives playing, for example in highly developed civilizations certain sections of the community are rewarded for playing (artists and scientists). This development leads to control over the external environment in humans to a remarkable extent.

An important function of nervous systems that greatly increases the ability of an organism to survive is that they are capable of learning. Learning, and its closely associated function of memory, allow an organism to change its behaviour as a result of experience.

The Nervous System and Communication

The nervous system is able to exert control over the internal and external environment because of its remarkable ability to communicate. Nerve cells, which make up the nervous system, communicate with each other and with muscle and gland cells. Not only that, nervous systems communicate with one another too. Thus in both invertebrate and vertebrate species highly organized communication about the external environment can occur, e.g. the well-known "dance" mechanism in honey bees for communicating the distance

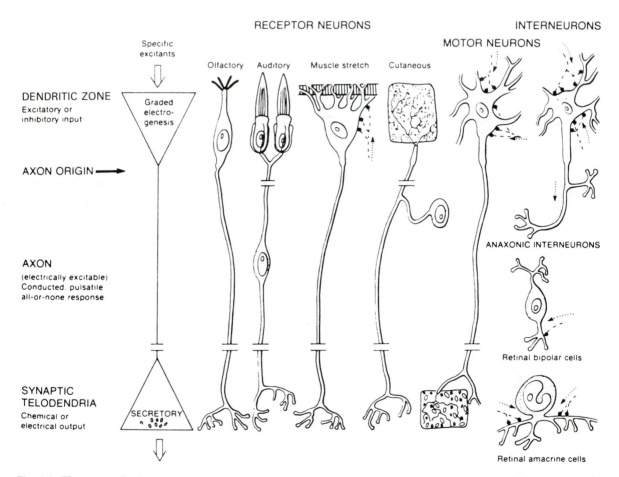

Fig. 1.1. The "generalized" neuron and a variety of neuronal types. On the *left* is a diagram of the generalized neuron that relates structural neuronal components to functional properties. On the *right* is a series of simplified diagrams of the structure of a variety of neurons. Note that the position of the cell body (soma), which contains the nucleus, does not have a constant relationship to the functional geometry of the generalized neuron. (Reproduced with permission from Bodian 1967.)

and direction of a source of nectar or pollen, or communication within a pack of wolves during a hunt. This communication is especially well developed in man. The evolution of language has allowed learned experience to be passed between members of the human race and between members of different generations in contact with one another (some other species can also pass on experience by example), but more than this, the development of written languages has meant that learning can be passed on to members of the species not yet born. The current important technological changes in information transmission using electronic communication methods will have even more far-reaching effects on human interactions across distance and time.

Nerve Cells

The active components of nervous systems are the individual nerve cells or neurons. The human nervous system contains somewhere in the order of 10^{20} neurons. These neurons are the units that communicate with one another and with the various effector organs. The essential aims of neuroscience are to understand (1) how single neurons operate, (2) how one nerve cell communicates with another or with an effector cell, (3) how groups of neurons are interconnected to form component parts of the nervous system, (4) how neurons within a group interact with one another, (5) how groups of neurons interact with one another, (6) how nervous systems develop and how the interconnections are made, and ultimately (7) how whole nervous systems operate and control animal behaviour. In the following chapters we shall consider these various problems. Considerable advances in knowledge have been made concerning items 1–3, some advances in items 4–6 and rather little as yet in item 7. Before considering these items in more detail, some basic background information about the structure and function of nervous systems will be required. An introduction to the experimental approaches available for studying the structure and function of single neurons and their interconnexions in nervous systems is indicated in Boxes 1.1 and 1.2.

The Generalized Neuron

Neurons, in order to carry out their function of communication, need to receive input from other neurons, to balance (integrate) this input, to produce a signal that reflects this balance, and to send

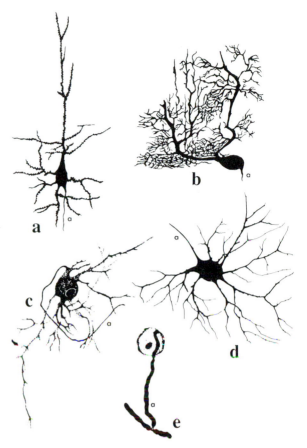

Fig. 1.2a–e. Examples of verbebrate neurons. **a** A pyramidal cell from the cerebral cortex. The dendrites are covered in spinous processes. In this, and the other parts of the figure, *a* is the axon. **b** A Purkinje cell from the cerebellar cortex. **c** A sympathetic postganglionic neuron. **d** An alpha-motoneuron from the spinal cord. **e** A dorsal root ganglion cell. Note the absence of dendrites. In all of these drawings the axon is incomplete. (Reproduced with permission from Willis and Grossman 1973.)

the signal to the neuron's contact points with other neurons or effector cells. Fig. 1.1 (left) shows a concept of a generalized neuron in which these various functions have been anatomically separated, and compares this generalized neuron with a variety of vertebrate neuronal types. As may be seen, such anatomical separation is indeed commonly found in some vertebrate neurons, but it is by no means standard in vertebrate nerve cells and is not found in invertebrate neurons (Figs. 1.2, 1.3).

Resting Membrane Potential

Like all other cells in an organism, neurons have a cell membrane which separates the contents of

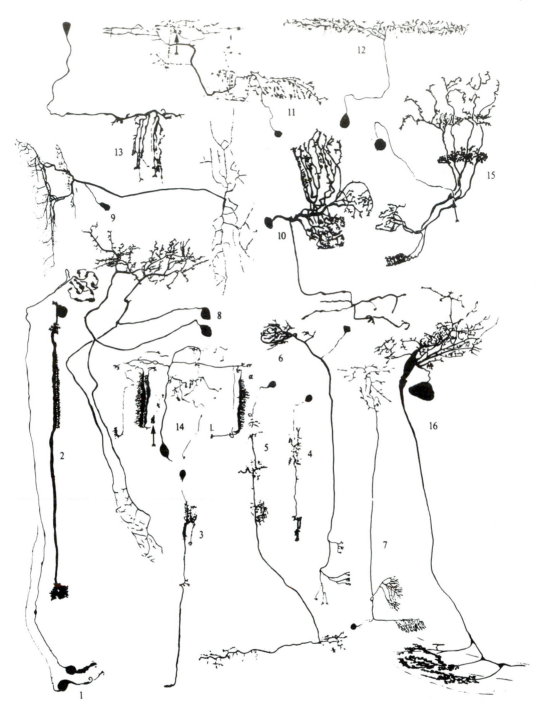

Fig. 1.3. Examples of invertebrate neurons, taken from the nervous systems of various flies. The numbers indicate different anatomical types of cells. Note the cell bodies (somata, perikaria) set off from the rest of the neurons. (Reproduced from Strausfeld 1976.)

the cell from the extracellular environment. There is a separation of electric charge (ions) across this membrane such that the inside of the cell is held at a negative potential (of some tens of milli-volts) compared with the outside, which is taken to be at earth (zero) potential. Most signalling in the nervous system involves changes in the membrane potential of neurons.

Receptive Function

Neurons contact each other at sites called synapses, where subcellular specializations occur in both the presynaptic and postsynaptic cell. Neurons communicate with each other in one of two ways, either by means of the passage of electrical current (produced by movement of ions) or by the release of chemical transmitters from the presynaptic neuron onto the postsynaptic target, which either cause changes in the permeability of the postsynaptic cell's membrane to ions or alternatively affect that cell's metabolism. These neuronal communications may have one of two actions on the target cell: they may increase the cell's excitability (excitation) or they may decrease its excitability (inhibition). Usually, excitation causes a depolarization of the target cell. Inhibitory action may cause a hyperpolarization, a depolarization or no change in membrane potential of the target cell, but in any event it effectively clamps the membrane potential at some level that makes excitation more difficult.

Integrative Function

The excitatory and inhibitory responses of neurons are summed. This activity, in vertebrate neurons, takes place within the receptive components of the neuron, the dendrites and the cell body or soma.

Impulse Initiation

In many neurons, but by no means in all and perhaps only in a minority, nerve impulses are set up if the neuron's membrane potential is depolarized sufficiently to reach a certain threshold level. These impulses are all-or-nothing events, that is they are all the same size and shape. In neurons that are capable of initiating impulses the information that such cells pass on to their targets is in the form of a frequency code.

Conduction

The nerve impulses travel (are conducted) actively along the neuron's axon or nerve fibre. In those nerve cells that do not produce impulses, the potential change caused by the input is conducted passively to the terminals of the axon.

Transmission

As mentioned above, transmission between two neurons can be either electrical or chemical in character. In electrical transmission one neuron influences another by passive electrical means. In chemical transmission the potential change in one neuron leads to the release of a chemical neurotransmitter that diffuses to the other neuron, combines with specific receptor molecules on its membrane and leads to changes in the permeability of the membrane to particular species of ions, or to changes in the cell's metabolism.

The Anatomy of Neurons

The generalized neuron discussed above is a convenient abstraction. Few neurons bear much resemblance to it. Perhaps the nearest are certain vertebrate neurons in the brain and spinal cord (see Fig. 1.2). These nerve cells consist of a cell body, or soma, that contains the nucleus of the cell. From the soma arises a tree-like series of branches, the dendrites, and also the nerve fibre or axon (the axon may arise from one of the dendrites). The first part of the axon, the initial segment, is usually the site of origin of the nerve impulses elicited by the cell. The dendrites and soma form the receptive surface for incoming messages from other neurones, and it is in the soma that the balancing of inhibitory and excitatory actions is performed. The axon may be short (a few tens of micrometres) or long (several metres in large animals), but ultimately breaks up into a series of branches that may divide repeatedly and finally, in their terminal arborization (telodendria), form synaptic boutons which are the sites of transmission to the next cell in the series.

The anatomy of vertebrate neurons may depart considerably from this form. There may be no obvious axon, or no obvious dendritic tree. Invertebrate neurons (see Fig. 1.3) have a different structure in that the soma is set off from the rest of the neuron and the neuronal processes carry out the receptive, integrative and transmission functions, and in many cases the impulse initiation and conduction functions too.

Ultrastructure of Neurons

Like all animal cells, neurons contain the machinery for life (Fig. 1.4). This machinery includes the usual organelles found in cells: a nucleus with a nucleolus, mitochondria, endoplasmic reticulum and Golgi apparatus, and a cytoskeleton of tubular structures – the neurofilaments, the microtubules and the microfilaments. The cytoskeleton is responsible for the shape of the neuron and also for the transport of many substances (proteins)

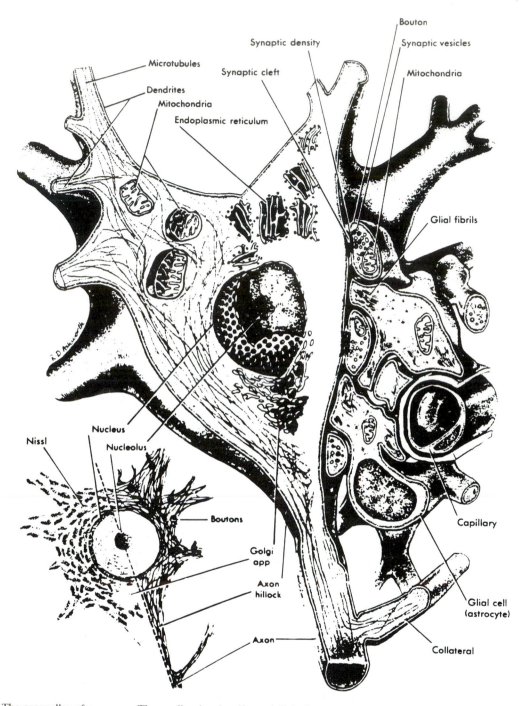

Fig. 1.4. The organelles of a neuron. The smaller drawing (*lower left*) indicates the organelles as seen using light microscopy after staining with basic aniline dyes (to *left* of broken line) or after staining with heavy metals (to *right* of broken line), which also indicates the synaptic boutons from other neurons. The larger drawing shows structures demonstrable with the electron microscope. (Reproduced with permission from Willis and Grossman 1973.)

and organelles from one part of the neuron to another. Neurons which communicate with their target cells by means of chemical transmission also contain synaptic vesicles, which can be of different sizes and shapes. Synaptic vesicles accumulate on the presynaptic side of synaptic contacts; indeed, their location may be used to determine which is the presynaptic component of a synapse.

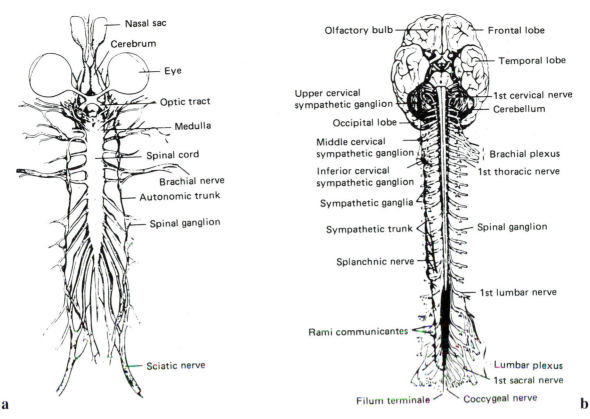

Fig. 1.5a,b. General plan of the vertebrate nervous system. **a** Frog; **b** human. Both are viewed from the ventral aspect. (Reproduced with permission from Eckert and Randall 1978.)

The General Plan of Nervous Systems

In all but the simplest multicellular animals the nervous system can be considered to consist of two main parts, the central nervous system and the peripheral nervous system. The central nervous system contains a large number of neuronal somata and their processes, which in vertebrates make up the brain within the skull and the spinal cord within the vertebral canal (Fig. 1.5). In invertebrates the central nervous system consists of a series of ganglia, containing nerve cells and their processes, that run in pairs along the length of the animal (Fig. 1.6). In the more complex invertebrates a number of ganglia at the head end of the animals fuse together to form a brain or head ganglion (Fig. 1.6). In all animals the brain or head ganglion is especially concerned with the special sense organs, including those for vision, audition, olfaction etc., situated on the head. Within the brain, spinal cord and (in inverte-

brates) the ganglia most of the neuronal processing takes place.

The peripheral nervous system consists of several sets of nerve fibres: those with cell bodies situated within the central nervous system and whose axons run to innervate muscles; or other neurons outside the central nervous system; nerve fibres running from peripheral sense organs and whose cell bodies are usually situated outside the central nervous system, often in ganglia such as the dorsal root ganglia or cranial nerve ganglia in vertebrates; and nerve cells whose cell bodies and processes are completely outside the central nervous system. Thus in mammals the peripheral nervous system consists of three parts, a somatic component, a visceral component and an enteric component. The somatic component is made up of (1) an afferent (or incoming) component consisting of nerve fibres that innervate sense organs in the skin, muscles, tendons and subcutaneous tissue and whose somata are located outside the central nervous system in ganglia and (2) an efferent (or outgoing) component consisting of nerve

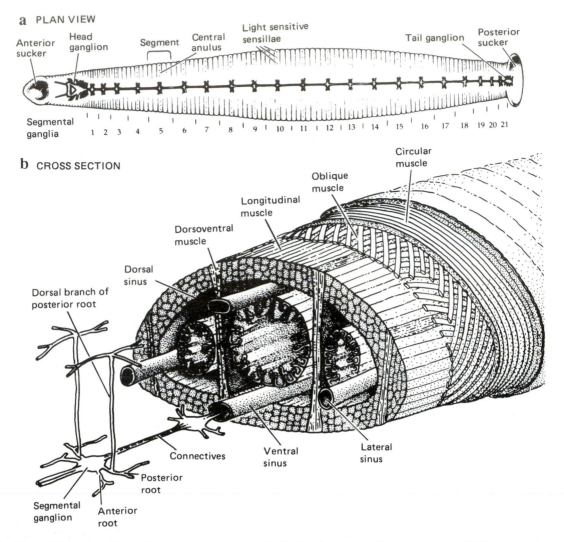

a PLAN VIEW

b CROSS SECTION

Fig. 1.6a–e. Examples of invertebrate nervous systems. **a,b** The leech. **a** Shows the general plan with 21 segmental ganglia, and head and tail ganglia; **b** Shows the ventral nerve cord running between the ganglia. **c,d,e** The sea snail, *Aplysia*. **c** Shows the general plan of the nervous system; **d** and **e** indicate identified neurons in the abdominal ganglia. (Reproduced with permission (**a**, **b**) and modified (**c**, **d**, **e**) from Kuffler et al. 1984.)

fibres that innervate somatic (skeletal) muscle and whose nerve cell bodies are located in the central nervous system. The visceral component likewise consists of a sensory or afferent part and a motor or efferent part, the sensory part running from sense organs in the viscera (the internal organs and tissues such as the heart, stomach, lungs, uterus etc.) and having somata in ganglia, and the motor part consisting of nerve fibres with cell bodies in either the central nervous system or in well-formed ganglia or in the viscera themselves. The efferent visceral component of the vertebrate peripheral nervous system is also known as the peripheral autonomic nervous system (Fig. 1.7). The enteric nervous system consists of several sets of neurons and their processes in the wall of the gastrointestinal tract and is capable, by itself, of regulating reflex activity of the gut, although it is normally under control from the autonomic nervous system.

The Neuroglia

The nervous system contains another group of cells in addition to neurons. These are the neuro-

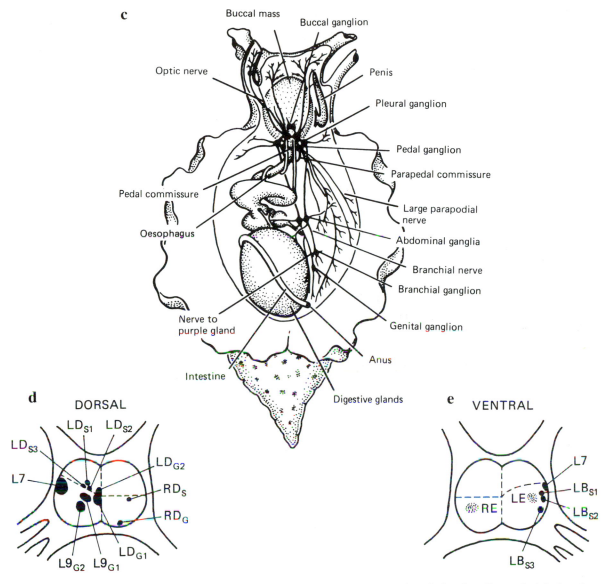

c

Buccal mass
Buccal ganglion
Optic nerve
Penis
Pleural ganglion
Pedal ganglion
Parapedal commissure
Pedal commissure
Large parapodial nerve
Oesophagus
Abdominal ganglia
Branchial nerve
Branchial ganglion
Nerve to purple gland
Genital ganglion
Intestine
Anus
Digestive glands

d DORSAL
LD_{S1} LD_{S2}
LD_{S3}
LD_{G2}
L7
RD_S
RD_G
LD_{G1}
$L9_{G2}$ $L9_{G1}$

e VENTRAL
L7
LB_{S1}
LE
LB_{S2}
RE
LB_{S3}

glia or glial cells. In the mammalian central nervous system they are far more numerous than the neurons. They are generally small cells and do not partake in the active generation of signals (impulses), nor do they have a direct role to play in the information processing functions of the nervous system. Some, however, are influenced by neuronal activity and help regulate the ionic environment of the neurons and also remove some transmitters released by neurons.

A number of functions for glia are known or suggested. These include:

1. Support for the neurons of the central nervous system, that is, to act in the same way as connective tissue in other parts of the body.

2. Phagocytosis of dead cells and debris after nervous system injury.

3. Ionic regulation and transmitter removal.

4. A role in development for guiding growing neurons along appropriate paths.

5. The formation of an insulating cover, the myelin sheath, around certain axons in the central nervous system.

The glial cells can be divided into two major classes, the macroglia (astrocytes, oligodendrocytes and ependymal cells) and the microglia, which act as phagocytes. Astrocytes are star-shaped cells which take up excess potassium (K^+) ions from the extracellular space. Other astrocytes

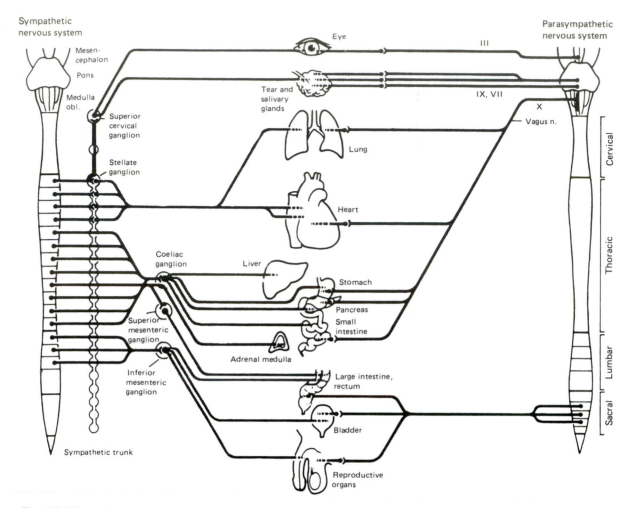

Fig. 1.7. The peripheral autonomic nervous system of mammals. The sympathetic component is on the *left* and the parasympathetic component on the *right*. The sympathetic innervation of blood vessels, sweat glands and piloerector muscles is not shown. (Reproduced from Schmidt and Thews 1983.)

are capable of removing neurotransmitters (gamma-aminobutyric acid and serotonin) from the region of the synaptic cleft. Astrocytes may also have other, nutritive, functions, but little is known about this. Oligodendrocytes are responsible for forming the myelin sheath around the axons of certain cells in the central nervous system. In the peripheral nervous system this role is carried out by Schwann cells, which have a different origin to the glia.

Regulation of the External Environment of Neurons

In order for neurons to carry out their functions of communication and control they need to be in

a relatively stable environment. But they also need an adequate supply of oxygen and metabolites and need to have carbon dioxide and waste products removed from their vicinity. In vertebrates the brain and spinal cord are surrounded by a special fluid – the cerebrospinal fluid (CSF) – formed from blood plasma by active secretory processes in special capillary loops, the choroid plexuses, which protrude into the cavities of the brain, the ventricles (Fig. 1.8). Unlike blood plasma, CSF is almost protein free. The CSF around the brain and spinal cord is in communication with the CSF in the ventricles (and their continuation in the spinal cord, the spinal canal). The CSF is continually formed and drains back into the blood via the arachnoid villi into the superior sagittal sinus and other venous sinuses.

The CSF surrounding the brain and spinal cord is contained within two connective tissue sheets,

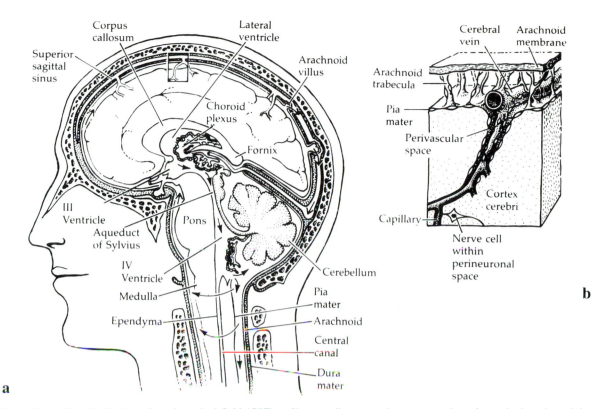

Fig. 1.8a,b. The distribution of cerebrospinal fluid (CSF). **a** Shows a diagrammatic representation of a sagittal section of the human skull. The CSF is formed in the choroid plexus and drains via the arachnoid villi into the venous blood in the sagittal sinus. The *arrows* show the direction of flow of the CSF. **b** Shows an enlarged view of the box outlined in **a**. (Reproduced with permission from Kuffler et al. 1984.)

an outer, thick, dura mater and an inner, thin, dual sheet, the pia-arachnoid. This outer CSF provides a shock-absorbing system that prevents mechanical injury to the nervous system during sudden accelerations and decelerations. The major blood vessels run between the two components of the pia-arachnoid, the arachnoid membrane and the pia mater, and give off smaller vessels that run into the central nervous system carrying a sheath of pia mater and CSF with them. The CSF does not bathe the neurons and neuroglia but is separated from it by a layer of basement membrane. The extracellular fluid of the brain is contained within very small intercellular clefts. Between the neurons and neuroglia, on the one hand, and the blood in the brain capillaries, on the other, there is (1) the extracellular fluid, (2) a basement membrane, (3) the CSF and (4) the endothelium of the capillaries.

There are barriers to the free passage of substances from the blood into the extracellular fluid of the brain. It is conventional to consider these as a blood–CSF barrier and a CSF–brain barrier. These barriers are not complete. In certain areas peptide hormones can gain access to the brain and

this is important in the communication between the endocrine and nervous systems. Infection of the meninges (the dura mater, arachnoid and pia mater) and encephalitis also lead to increased permeability of the barriers, as may tumour formation in the brain. This increased permeability can aid treatment by allowing drugs, which are normally kept out of the nervous system, into the affected parts.

Summary

1. The essence of nervous system function is control by communication. The nervous and endocrine systems together control the internal environment of the organism and allow the organism to interact with the external environment.

2. The active components of nervous systems are the individual nerve cells or neurons. Neurons are of many different shapes and sizes but all have receptive, integrative and transmission func-

tions that allow them to communicate with other neurons and with the effector cells – muscle fibres and gland cells. Many neurons are also able to initiate and conduct nerve impulses, allowing them to communicate efficiently over relatively long distances within an animal. Transmission between neurons or between neurons and effector cells may be electrical or chemical, and may have excitatory or inhibitory actions.

3. In all but the simplest multicellular animals, the nervous system consists of central and peripheral components. The central nervous system of vertebrates consists of the brain and spinal cord. In invertebrates the central nervous system consists of a chain of paired ganglia, some of which may be fused together at the head end to form a brain. The cell bodies of neurons are generally located in the central nervous system. The peripheral nervous system consists of nerve fibres (axons) passing to the central nervous system (afferent fibres) or away from it (efferent fibres). The afferent fibres arise from sensory receptors on the surface and within the body. Their cell bodies are usually outside the central nervous system in ganglia. The efferent fibres consist of motor fibres supplying the skeletal muscles and other fibres forming part of the peripheral autonomic nervous system that controls the activity of cardiac and smooth muscle and gland cells. The peripheral autonomic nervous system contains ganglia where connexions are made between different neurons and where the cell bodies of (postganglionic) neurons are located. The enteric nervous system in the wall of the gut is a third component of the peripheral nervous system.

4. In addition to neurons, there are other cells in the nervous system – the neuroglia. The neuroglia have important functions during the development of the nervous system and following injury, and also play a role in maintaining the ability of the neurons to function by controlling their ionic environment and removing excess neurotransmitters.

5. The ionic environment of neurons is also controlled by a system of barriers that prevents free passage of substances from the blood into the extracellular space of the brain and spinal cord. CSF is formed within the cavities of the brain and also surrounds it, forming a shock-absorbing system. CSF is formed by epithelial cells surrounding special capillaries (the choroid plexus), and the cells act as a barrier for ions and various molecules. Necessary substances are brought to the brain by arterial blood, and waste

products are removed in venous blood. The endothelial cells of the brain capillaries provide another barrier to free passage of substances.

BOX 1.1

EXPERIMENTAL METHODS FOR STUDYING THE STRUCTURE OF NERVOUS SYSTEMS

The microscopical structure of nerve cells may be examined after staining thin sections of fixed nervous tissue with a variety of stains. The Nissl method, using basic aniline dyes, stains the ribosomal RNA of the rough endoplasmic reticulum and is useful for examining the sizes, shapes and densities of neuronal cell bodies. Staining with silver or gold salts (the Golgi method is a powerful technique of this type) allows visualization of the dendritic tree and the axon and its branches of single neurons. Furthermore, preparations stained with the Golgi method can be examined under the electron microscope after light microscopical examination, thus providing a bridge between these two methods. The Golgi method stains only a random sample of cells. Recently, a variety of dyes has been used to stain individual neurons by direct intracellular injection through a micropipette that can also be used for physiological recording, thus combining study of single neuron structure and function. The development of antibody techniques and their application to histochemistry has allowed the presence of particular substances, such as neurotransmitters, to be localized to individual neurons.

A variety of experimental anatomical methods has provided important information about the connexions between neurons. If an axon is transected its peripheral parts undergo degeneration – anterograde degeneration – and these can be seen using particular techniques. Thus the Marchi method stains degenerating myelin, and a variety of methods can demonstrate degenerating axons and terminals. Degenerating synaptic boutons may also be identified under the electron microscope. After axonal section those parts of the neuron proximal to the section also undergo changes – retrograde degeneration – and these

Continued

Continued

can also be demonstrated microscopically. More recently there has been an explosion in our knowledge of neuronal connexions due to the development of techniques that utilize a neuron's ability to transport substances both from the cell body to its terminals (anterograde transport) and from its terminals to its cell body (retrograde transport). The enzyme horseradish peroxidase (HRP) has been especially useful for retrograde transport studies, and if it is conjugated with various other substances it can also be used for anterograde transport studies. If HRP is injected around nerve terminals it is taken up by them and transported back to the cell bodies, thus allowing the origins of particular terminals to be identified. Likewise, injection of conjugated HRP into a region containing cell bodies of neurons (a nucleus, for example) results in transport of the conjugate to the neurons' terminals, allowing their targets to be identified. Radioactive amino acids may also be used to determine neuronal pathways since they are taken up by neurons and incorporated into proteins, which are then transported to the nerve terminals, where they can be detected by exposing the histological slide to a photographic emulsion (autoradiography). Recently, viruses and various toxins have been shown to cross synapses and have been used to delineate chains of connected neurons.

Finally, electrophysiological methods can be used for neuronal tract tracing. Thus, if a recording is made from a neuronal soma, then the location of its axon and its axon terminals may be determined by systematic electrical stimulation in other parts of the nervous system to find those locations from which the neuron may be excited antidromically, that is, back-fired. Also, by examining those regions of the nervous system that respond orthodromically (that is, usually transsynaptically) to electrical stimulation of another part, then neuronal pathways may be delimited.

BOX 1.2

EXPERIMENTAL METHODS FOR STUDYING THE FUNCTION OF NERVOUS SYSTEMS

Classically there are three techniques for studying neuronal function: by making lesions, by stimulation and by recording. Lesions may be made surgically or by injecting particular chemicals into the nervous system. Following such lesions, the behaviour of the animal is examined. Any behavioural deficits following such interference are usually interpreted to mean that the lesioned part had a role to play in the behaviour. But there are difficulties of interpretation of such experiments. It is the remaining ability of the nervous system which is really being tested under these conditions. Stimulation, either by electrical or chemical means, has also been much used and has been important in human studies (the brain can be stimulated in conscious patients under local anaesthesia) as well as in animal preparations. The original recognition and demarcation of motor areas in the cerebral cortex was determined in this way. Undoubtedly the most powerful techniques for studying the behaviour of neurons have been to record their electrical activity. These techniques range from gross recordings of massed neuronal activity using coarse surface electrodes to the recording of single neuron activity using microelectrodes. Microelectrodes may be placed just outside of a neuron (extracellular recording) or placed inside a single neuron (intracellular recording). Such microelectrodes may be fine wires, insulated except at the tip, used for extracellular recording, or fine glass capillaries filled with an electrically conducting fluid, such as sodium chloride or potassium citrate, and used for either extra- or intracellular recording. By including a dye or an enzyme such as HRP in the microelectrode the anatomy of the recorded neuron may be determined, if the dye is injected into the neuron.

2 The Cell Membrane and Ionic Permeability

All living cells are surrounded by a cell membrane which separates the cellular contents from the outside medium. The organized contents of the cell, including the nucleus and such organelles as the mitochondria, Golgi apparatus, lysosomes, the endoplasmic reticulum, as well as the components of the cytoskeleton, exist in a watery medium – the intracellular fluid (or cytoplasm) – which differs in composition from the fluid bathing the cell – the extracellular fluid or interstitial fluid. There are differences in the compositions of these fluids between different cells and different species, but in general the intracellular fluid contains less sodium and chloride than the extracellular fluid but more potassium, and also contains various negatively charged ions of a protein nature. The fact that there are these differences in composition between the intracellular and extracellular fluids is, of course, evidence for the existence of the cell membrane. Table 2.1 lists the distribution of the major ions across the cell membranes of a number of different cells.

The Structure of The Cell Membrane

The cell (or plasma) membrane is essentially a double (bimolecular) layer of lipid molecules embedded in which are many different kinds of protein molecules. The membrane is about 8–10 nm (8–10 $\times$ 10^{-9} m) thick. The evidence for a bimolecular layer structure of the cell membrane originated in some beautiful experiments of Gorter and Grendel as long ago as 1925. These workers extracted the lipid from red blood cells and floated it on water so that it formed a monomolecular layer. They then reduced the surface area of the water until the force required to compress the layer began to increase, at which point the molecules formed a coherent layer. It turned out that the area of the coherent monomolecular layer was very close to twice the original (calculated) surface area of the red blood cells (see Box

Table 2.1. Distribution of the major ions across cell membranes

| | Approximate electrolyte concentrations in mmol/litre | | | | | | Resting potential (mV) |
| | Extracellular fluid | | | Intracellular fluid | | | |
	Na$^+$	K$^+$	Cl$^-$	Na$^+$	K$^+$	Cl$^-$	
Squid axon	440	20	560	50	400	40	−70
Frog muscle	120	2.5	120	9	140	3	−90
Cat motoneuron	150	5.5	125	15	150	9	−70

2.1 for details of the Gorter and Grendel experiment).

Continued

BOX 2.1

EVIDENCE FOR A BIMOLECULAR ARRANGEMENT OF MEMBRANE LIPIDS

Gorter and Grendel (1925) extracted the lipid from red blood cell ghosts – the membrane left after haemolysis in hypotonic solutions – and spread it as a monolayer on a trough containing water. The area of the trough was then progressively reduced by sliding a glass barrier to the point where a measurable resistance was exerted (Fig. 2.A).

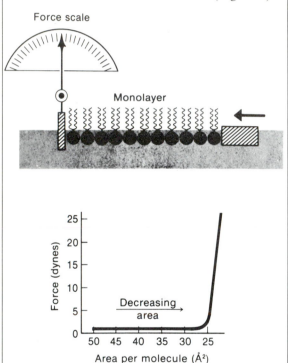

Fig. 2.A. Determination of the area of a monolayer of lipid. The *upper diagram* shows the schematic experimental arrangement. The lipid is spread on the surface of water in a trough and the resistance to movement of one wall of the trough is measured. The area of the trough at which measurable resistance to movement of the wall is first noted is the area formed by a coherent monolayer. (Reproduced with permission from Eckert and Randall 1978.)

At this point the molecules form a coherent film with the polar ends of the lipid molecules attached to the water and the non-

_____ *Continued*

polar, hydrophobic, ends sticking out. The area of the lipid-covered water was measured, and the figure gave the total area the molecules could cover if organized in this way. The number of red blood cells used was determined from blood cell counts, and the mean surface area of a single blood cell was estimated. From these values the total surface area of the red blood cells used in the trough was calculated. The ratio of the area of the lipid film to the area of the cells was approximately 2. Thus, the idea that the lipid was arranged in a bimolecular leaflet was born.

The lipids of the bimolecular layer are mainly phospholipids which consist (Fig. 2.1a) of a hydrophilic (water-loving) head group made up of a phosphate linked to a residue that can be choline, serine, inositol or ethanolamine, and this hydrophilic head group is attached to two hydrocarbon chains that form a hydrophobic (water-hating) tail to the molecule. The phospholipids, when in a watery medium, organize themselves into a bimolecular layer such that the hydrophobic tails are as far from the watery medium as possible and the hydrophilic heads are interposed between the hydrophobic tails and the water (Fig. 2.1b). Such a fatty bimolecular layer is essentially impermeable to most biologically active molecules, like amino acids and sugars, and also to charged particles (ions). Obviously the cell membrane cannot be impermeable to such molecules, although relative impermeability to them does exist. It is the proteins embedded within the bimolecular lipid layer (Fig. 2.1c) that provide the membrane with its permeability to many substances and also are responsible for the functional activity of the living membrane.

The proteins of the cell membrane are of two main types: rod-like alpha helix proteins and globular proteins. It is thought that the alpha helix proteins act as receptors for various extracellular messengers such as hormones and neurotransmitters and also recognize antibodies. The globular proteins act as channels through which ions can cross the membrane. As will be discussed later, ion channels are of supreme importance in the function of nerve cells and can be classified as non-gated, voltage-gated and chemically gated, that is, the channels may be opened or closed by voltage or chemical changes or may not be controlled (non-gated). Ion channels provide a suit-

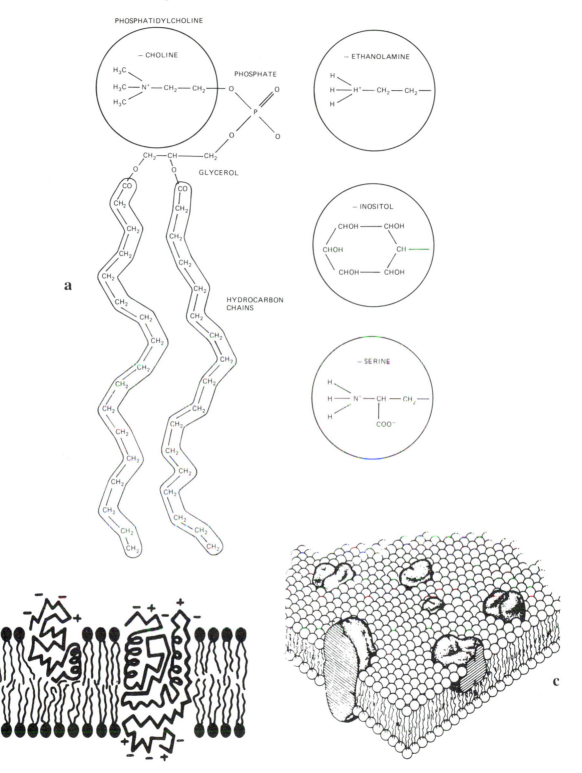

Fig. 2.1a–c. The structure of cell membranes. **a** Phospholipids of cell membranes. There are four main kinds, differing only in their hydrophilic head groups. Each head group is attached by a glycerol group to two hydrocarbon chains which are hydrophobic. **b** Bimolecular arrangement of cell membrane lipids. **c** Fluid-mosaic model of the cell membrane showing bimolecular lipid layer with protein molecules embedded in it. (Reproduced with permission from Bretscher 1985 (**a**) and from Singer and Nicolson 1972 (**b**, **c**).)

able environment in the membrane to allow ions (together with their accompanying water molecules – water of hydration) to pass through because they are made up of a series of transmembrane segments that consist of alpha helixes of a protein backbone with amino acid side-chains projecting from it, the alpha helix segments being arranged close together to form a globular structure. The channels thus provide a polar medium through which the ions can pass, especially as the channel is large enough to allow the ions and their accompanying water of hydration through.

Non-gated Channels and the Resting Membrane Potential

An electrical potential difference is maintained across the membrane of living cells such that the inside of the cell is negative to the outside (which is conventionally considered to be at earth – zero – potential). In nerve and muscle cells this resting potential is of the order of several tens of millivolts and is due to the unequal distribution of ions across the cell membrane, the unequal distribution being maintained by the metabolic activity of the cell.

Resting Potential of an Ideal Cell

The Nernst Equation

Given a cell, containing a relatively large concentration of potassium ions (cations) and large protein anions, surrounded by a membrane containing non-gated channels that are permeable only to potassium ions, then potassium will diffuse out of the cell down its chemical concentration gradient (Fig. 2.2). For every potassium cation that diffuses out, an anion remaining behind becomes uncovered and the inside of the cell develops a negative potential with respect to the outside (the outside medium is considered to be infinite in volume and the addition of potassium ions to it does not alter the external concentration

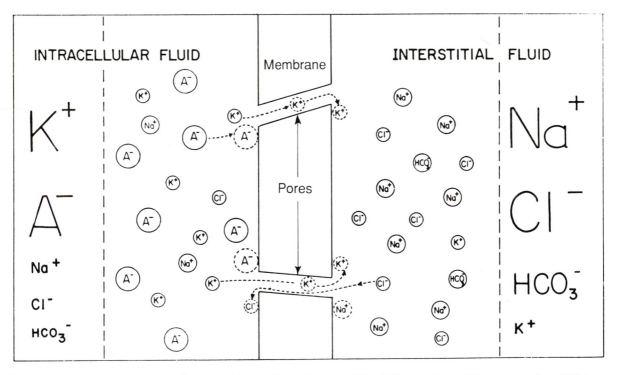

Fig. 2.2. The development of a resting potential in an ideal cell. Intracellular fluid containing a high concentration of K^+ ions and large anions (A^-) separated from the extracellular fluid containing a high concentration of Na^+ and Cl^- ions. The membrane is freely permeable to K^+ ions, but not to Na^+, Cl^-, and A^- ions. K^+ diffuses out of the cell (through nongated channels) down its concentration gradient leaving behind uncovered negative charges on the A^- ion. K^+ diffuses out until the chemical gradient forcing it out is balanced by the increasing internal negativity which attempts to pull K^+ back down the electrical gradient. (Reproduced with permission from Ruch and Fulton 1960.)

of these ions). Potassium ions will continue to pass out of the cell until the diffusion gradient down which they are moving is exactly balanced by the negative charge inside the cell which attempts to pull the potassium ions back. At such a time the potassium ions are said to be in electrochemical equilibrium across the membrane. At this point the potential across the membrane (the Equilibrium Potential) is given by the Nernst Equation (Box 2.2) for potassium ions:

$$E_K = \frac{RT}{FZ} \log_e \frac{[K^+]_o}{[K^+]_i}$$

where R is the gas constant, T the absolute temperature, F the Faraday, Z the valence of the ion (+1 for potassium), $\log_e$ the natural logarithm, $[K^+]_o$ and $[K^+]_i$ the concentrations of potassium outside and inside the cell respectively. In other words, the equilibrium potential for a cell whose membrane is permeable to potassium ions only is determined by the ratio of the potassium ion concentration across the membrane, increasing (becoming less negative) as the potassium concentration outside increases.

BOX 2.2

DERIVATION OF THE NERNST EQUATION

The original derivation of the Nernst equation was based on thermodynamic principles concerned with the electrical work required to move a small number of ions across a barrier and with the osmotic work required to move the same quantity of ions across the barrier in the opposite direction.

The electrical work, W, required to move 1 mole of univalent ions (say potassium) against an electrical potential difference, E, is given by:

$$W = EF \qquad (1)$$

where F is the Faraday (the charge per mole of univalent ion). The osmotic work required to move 1 mole of potassium from a concentration $[K^+]_o$ on one side of the barrier to a concentration $[K^+]_i$ on the other side, where the concentration is greater, can be considered from the point of view of compressing 1 g equivalent of a gas. For example, mechanical work is force times distance, and, if the gas is in a cylinder, then the force

---

Continued

is equal to the gas pressure, P, multiplied by the cross-sectional area of the cylinder, A, for small compressions which move the piston in the cylinder by an amount δl. That is,

$$\delta w = PA\delta l \text{ or } P\delta V$$
$$\text{where } V \text{ is the volume of gas.}$$

The work done in compressing the gas from a volume V_1 to a volume V_2 is given by:

$$W = \int_{V_2}^{V_1} P\delta V \qquad (2)$$

For an ideal gas Boyle's Law states that pressure is inversely related to volume at constant temperature:

$$P \propto \frac{1}{V}$$

Charles's Law states that volume is proportional to temperature at constant pressure:

$$V \propto T$$

Avogadro's Law states equal volumes of gas at the same temperature and pressure contain equal numbers of molecules. The Ideal Gas Law combines the above three laws and gives the following relation (for 1 g molecule of gas)

$$PV = RT$$

Hence:

$$P = \frac{RT}{V}$$

and by substituting in equation (2)

$$W = RT \int_{V_2}^{V_1} \delta V = RT(\log_e V - \log_e V)$$
$$= RT \log_e \frac{V_1}{V_2}$$

By compressing the gas its molecules have been concentrated, and the same argument may be applied to the work done in concentrating solute molecules in moving them from a region of lower, C_1, to a region of higher, C_2, concentration. Thus:

$$W = RT \log_e \frac{C_1}{C_2}$$

Continued

Continued

and for a living cell where $[K^+]_o$ and $[K^+]_i$ are the concentrations of potassium ions outside and inside the cell respectively the relationship becomes:

$$W = RT \log_e \frac{[K^+]_o}{[K^+]_i} \qquad (3)$$

At equilibrium the electrical and osmotic work balance out; therefore, from equations (1) and (3):

$$EF = RT \log_e \frac{[K^+]_o}{[K^+]_i}$$

and

$$E = \frac{RT}{F} \log_e \frac{[K^+]_o}{[K^+]_i}$$

which is the Nernst equation for potassium ions.

At 18 °C and converting to logarithms to the base 10, the equation becomes:

$$E_k = 58 \log \frac{[K^+]_o}{[K^+]_i}$$

It is instructive to ask whether a real cell behaves like this, for, if it does, then the resting potential will be a potassium equilibrium potential. Many different types of cells have been studied, but one of the earliest preparations used was the giant axon of the squid, which was introduced to experimentalists by J. Z. Young. Giant axons can be up to 1 mm in diameter and their size makes them particularly useful for many types of manipulation. The membrane potential of a giant axon may be measured by inserting a fine glass capillary tube filled with a concentrated KCl solution into the axon and using this microelectrode as a probe to measure the potential difference between the inside and outside of the axon. The external potassium concentration may then be changed and the relationship between membrane potential and external potassium concentration determined. The results of a

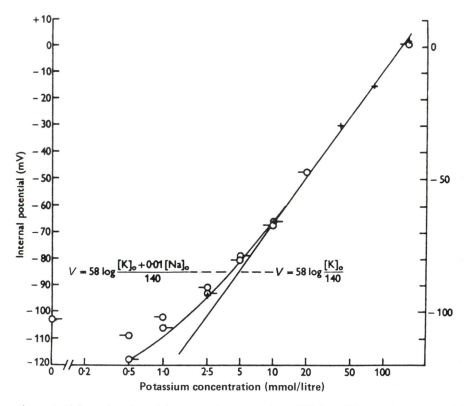

Fig. 2.3. The resting potential as a function of the external concentration of K^+ ions. The membrane potential was recorded from frog striated muscle fibres (*open circles, curved line*) and is compared with the theoretical predictions from the Nernst equation for K^+ ions (*straight line*). At low external K^+ concentrations the experimental points deviate from the predicted line. (Reproduced with permission from Hodgkin and Horowicz 1959.)

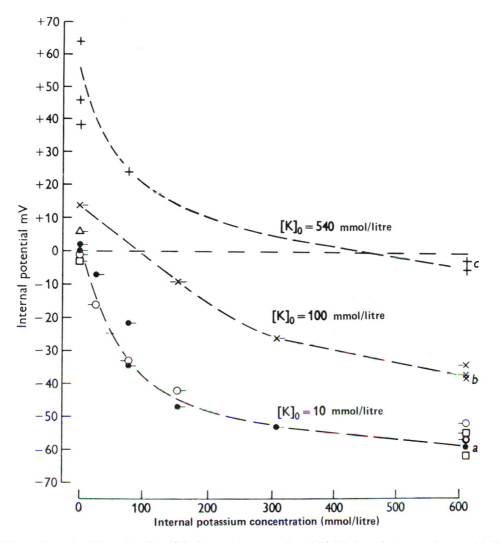

Fig. 2.4. The resting potential as a function of the internal concentration of K^+ ions in a giant axon of the squid. The internal K^+ concentration was changed by replacing the axoplasm with solutions containing different concentrations of K^+ ions. The three sets of data show the relationship between internal K^+ concentration and membrane potential recorded from inside the axon at different external K^+ concentrations. The membrane potential depends on the ratio of K^+ concentrations across the membrane: with large concentrations of K^+ inside compared with outside the potential is positive. (Reproduced with permission from Baker et al. 1962.)

similar experiment on frog muscle fibres are shown in Fig. 2.3. The expected relation between the two measurements is realized only at high concentrations of external potassium. As the external potassium is lowered the experimental points deviate more and more from the line predicted by the Nernst equation until at very low values the deviation is considerable. These experiments suggest, therefore, that the Nernst equation provides only a first approximation to a description of the factors determining the membrane potential. Nevertheless, it appears that the distribution of potassium across the cell membrane is an important factor. That this is the case was shown by Baker et al. (1962) in some remarkable experiments in which they squeezed the cytoplasm (axoplasm) out of a squid axon and replaced it with fluid of controlled compositions. In this way they were able to alter the internal potassium concentration and showed that the membrane potential varied according to the ratio of $[K^+]_o$ to $[K^+]_i$ (Fig. 2.4).

In some cells, e.g. glial cells, the cell membrane contains only potassium channels (non-gated potassium channels; see below for the significance of non-gated and gated channels), and the mem-

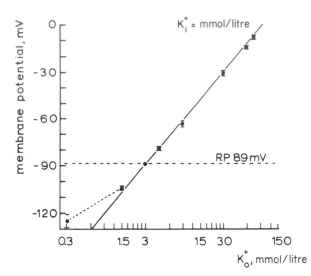

Fig. 2.5. The membrane potential of glial cells is predicted exactly by the Nernst equation for K^+. Glial cell membranes contain only non-gated K channels. *RP*, resting potential. (Modified from Kuffler et al. 1966.)

brane potential measured in glial cells is predicted perfectly by the Nernst equation for potassium over a wide range of external potassium concentrations (Fig. 2.5). In nerve and muscle cells, however, there are considerable deviations from the Nernst equation and we must consider the reasons for such deviations.

Deviations from the Nernst Equation

The deviations of the membrane potential in nerve and muscle cells from the values predicted by the Nernst equation are largely due to the fact that the cell membranes of these cells are permeable to other ions in addition to potassium. Experiments in which radioactively labelled ions have been used to measure the flux of these ions across membranes have shown that the membrane is permeable to sodium and chloride ions. The Nernst equation predicts that the equilibrium potential for sodium is of the order of 55–60 mV (inside positive), a long way from the measured resting membrane potential of −70 to −80 mV. Since the concentration of sodium in the extracellular fluid is much greater than its concentration inside the cell, there are both chemical and electrical gradients attempting to force sodium ions across the membrane and into the cell. So, even though the membrane is much less permeable to sodium than to potassium, sodium ions do enter the cell at rest, and the membrane is said to have a con-

ductance to sodium. The membrane conductance (g) of an ion is the ratio of the current (carried by the charged ions) flowing across the membrane to the driving force (potential difference) across the membrane, that is, conductance is the reciprocal of resistance. At resting potential the membrane has a conductance for potassium about 10–25 times that for sodium.

As the positively charged sodium ions enter the cell, the resting membrane potential becomes less negative and this, in turn, drives out some potassium ions. In the short term these "leaks" of sodium and potassium balance each other out and the resting potential settles at a value slightly less than the equilibrium potential for potassium. When the concentration of potassium outside the cell is artificially lowered, the deviation from the values predicted by the Nernst equation become larger. Further, at very low external potassium concentrations the efflux of potassium becomes significant in determining the potassium concentration very close to the membrane and leads to errors in concentration measurement.

Active Transport of Sodium and Potassium

These passive net movements of sodium and potassium cannot be allowed to continue for any length of time because continued gain of sodium and loss of potassium would lead to a run-down of the transmembrane potential difference. Such dissipation of the membrane potential is prevented by active pumping of sodium and potassium ions across the membrane in a process that requires metabolic expenditure of energy. The sodium – potassium pump is an adenosine triphosphate (ATP) dependent system (Fig. 2.6). When the cell is at rest the active extrusion of sodium and influx of potassium balance the passive influx and efflux of these two ion species. The presence of the pump in the membrane may be demonstrated by loading a cell with radioactively labelled sodium ($^{24}Na^+$) and measuring its efflux. Cooling or poisoning the preparation show that the efflux is dependent on metabolic activity (Fig. 2.7). More specifically, drugs such as the digitalis glycosides (used therapeutically in heart failure) and ouabain specifically block the pump but do not affect the oxidative metabolism of the cell.

The extrusion of sodium by the pump is linked to the influx of potassium. If the external potassium is removed from the external bathing medium pump activity is blocked. For every three sodium ions pumped out, two potassium ions are pumped in – the sodium to potassium pump ratio is 3:2.

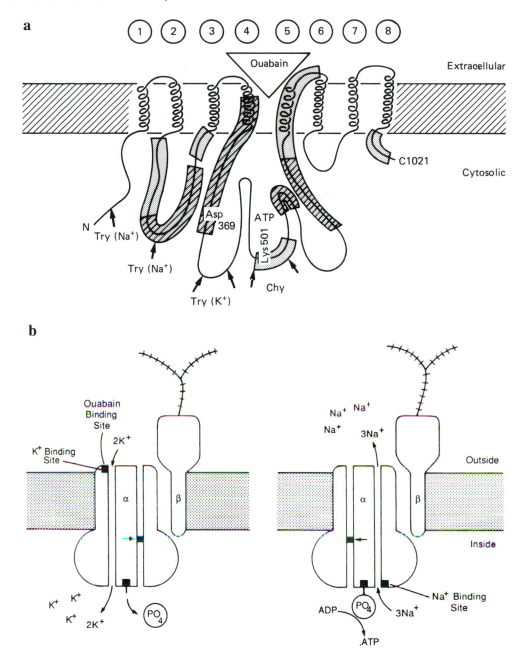

Fig. 2.6a,b. The sodium–potassium pump. **a** Model of the alpha catalytic subunit of sodium-potassium ATPase. The hydrophobic alpha helical chains (*1–8*) are embedded in the cell membrane with most of the molecule inside the cell. The ATP hydrolysis site is at the lysine 501 position. The ouabain receptor site is on the outside of the membrane. **b** Model of the pump mechanisms. In the presence of external K^+ ions the ATPase takes up a certain configuration that leads to the dephosphorylation of ATP and the K^+ moves into the cell. Internal Na^+ ions attach to the molecule, leading to phosphorylation of ADP, a conformational change in the molecule and the extrusion of Na. (Reproduced with permission from Cantley 1986 (**a**) and from Shepherd 1988 (**b**).)

Therefore, the pump is not electrically neutral, because more positive ions are pumped out than are pumped in. The pump activity makes a contribution to the resting potential of the cell, bringing the potential closer to the potassium equilibrium potential. At rest the rates of ion transfer by passive ionic leakage and by pump action are matched.

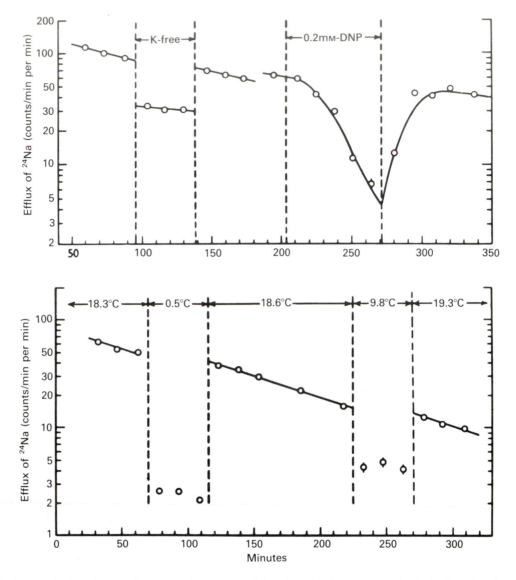

Fig. 2.7. Demonstration of the sodium–potassium pump activity. A squid giant axon was loaded with radioactive Na$^+$ ions and its efflux measured. The efflux was inhibited by removing K$^+$ ions from the bathing solution, by adding the metabolic inhibitor dinitrophenol (DNP) and by cooling. (Reproduced with permission from Hodgkin and Keynes 1955.)

Distribution of Chloride Ions Across the Membrane

As described above, the distribution of sodium and potassium ions across the membrane is determined by the sodium–potassium pump. In many nerve cells chloride ions are relatively free to move across the membrane, and this ion is distributed passively. The Nernst equation for chloride predicts an equilibrium potential close to the resting potential. In many nerve cells there is a chloride pump which is outwardly directed and which balances a steady inward leak of chloride (the equilibrium potential for chloride is more negative than the resting membrane potential).

The Goldman–Hodgkin–Katz Equation

As described above, the value of the membrane potential is only given to a very rough first approximation by the Nernst equation and this is because the cell membrane is permeable to ions in addition to potassium. Each ion species involved has an effect on the membrane potential determined by its concentrations on each side of the

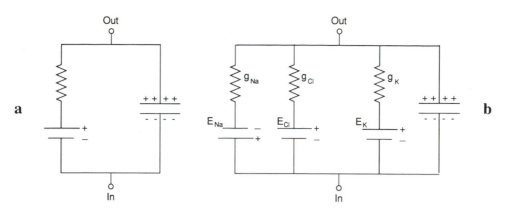

Fig. 2.8a,b. Simple equivalent electrical circuits of the passive properties of the cell membrane. **a** The membrane can be considered to have a battery (responsible for the resting potential) in series with a resistance (or conductance) to current flow, and a capacitance in parallel with the battery and resistance. **b** Each non-gated ion channel (to K^+, Na^+ and Cl^- ions) can be represented separately.

membrane and the permeability of the membrane to the ion. The membrane potential is accurately predicted by the Goldman–Hodgkin–Katz, or Constant Field, equation:

$$V_m = \frac{RT}{F} \log_e \frac{P_k[K^+]_o + P_{Na}[Na^+]_o + P_{Cl}[Cl^-]_i}{P_k[K^+]_i + P_{Na}[Na^+]_i + P_{Cl}[Cl^-]_o}$$

where v_m is the membrane potential and P the membrane permeabilities to the various ions.

Passive Electrical Properties of Nerve Cells

Nerve cells have a resting membrane potential which is maintained by the activity of the sodium–potassium pump in the membrane. The membrane may be considered to have an electrical battery within it. Further, the membrane separates charged particles (ions) and therefore acts as a capacitor and has capacitance. The capacitance is largely due to the bimolecular lipid layer of the membrane. Finally, the membrane is permeable to ions and has conductance (or resistance, which is the reciprocal of conductance). At rest the permeability is due to the presence of non-gated ion channels in the membrane. The electrical properties of the membrane may, therefore, be modelled by a simple electrical circuit (Fig. 2.8a).

Non-gated Ion Channels

The passive movement of ions across the cell membrane at rest takes place through non-gated ion channels which remain open at all times (other,

gated, ion channels may be opened or closed by voltage changes across the membrane, or by neurotransmitters or by other physical or chemical means). It is convenient to consider that there are separate non-gated channels for each of the major species of ions to which the membrane is permeable, i.e. channels for K^+, Na^+, and Cl^-, although this is an oversimplification as the channels are not exclusively selective for a single ion species. Because the ions are distributed unequally across the membrane, each channel (each set of like channels) may be considered to contribute to the membrane potential of the cell. In addition, each channel has a conductance, since it allows ions to move through it, and it therefore also has a resistance. Each channel may be represented by a battery in series with a conductance (Fig. 2.8b).

Membrane Capacitance

When two electrical conducting materials are separated by an insulator and a voltage is applied across the insulator, then capacitance results. The cell membrane, which acts as a leaky insulator, separates two conducting media, the intracellular and the extracellular fluids. It therefore has capacitance. When a potential difference exists across a capacitor, electrical charges of opposite sign are stored on its two surfaces. The value of a capacitance (in farads) is given by the ratio of the amount of charge separated (in coulombs) to the voltage across the capacitor (in volts). A typical nerve cell membrane has a capacitance of about $10^{-6} F/cm^2$.

What effect does membrane capacitance have on the function of cells? The answer is that it slows down the rate of change of potential across

Applied current

Membrane response

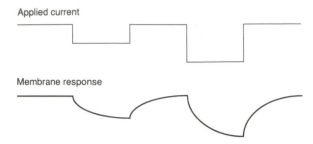

Fig. 2.9. Response of a passive membrane to a hyperpolarizing square wave of current. The current applied across the membrane resistance leads to a voltage change (ΔV_m). Because of the membrane's capacitance the time course of the voltage change is slowed down, since it takes time to charge and discharge the membrane capacitance.

the membrane in response to the passage of ions across the membrane. If a microelectrode is inserted into a nerve cell, or a squid giant axon, and used to pass a rectangular pulse of current across the membrane (Fig. 2.9), then the change in membrane potential produced by the current pulse lags behind the current pulse, at both the beginning and end of the pulse. (The current pulse considered in Fig. 2.9 is in the hyperpolarizing – negative – direction. Depolarizing (positive) current pulses will, in excitable cells – those with voltage-gated channels in their membrane – lead to more complex responses in the cell.) When current flows across the membrane it is made up of two components: the ionic current, which is the movement of ions through the ion channels, and the capacitative current, which is the change in the net charge stored on the membrane capacitance. It takes time to charge a capacitor and likewise it takes time to discharge it (Fig. 2.9).

The waveform of the potential change (ΔV_m) occurring in response to a rectangular current pulse (I_m) is given by the following equation:

$$\Delta V_m(t) = I_m R^{(1-e^{t/\tau})}$$

where e is the base of the system of natural logarithms, τ is the product of R and C, the resistance and capacitance of the membrane, and is called the membrane time constant. The time constant is the time taken for the membrane potential to reach 63% (that is $(1^{-1/e}) \times 100$) of its final value. In different nerve cells time constants vary over a range of about 1–20 ms. Therefore, injection of current into nerve cells, as happens during synaptic activity, produces membrane voltage changes in the cells and these changes will last different times according to the membrane time constant of the particular cell, the longer the time constant the longer the synaptic potentials last. Because of this effect, temporal summation, i.e. the addition over time of several potential changes, can take place (Fig. 2.10).

Membrane Conductance

A length of neuronal membrane, part of an axon or dendrite for example, can be considered as a series of equivalent circuits (Fig. 2.11a). Furthermore, as the cross-sectional area of a neuronal process is relatively small, there is a considerable electrical resistance to current flow within the process (flow along the process), and this resistance is shown in the circuit of Fig. 2.11 as axoplasmic resistance. Now consider what happens if a rectangular pulse of current is injected at a point on such a neuronal process by either a microelectrode or at a synapse (Fig. 2.11b). If the pulse

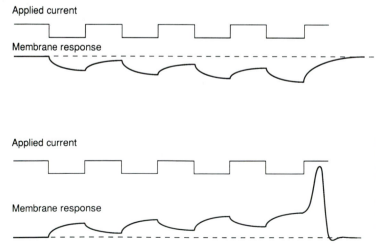

Applied current

Membrane response

Applied current

Membrane response

Fig. 2.10a,b. Temporal summation of membrane voltage changes produced by small current pulses. If the current pulses are close together in time, then the membrane potential changes may overlap and summate, producing larger voltage changes (**a**). If depolarizing current pulses are applied, this temporal summation may be sufficient, in an excitable cell, to generate action potentials (**b**).

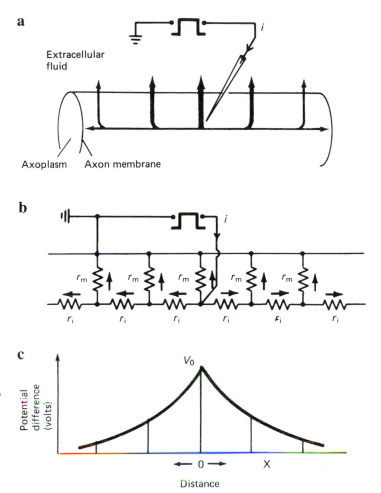

Fig. 2.11a–c. A length of neuronal membrane may be considered as a series of equivalent circuits (**b**), ignoring membrane capacitance. r_m is membrane resistance, r_i is the longitudinal resistance of axoplasm per unit length. In **a** current injected at one point in the membrane produces a voltage change (V_m) that is greatest at the point of current injection (V_o) and which decays, exponentially, with distance along the length of the membrane (**c**) (Modified from Kuffler et al. 1984.)

of current is of long duration relative to the time constant of the membrane, i.e. we are considering a steady injection of current at the point, then the capacitive components may be ignored, since all the capacitors have been charged. All the current is now ionic. Current flows from the point of injection back out across the membrane (through the channels) and also flows along the length of the process. The path of current flow is that of least resistance. Since resistances in series add, most of the current flows out across the membrane near to the point of injection with less and less current flowing with distance from that point. Since by Ohm's Law ($V = IR$) the voltage at any point is proportional to the current across the membrane, then the membrane voltage decreases with distance from the point of current injection. This decrease is of an exponential nature (Fig. 2.11b) and is given by the following equation:

$$\Delta V_m(x) = \Delta V_o e^{-x/\lambda}$$

λ is the length constant of the membrane (the length constant is often called the space constant) and is the distance along the neural process at which the membrane potential has fallen to $1/e$ (37%) of its value at the point of current injection. This property of nerve cell membranes has important consequences. Thus the passive spread of potential along a membrane forms the basis for the phenomenon of spatial summation, whereby two or more events taking place at different points on the membrane may add together. Also, the passive spread of potential change along an axon is necessary to allow the propagation of an action potential (nerve impulse), as will be described in the next chapter. The length constant of a neuronal process depends on the ratio of the membrane resistance (r_m) and the cytoplasmic resistance (r_i) and is given by:

$$\lambda = \sqrt{\frac{r_m}{r_i}}$$

Thus the greater the membrane resistance (the better the insulating properties of the membrane) and the lower the cytoplasmic resistance, then the greater is the length constant. If membrane resistance is constant, then the length constant increases as the square root of the reciprocal of cytoplasmic resistance. Therefore, as the diameter of the process decreases, the length constant increases, since the cytoplasmic resistance, r_i, is inversely proportional to the square of the diameter of the process, if the membrane resistances in the two processes are the same.

Summary

1.   Like all living cells, nerve and muscle cells are surrounded by a cell membrane consisting of a bimolecular layer of lipid molecules in which are embedded many different kinds of protein molecules. One set of functions of the protein molecules is to provide the membrane with its selective permeability to many substances, including inorganic ions.

2.   An electrical potential difference – the resting or membrane potential – is maintained across the membrane of living cells, the inside of the cell being held negative with respect to the outside. This is due to the unequal distribution of ions across the membrane.

3.   To a first approximation the size of the resting potential is given by the Nernst equation for K^+ ions. The Nernst equation for K^+ ions predicts the potential occurring when the K^+ is in electrochemical equilibrium across the membrane.

4.   An excellent fit of theoretical to observed potential is given if other ions (Na^+ and Cl^-) are also considered, together with the cell's selective permeability to them (Goldman–Hodgkin–Katz or Constant Field equation).

5.   Nerve and muscle cells allow K^+, Na^+ and Cl^- ions to pass through the membrane. This passive movement of ions occurs through non-gated ion channels that remain open at all times. Because of this resting movement of ions the membrane potential would run down unless an active process were to oppose it. Active transport of Na^+ and K^+ by the metabolic expenditure of energy prevents this run-down in membrane potential.

6.   Nerve and muscle cell membranes have resistance (or conductance) and capacitance and act like electric cables. The cable properties of the membranes allow, among other things, small potential changes to be added in both space (spatial summation) and time (temporal summation).

3 The Action Potential and Voltage-Gated Channels

Electrically Excitable Cells

Many nerve cells communicate with one another by means of nerve impulses. The mechanism underlying the nerve impulse is the action potential. Action potentials, which are brief (usually in the order of milliseconds) changes in the membrane potential of a cell produced by flow of ionic current across the membrane, are not limited to neurons but can occur in other types of cells, such as striated, cardiac and some smooth muscle cells, eggs and even plant cells. Generally, action potentials occur in cells whose membrane contains voltage-gated ion channels and which, in the terminology of Grundfest (1957) are said to be electrically excitable.

Experimentally an action potential may be elicited in an electrically excitable cell by depolarization, i.e. by passing (conventional) current outwards across the cell membrane. In living cells current is carried by ions (as opposed to the electrons in physical electrical circuits) and depolarization may be achieved by either the direct injection of positive ions into the cell by means of an intracellular microelectrode or under the cathode (negative) if extracellular stimulating electrodes are used. In electrically excitable cells the responses to hyperpolarizing current are governed by the passive cable properties of the cell membrane (see Chap. 2). Responses to depolarizing current, however, are more complicated, especially as the depolarizations increase in amplitude. With very small depolarizations (Fig. 3.1) the responses also behave according to predictions from cable theory. Slightly larger depolarizations result

in responses greater than expected. There is an additional local response of the membrane. As the depolarizations increase, the local responses increase until, at threshold, an action potential is elicited. The action potential is a self-regenerating (or regenerative) process due to the fact that depolarization leads to an increase in the permeability of the cell membrane to sodium ions which, as more sodium ions enter, leads to further depolarization and a greater increase in the permeability of the membrane to sodium.

Ionic Basis of Action Potentials in Nerve

Like much of our basic knowledge of biophysical mechanisms in cells, understanding of the action potential comes from work performed on the squid giant axon. Modern experimental results can be said to have started in 1939, when Hodgkin and Huxley in the UK, and Curtis and Cole in the USA, using intracellular microelectrode recording, reported that the action potential is a brief reversal of the membane potential such that the inside of the axon becomes positive by about 40 mV compared with the outside (Fig. 3.2) (see Hodgkin and Huxley 1939; Curtis and Cole 1940). In order for such a reversal of membrane potential to take place, either positive ions would have to enter the cell or negative ions would have to leave. Since the major anions inside the cell are large protein ions and unable to cross the cell membrane, it seemed likely that an influx of cations was the

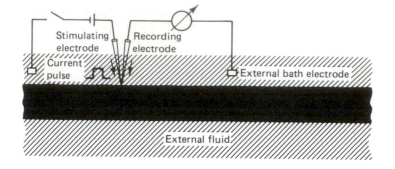

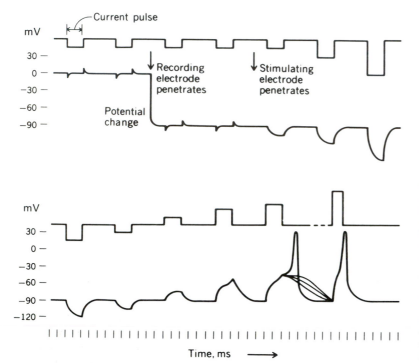

Fig. 3.1. Electrotonic potentials and
local responses in excitable cells. The
diagram shows the responses of an
excitable cell (nerve or muscle) to
rectangular current pulses of 2 ms
duration but different amplitudes and
polarity. Hyperpolarizing pulses produce responses governed by the passive
electrical properties of the cell membrane (note the delayed response at the
beginning and end of the pulse due to
the capacitance of the membrane).
Small depolarizing pulses produce
mirror images of the same amplitude
hyperpolarizing pulses. With depolarizing pulses of larger amplitudes, however, the responses exceed those
expected from the passive properties
of the membrane. The extra components
are the local responses of the membrane. With the largest depolarizing
pulses the response passes threshold
and an action potential is produced.
(Reproduced with permission from
Katz 1966.)

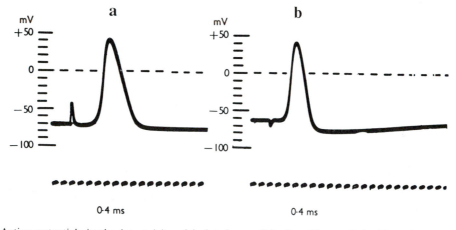

Fig. 3.2a,b. Action potentials in the intact (**a**) and isolated axon (**b**) of squid recorded with an intracellular micropipette
electrode. The time marks are at 0.4 ms intervals and the temperature in **a** was 8.5 °C and in **b** 12.5 °C. Note the resting
potential of about −65 to −70 mV and the overshoot to about +40 mV. (Reproduced with permission from Hodgkin 1964.)

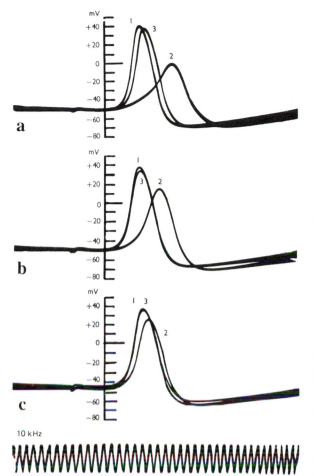

a

b

c

10 kHz

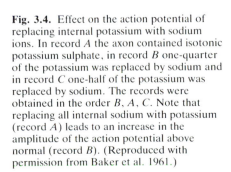

Fig. 3.3a–c. The effects of alterations in the concentration of sodium in the external solution on the action potential in a squid axon. In records labelled *1* and *3* the axon was in sea water. In **a**2 the external sodium was reduced to one-third normal, in **b**2 to one-half normal and in **c**2 it was seven-tenths normal. The records *1* and *3* in each panel were taken before and after the reduction in external sodium. (Reproduced with permission from Hodgkin and Katz 1949.)

cause of the potential reversal. The major external cation is sodium, and it was shown by Hodgkin and Katz (1949) that changes in external sodium concentration affected the level of the peak of the action potential in a direction predicted by the Nernst equation for sodium (Fig. 3.3). Later, Baker et al. (1962) replaced the internal potassium with increasing amounts of sodium and showed that the height of the action potential was reduced (and its width increased) as the internal sodium was raised. Removing all internal sodium increased the height of the action potential (Fig. 3.4). Thus, entry of sodium ions is responsible for the membrane potential reversal in squid axon, but unless some further changes occur in membrane permeability entry of sodium *per se* would leave the cell with a positive membrane potential at or near the sodium equilibrium potential. This does not happen: the membrane potential returns to a negative level (before reaching the sodium equilibrium potential), and this must be due to either influx of negatively charged ions or efflux of positively charged ions. The experimental determination of the ionic changes underlying the action potential was a most important advance in knowledge.

In order to study the ionic basis of the action potential it is necessary to measure the changes in membrane conductance that occur and to relate these changes to the flow of ionic current that they cause. This is not an easy matter for the following reasons:

1. When ions flow across the cell membrane the membrane potential changes, and when the membrane potential changes the conductance of the membrane changes too. The changes in

Fig. 3.4. Effect on the action potential of replacing internal potassium with sodium ions. In record *A* the axon contained isotonic potassium sulphate, in record *B* one-quarter of the potassium was replaced by sodium and in record *C* one-half of the potassium was replaced by sodium. The records were obtained in the order *B*, *A*, *C*. Note that replacing all internal sodium with potassium (record *A*) leads to an increase in the amplitude of the action potential above normal (record *B*). (Reproduced with permission from Baker et al. 1961.)

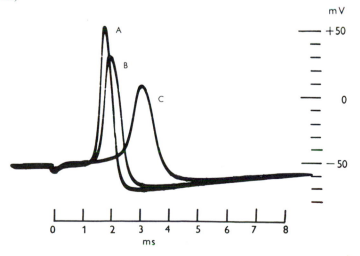

conductance will lead, in turn, to further changes in ionic current, and so on. (This is because of the existence of voltage-gated channels in the membrane, which will be discussed later.) Obviously, it is therefore difficult to determine the relationship between membrane potential and membrane conductance.

2. Not all membrane current during an action potential is ionic current: some of the current is capacitative current and will alter the net charge stored in the membrane. It is necessary to distinguish capacitative current from ionic current.

3. In order accurately to describe the ionic mechanisms underlying the action potential it is necessary to be able to identify the currents carried by separate species of ions.

Voltage Clamp Experiments

The development of the voltage clamp technique (Box 3.1) by Cole provided the experimental means to overcome the first problem and paved the way for Hodgkin and Huxley to determine the ionic mechanisms of the action potential. The voltage clamp is essentially a current pump that connects an electrode inside a cell with one outside and, by means of a negative feedback

circuit, allows the experimenter to set the membrane potential of the cell at any required level (command potential) and hold it there despite the membrane conductance changes that would otherwise tend to bring the membrane potential to a new equilibrium level. After a step change in the command potential to a new clamped level, ionic current flows across the membrane and can be determined. By altering the ionic concentrations in the bathing medium the contributions of different ion species to the total current may be determined.

BOX 3.1

THE VOLTAGE CLAMP TECHNIQUE

In order to determine the time course of the ionic conductance change and the current flow across an excitable membrane during an action potential it is necessary to set the membrane potential to different levels and examine how the currents vary. This requires that an action potential is held stationary over a length of axon (space clamp) and that the membrane voltage is changed to different

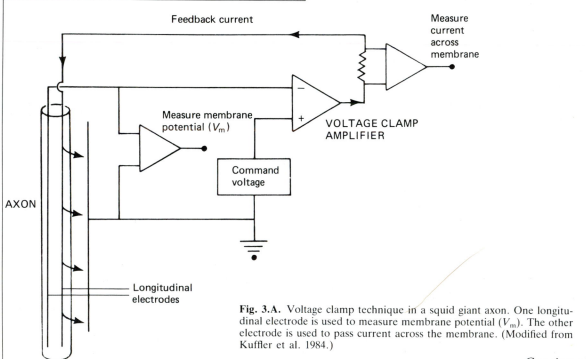

Fig. 3.A. Voltage clamp technique in a squid giant axon. One longitudinal electrode is used to measure membrane potential (V_m). The other electrode is used to pass current across the membrane. (Modified from Kuffler et al. 1984.)

Continued

Continued

values and held at those values during ionic current flow (voltage clamp). The technique is shown diagrammatically in Fig. 3.A.

Two long fine metal electrodes are placed inside a squid giant axon, parallel to the long axis of the axon. One electrode is used to measure the membrane potential of the axon by connecting it to the negative input of the voltage clamp amplifier. The other input of the voltage clamp amplifier is connected to a voltage source which can be varied (the command voltage). The second electrode is connected to the output of the voltage clamp amplifier and is used to pass current across the axon's membrane, and this current is measured. During a voltage clamp experiment a command voltage is fed to the axon and the membrane potential is held constant by means of feed-back current which opposes exactly the currents that would normally flow due to the voltage change. By recording the current that must be generated to keep the membrane potential from changing, the membrane current can be measured directly.

Let us consider what happens if, in the squid giant axon, the membrane potential is changed rapidly from a clamped potential of −65 mV to another clamped potential of −9 mV (Fig. 3.5). Following such a step change in membrane potential there are current changes. During the step change in potential there is a brief positive surge of current that is the capacitative current. This capacitative current occurs because during the membrane potential change the membrane capacitance is changed as the membrane is charged to the new level. Following the capacitative current there are two phases of current flow, an initial inward current that lasts about 1.5 ms and then an outward current that lasts as long as the new membrane potential is maintained. By altering the amplitude of the step change in voltage (from the holding potential of −65 mV) Hodgkin et al. (1952) were able to gain insight into the nature of the ionic currents (Fig. 3.6). As the membrane was depolarized more and more the initial inward current became smaller and smaller until, at a potential of about +52 mV it disappeared, and with further depolarizations the initial current reversed to an outward current. The later current increased as the membrane was hyperpolarized.

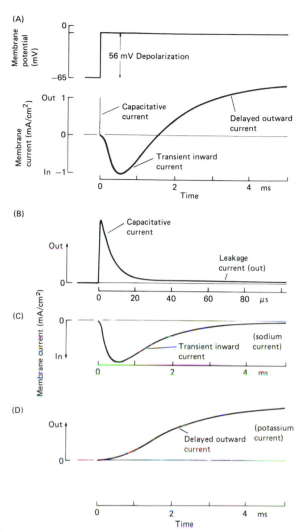

Fig. 3.5a–d. Current flow across the membrane of the squid axon during depolarization. **a** Shows membrane currents during a 56 mV depolarization produced by voltage clamp. The currents consist of an initial brief outward current due to the discharge of the membrane capacity, then a phase of transient inward current, followed by a delayed, maintained outward current. **b** Shows the capacitative current in more detail and also indicates the small leakage current (due in part to movement of chloride) that follows it. **c,d** Show the transient inward and the delayed outward current separately. (Modified from Kuffler et al. 1984, after Hodgkin and Huxley 1952a,b.)

The Initial Inward Current Is Due To Movement of Sodium Ions

The above experiment showed that if the initial current was due to movement of a single ion species then that ion would have an equilibrium potential at about +52 mV. Sodium has an equilibrium potential of this level in the squid giant

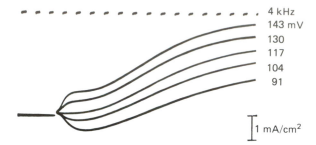

Fig. 3.6. Membrane currents for different displacements of the membrane potential in a squid giant axon at 3.5 °C. Outward currents are upwards. The figures on the *right* give the change in internal potential from a resting (holding) potential of −65 mV. Note that the early transient current reverses in sign at 117 mV corresponding to a membrane potential of +52 mV (the equilibrium potential for sodium). The delayed, maintained current increases monotonically with increased depolarization. (Reproduced with permission from Hodgkin 1964, after Hodgkin et al. 1952.)

axon bathed in sea water. This is good evidence that the initial inward current is indeed due to movement of sodium into the axon. Further confirmation was provided by removing the sodium from the external medium (replacing it with the impermeant choline ion, as choline chloride, to maintain osmotic equilibrium), when the inward current was eliminated (Fig. 3.7).

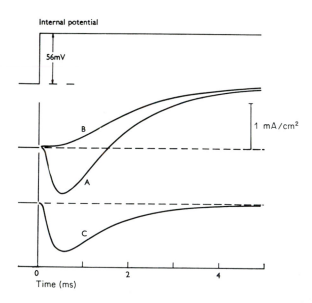

Fig. 3.7. Separation of membrane currents into components carried by sodium and potassium ions; outward current upwards. Record *A* shows the current with the axon in sea water. Record *B* is with most of the external sodium replaced with choline and therefore shows the potassium current. Record *C* is the difference between *A* and *B* and shows the current due to sodium. (Reproduced with permission from Hodgkin 1964, after Hodgkin and Huxley 1952a.)

The Later Outward Current Is Due To Movement of Potassium Ions

That the later outward current was due to potassium was confirmed by Hodgkin and Huxley. They loaded an axon with radioactive potassium and then performed a combined voltage clamp and radioactive efflux experiment. When the membrane was clamped at a depolarized level the total charge carried across the membrane by the outward current was calculated and was compared with the amount of potassium carried out across the membrane during the period of the outward current. The agreement was excellent between the two values and provided convincing evidence that the outward current was indeed carried by potassium ions. Furthermore, it was shown that the inward and outward currents were independent of one another – the potassium current was not affected by changes in the external concentration of sodium – and therefore the sodium and potassium ions passed through different channels in the membrane.

The Inward and Outward Currents Can Be Separated by Drugs

More recently it has been possible to separate the sodium and potassium currents by pharmacological means. Tetrodotoxin (TTX), a poison found in certain species of fish, selectively blocks the voltage-sensitive sodium channels, and tetra-ethylammonium (TEA) selectively blocks the voltage-sensitive potassium channels. TTX binds to the outer mouth of the sodium channel, and is only effective when applied to the outside of the membrane, whereas TEA binds to the inner mouth of the potassium channel and is only effective from the inside of the axon (Fig. 3.8).

The Separate Sodium and Potassium Conductances Can Be Determined

By use of the voltage clamp technique Hodgkin and Huxley were able to determine the dependence of the amplitude and time course of both the sodium and potassium currents on the membrane potential and to determine the equilibrium potentials for both ions. From this data they were able to calculate the conductances for each ion (Fig. 3.9). In response to depolarizing voltage steps from the level of the resting potential the two conductances were shown to have quite different time courses (although similar ampli-

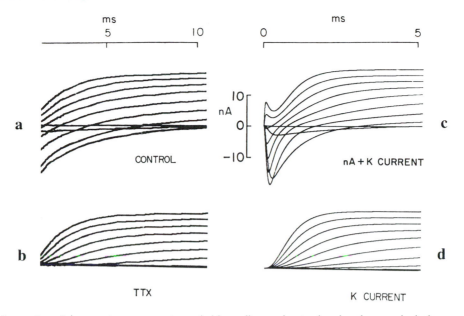

Fig. 3.8a–d. Separation of the membrane currents carried by sodium and potassium by pharmacological means. The records are from a frog myelinated nerve fibre in which the membrane potential is displaced to various levels between −60 and +75 mV. **a,c** Records which are controls. **b** Shows that addition of 300 nmol/litre TTX blocks the sodium current leaving the potassium current intact. **d** Shows that addition of TEA blocks the potassium current leaving the sodium current intact. (Reproduced with permission from Hille 1970.)

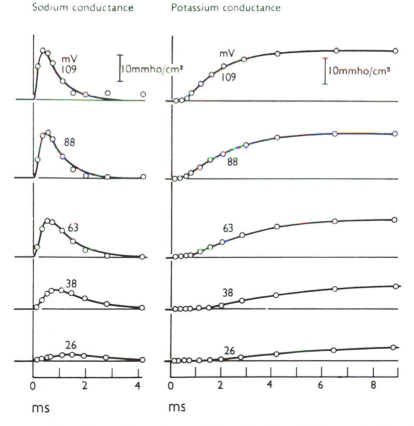

Fig. 3.9. The time course of the sodium and potassium conductances for different displacements of membrane potential from −65 mV by the amounts indicated. (Reproduced with permission from Hodgkin 1964, after Hodgkin and Huxley 1952d.)

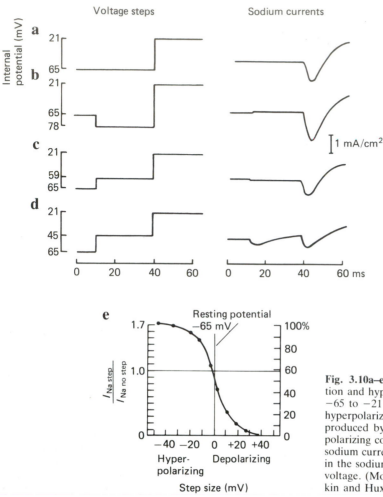

Fig. 3.10a–e. Effect on sodium current of depolarization and hyperpolarization. If a depolarizing step (from −65 to −21 mV as shown in **a**) is preceded by a small hyperpolarizing conditioning step (**b**) the sodium current produced by the later depolarization is increased. Depolarizing conditioning steps produce a reduction in the sodium current (**c** and **d**). **e** Shows the fractional change in the sodium currents as a function of the conditioning voltage. (Modified from Kuffler et al. 1984, after Hodgkin and Huxley 1952c.)

tudes at similar membrane potentials). The sodium conductance increased before the potassium conductance and was not maintained during the voltage step. The potassium conductance, on the other hand, was delayed in onset and was maintained at its maximal value throughout the voltage step.

Sodium Inactivation Is a Distinct Process

The decline of the sodium conductance back to its initial value, even though the voltage step in the voltage clamp experiment was maintained, was termed inactivation. Inactivation is an interesting phenomenon. Obviously, the sodium conductance is quite abruptly reduced after about 1–2 ms, even though the axon is still depolarized. Hodgkin and Huxley investigated the inactivation of the sodium conductance by determining the effects of small depolarizations and hyperpolarizations just before the standard voltage clamp step. It turned out that small depolarizations decreased the peak level attained by the sodium conductance, whereas small hyperpolarizations had the opposite effect – an increase in the peak sodium conductance (Fig. 3.10). Hodgkin and Huxley concluded that inactivation is a distinct process. That this conclusion was correct has been shown by Armstrong et al. (1973), who perfused a solution containing the proteolytic enzyme pronase through a giant axon. Such treatment led to a selective abolition of the inactivation process. Normally inactivation is removed by the repolarization of the membrane to near its resting potential level, but the removal takes several milliseconds, and during this time a depolarization of the membrane results in a reduced increase in sodium conductance.

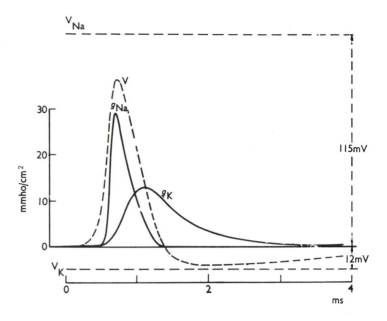

Fig. 3.11. Theoretical solution for the propagated action potential and the underlying sodium and potassium conductances for the squid giant axon. (Reproduced with permission from Hodgkin 1964, after Hodgkin and Huxley 1952d.)

Action Potential Shape and Propagation Can Be Predicted on a Theoretical Basis

Finally, once Hodgkin and Huxley had characterized the sodium and potassium conductances they were able to compute the predicted shape (and also the conduction velocity – the speed of propagation along the axon; see below) of the action potential in the squid giant axon. The prediction was remarkably accurate (Fig. 3.11).

Summary of the Action Potential

Thus, during an action potential the following events take place: (1) activation of a sodium conductance mechanism, (2) inactivation of the sodium conductance, and (3) activation of a potassium conductance mechanism. These underlying mechanisms explain why the action potential is an all-or-nothing event and why it has associated refractory periods and a threshold. An all-or-nothing event is one that either occurs or does not occur and when it does it is always the same (under the same set of conditions). The absolute refractory period lasts during the falling phase of the action potential at a time when the sodium conductance is inactivated and when potassium conductance is high. At this time it is impossible to elicit another action potential. Following the absolute refractory period is the relative refractory period. During the relative refractory period it is possible to elicit another

action potential, but greater depolarizations than normal are required (the threshold is increased) because sodium inactivation has not been completely turned off and potassium conductance is still increased. Threshold is determined by the balance of currents across the cell membrane. Thus at rest the passive fluxes of ions across the membrane are exactly balanced by their active transport. In an electrically excitable cell a depolarization leads to an increase in the sodium conductance (an opening of voltage-gated sodium channels – see below); this can be balanced, at small levels of depolarization, by increased potassium efflux due to the increased driving force for potassium produced by the depolarization, and also by the gradual increase in potassium conductance due to the opening of voltage-gated potassium channels. At threshold these various conductances are just balanced but the system is unstable. A slight further depolarization leads to the opening of additional voltage-gated sodium channels, more depolarization and the onset of the self-regenerating action potential. For a deeper understanding of these events we must consider voltage-gated channels in more detail.

Voltage-Gated Channels in Electrically Excitable Membranes

The reason certain cells can generate action potentials is because their membranes contain voltage-gated channels in addition to the non-gated channels responsible for the resting potential. As we shall see, the distribution of voltage-gated channels may not be uniform in the membrane of individual cells – only certain parts of the cell may generate action potentials. We shall begin by considering the sodium and potassium voltage-gated channels that are responsible for the action potential in the squid giant axon. Later it will be necessary to consider other voltage-gated channels.

Not only did Hodgkin and Huxley describe the changes in conductance that occurred during the action potential and predict its form and threshold etc., but they also provided insights into how sodium and potassium might cross the membrane. They suggested a model in which sodium and potassium channels in the membrane were controlled by "gates" whose opening and closing were voltage dependent. The sodium channel was suggested to have two gates: one (m-gate) closed at rest and opened by depolarization, which is responsible for activation, and the other (h-gate) open at rest and closed by depolarization, which is responsible for sodium

inactivation. The potassium channel was suggested to have one gate (n-gate) which opens on depolarization.

Much more is now known about the voltage-gated channels, especially the sodium channel. By using TTX and other toxins that bind to the sodium channel it has been possible to isolate the channel protein and show that the channel is a large glycoprotein consisting of three subunits, a glycoprotein and two polypeptides (Box 3.2). The amino acid sequence of the channel has been determined by Noda and Numa and their colleagues (Noda et al. 1986) (Box 3.2).

BOX 3.2

THE VOLTAGE-GATED SODIUM CHANNEL

The voltage-gated sodium channel is a transmembrane protein surrounding a pore in the membrane. The diameter of the pore is controlled by the membrane potential. Fig. 3.Ba indicates the general organization and the functional characteristics of the channel. The channel contains four repeated units (I – IV

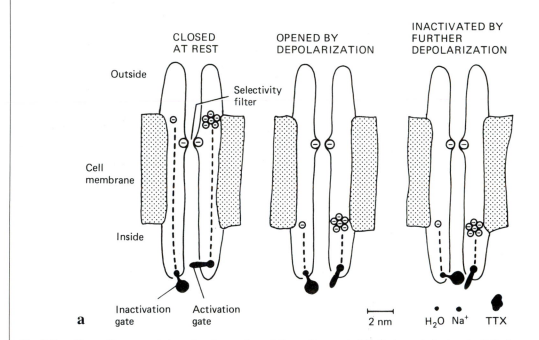

Fig. 3.B. a Shows the suggested mode of operation of the voltage-gated Na$^+$ channel. Ionic selectivity is provided by a constriction lined with negative charges near the outer surface of the membrane. The activation gate near the inner surface opens in association with movement of negative ions from outside to inside. The inactivation gate blocks the inner mouth of the channel, preventing closure of the activation gate. **b,c** Show the proposed structure of the channel. Four similar units span the membrane; they are arranged so as to surround a central pore which provides the channel for Na ions. (Modified from Kuffler et al. 1984(**a**) and reproduced with permission from Noda et al. 1986 (**b, c**).)

Continued

Continued

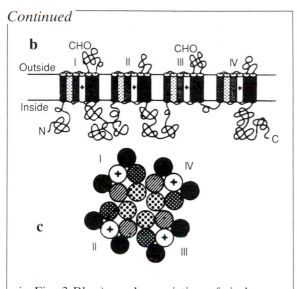

b

CHO

I   II   III   IV

Outside

Inside

N

C

c

I

IV

II

III

in Fig. 3.Bb,c), each consisting of six homologous transmembrane segments. The segments labelled (+) each contain a high proportion of positively charged residues and these are believed to act as the voltage sensor. The four repeated units are arranged around the central pore, which is the sodium channel.

Gating Currents

The Hodgkin–Huxley model predicted that charge movements associated with the opening and closing of the gates should lead to capacitive gating currents. It was 20 years before these predictions could be tested experimentally, but in the 1970s C. M. Armstrong and his colleagues confirmed their presence and provided detailed analysis (Fig. 3.12). It was shown that before the sodium channel opens in response to depolarization several steps occur in which charge moves and that these steps have different kinetics. Also, it was shown that the inactivation process was somehow linked to the activation process – a somewhat surprising result. It appears that the activation (m) gate cannot close as long as the inactivation (h) gate is closed, an observation that suggests the two gates are located close enough to one another to interfere with each other's action.

Density of Sodium Channels

Because the voltage-gated sodium channel binds TTX selectively it has been possible to determine

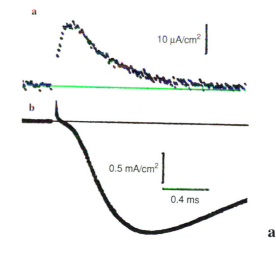

a

$10\ \mu A/cm^2$

b

$0.5\ mA/cm^2$

$0.4\ ms$

a

Fig. 3.12a,b. Gating current in a squid gaint axon. **a** The *upper curve* shows the gating current produced by a depolarization of 70 mV. Ionic currents were eliminated by placing the axon in sea water containing tris (hydroxymethyl) aminomethane (Tris) instead of sodium, to remove the sodium current, and by perfusing the axon with a caesium fluoride solution, to remove the potassium current. The *lower curve* in **a** shows the sodium current from the same axon in sea water. **b** A diagrammatic representation of gating. Capacitative current is shown on the *left*. In response to a depolarization, charge is displaced from the surface of the membrane (*a*), and electrons are redistributed within the membrane (*b*); charge (*c*) or bipolar (*d*) molecules become realigned. Ionic currents are shown to the *right*. (Reproduced with permission from Armstrong and Bezanilla 1974.)

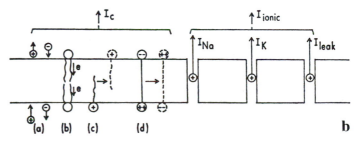

$\uparrow I_c$ $\uparrow I_{ionic}$

$\uparrow I_{Na}$ $\uparrow I_K$ $\uparrow I_{leak}$

(a) (b) (c) (d)

b

the density of the channels in the membrane by measuring the amount of tritiated TTX bound at saturation, since each channel binds a single TTX molecule. Values vary from tissue to tissue, e.g. for squid giant axon it is about 550 channels per square micrometer; figures for other axons range down to $35/\mu m^2$ and up to $12\,000/\mu m^2$ at the nodes of Ranvier in mammalian sciatic nerve. These figures show that the density of sodium channels is quite low. Since it is known, from electrophysiological experiments, how much current flows during an action potential, it is possible to calculate how much current flows through each channel. For the squid giant axon the sodium channel has a maximum conductance of $1200\ pS/\mu m^2$, so each channel has a conductance of about 2.2 pS. Slightly higher values have been found for vertebrate skeletal muscle (which is also electrically excitable) and vertebrate nerve.

Activity of Single Voltage-Gated Sodium Channels

It is now possible to examine the activity of single channels due to the development of an ingenious technique by Neher and Sackmann and their colleagues (Box 3.3). The technique is called patch clamping and involves attaching a fire-polished microelectrode to a cleaned cell membrane such that an electrically very tight (very high resistance – gigaohm) seal is formed. There are various ways in which the technique may be used with either whole cells or small pieces of cell membrane attached to the microelectrode. However, once the seal is attained and if the membrane contains the appropriate channels, then current passage through the channels may be recorded in the cell attached or patch configurations. When the membrane under the microelectrode contains a single sodium channel (and voltage-gated potassium channels are blocked with TEA) then depolarizing voltage pulses applied across the patch lead to openings of the sodium channel. Under these conditions (Fig. 3.12) it can be shown that the channel is either open or closed, and when it is open the magnitude of current flow is always the same, although the duration of opening varies. Thus, the single voltage-gated channel behaves in an all-or-nothing manner. The experiment of Fig. 3.13 also shows another important point. When 300 individual responses to the depolarizing voltage pulse were summed it was revealed that (1) the total current reached a maximum in 1–2 ms and (2) after this maximum the current declined

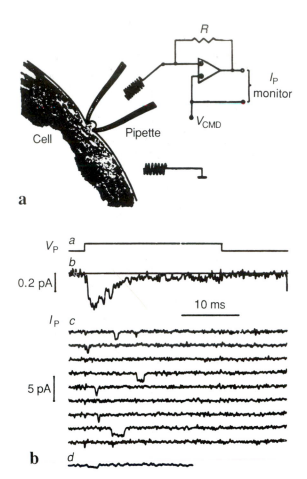

Fig. 3.13a,b. Sodium channel currents recorded with the patch clamp technique. **a** Shows the recording arrangement of a cell-attached patch of a cultured rat muscle fibre. **b** Shows the effect of voltage pulses (trace *a*) applied to the patch. Current pulses are produced in the patch (downward deflections in trace *c*, which shows nine successive records) and these pulses, which are channel openings, behave in an all-or-nothing manner. The sum of 300 responses is shown in trace *b*, which illustrates that most channels open within 1–2 ms of the onset of the voltage pulse and after this the probability of channel openings decays with a time constant the same as that of sodium inactivation. (Reproduced with permission from Sigworth and Neher 1980.)

with a time course identical to that of sodium inactivation. In other words, the sodium current recorded in a conventional voltage clamp experiment can be accounted for by the summed activity of the opening and closing of individual sodium channels. This means, of course, that the sodium conductance change during an action potential can also be accounted for in the same way.

BOX 3.3

THE PATCH CLAMP TECHNIQUE

A small glass micropipette (inside tip diameter 3μm or less) is brought up to the surface of a cell under visual control (A in Fig. 3.C). The tip is highly polished and when slight suction is applied through the electrode a very high resistance seal (gigaohm seal) may develop between the electrode and the cell (B in Fig. 3.C). Once such a seal is attained, then currents flowing through this cell-attached patch of membrane can be recorded. Further suction (in a low calcium medium) may pull the patch away from the rest of the cell, resulting in an inside-out patch (C in Fig. 3.C) which is cell-free. Alternatively, suction may break the patch leading to whole cell recording (D in Fig. 3.C), in which currents across the whole cell membrane may be recorded, and, by pulling the electrode away from the cell, a cell-free outside-out patch can be obtained (E in Fig. 3.C). These various preparations allow different solutions to be applied either to the inside or outside surfaces of the cell membrane.

Selectivity of the Sodium Channel

How is it that the sodium channel only allows sodium to enter? The relative permeability of the sodium channel to various ions has been examined by Hille (see Hille 1970), who found that the channel behaves as a filter with a pore size of 0.3–0.5 nm. This will limit the entrance of ions to those of appropriate hydrated diameter. Further, the channel selects against anions, even those of appropriate size, and Hille suggested that there were negatively charged carboxyl groups on the outer mouth of the channel that attract cations and repel anions. Finally, because of the ease with which cations with good hydrogen-bonding characteristics can pass through the channel, Hille suggested that only cations (of suitable size) that can lose their water of hydration to the carboxyl groups and oxygen radicals lining the channel can pass through.

Fig. 3.C. Patch clamp recording configurations. (Modified from Kuffler et al. 1984, after Hammill et al. 1981.)

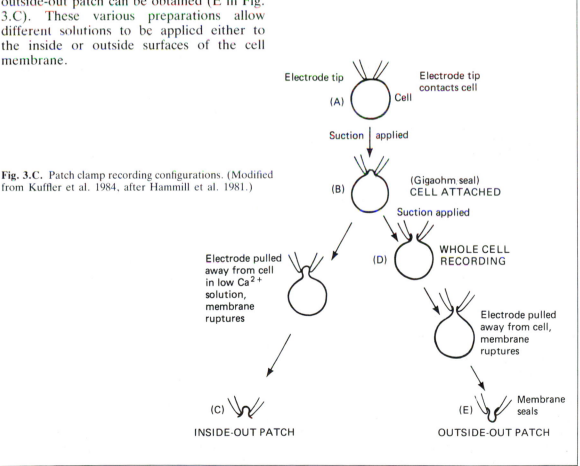

Voltage-Gated Potassium and Calcium Channels

Rather less is known about the voltage-gated potassium channels than about the sodium channel. Potassium channels have been patch clamped and shown to have a rather higher conductance than sodium channels, but a lower density, in squid axon.

Hodgkin and Huxley were rather lucky in that squid giant axons have relatively few types of voltage-gated channels, and the action potential is essentially due to sodium and potassium. In some nerve fibres calcium is much more important, and it is calcium, rather than sodium, which is responsible for the conductance change underlying the ascending limb of the action potential. But even in the squid giant axon some calcium enters during the action potential (through the sodium channel) as well as through separate calcium channels. These voltage-gated calcium channels are concentrated at the nerve terminals, where calcium entry is responsible for transmitter release (see Chap. 6). Calcium also has a role in affecting the excitability of the nerve membrane. A fall in extracellular calcium concentration leads to an increase in the excitability of the axon, whereas a rise in extracellular calcium has the opposite effect, causing the action potential threshold to fall.

Action potentials in which calcium plays a major role have been observed in a wide variety of invertebrate and vertebrate nerve cells. The voltage-gated calcium channels may be blocked by adding cobalt, manganese or cadmium ions to the extracellular medium, and barium ions can substitute for calcium and move through the calcium channel. A single nerve cell can have calcium and sodium action potentials in different parts of its membrane. For example, in the cerebellum (a major part of the brain concerned with learned movements) the only output neuron is the Purkinje cell. The Purkinje cell, which has inhibitory actions on its target neurons, is capable of generating action potentials in its dendrites, and these are calcium action potentials. Like many other vertebrate neurons the Purkinje cell has a sodium action potential in its cell body (soma) and axon. These differences are due to the selective localization of calcium and sodium voltage-gated channels (see Chap. 9).

It is now known that there is a variety of potassium channels in nerve cells. Some are activated by depolarization, some by depolarization after hyperpolarization, and some by the level of intracellular calcium. Further consideration of some of these channels will be given in later chapters.

Changes in Internal Ion Concentrations Due To the Action Potential

With each action potential some sodium enters the cell and some potassium leaves. In the squid giant axon, for every square centimetre of membrane between 3 and 4 pmol enter and leave during an action potential. These are very small amounts, but in axons with diameters of a few micrometres, with a low internal volume, repetitive firing could lead to a run-down of the sodium gradient after a few thousand action potentials. The changes in internal sodium and potassium concentrations, and the build-up of external potassium that might occur, are counteracted by the active transport of sodium out of the cell and of potassium into the cell by activity of the sodium–potassium pump. It is important to realize that the sodium–potassium pump plays no part in the mechanism of the action potential and is not responsible for any of the potential changes of the action potential (except for certain potentials occurring at the end of the action potential – after-potentials – in certain cells). The sodium–potassium pump has been considered in Chapter 2.

Summary

1.   Action potentials occur in cells whose membrane contains voltage-gated ion channels. Such cells, which include nerve and mammalian striated muscle cells, are said to be electrically excitable.

2.   During an action potential there is a brief reversal of the membrane potential such that the inside of the cell becomes positive. This is due, in most cells, to the entry of Na^+ ions followed by the exit of K^+ ions.

3.   The Na^+ and K^+ ions flow through separate voltage-gated channels in the membrane. Both channels open when the membrane is depolarized from its resting level. The Na^+ channel opens first and this leads to more depolarization and further Na^+ entry (a positive feed-back pro-

cess). The K^+ channel opens after the Na^+ channel and leads to efflux of K^+ ions and the restoration of the resting potential. Accompanying K^+ efflux there is inactivation of the Na^+ conductance.

4. The activity of single voltage-gated channels can be studied by patch clamp techniques. The single voltage-gated channels behave in an all-or-nothing manner; this accounts for the all-or-nothing behaviour of the action potential.

5. After the occurrence of a single action potential the cell has gained a very small amount of Na^+ ions and lost a very small amount of K^+ ions. These changes are compensated for by the efflux of Na^+ and the influx of K^+ due to the activity of the sodium–potassium pump.

4 Propagation of the Action Potential – The Nerve Impulse

It is worth differentiating between the action potential and the nerve impulse. To make this differentiation might be thought of as semantic quibbling. Many types of cells can generate action potentials, for example oocytes, some gland cells, and even plant cells. Few cells have action potentials that propagate from a point of origin in the cell to a particular terminal site or sites. Among those that do are striated muscle fibres, where the action potential is set up at the point of innervation by the motor nerve as a consequence of neuromuscular transmission (see Chap. 8) and propagates along the muscle fibre to its ends; and nerve cells, where the nerve impulse is set up, usually, at the region between the cell body of the cell (soma) and the nerve fibre (axon) at a site known as the initial segment (see Chap. 9) in response to excitatory input to the cell at points of contact between neurons (the synapses) and propagates along the axon to the axon terminals. Certain other types of muscle cells or modified muscle cells that form a functional syncitium also have the capability of propagating action potentials. It is also useful to note that giant nerve fibre systems (including the squid giant axon) are not single cells but consist of a large number of cells fused together.

Passive Electrical Properties of the Cell Membrane

The passive (cable) properties of the cell membrane have been considered earlier (Chap. 2) for electrically inexcitable cells, i.e. for cells incapable of generating action potentials. As described in Chapter 3, electrically excitable cells differ in the presence of voltage-gated channels in their membrane and depolarization leads to opening of the sodium (or calcium) channels followed by the all-or-nothing action potential. Propagation of the nerve impulse depends on the passive electrical properties of the axonal membrane.

It will be remembered that injection of a positive (or negative) pulse of charge at a point in an axon leads to spread of the potential changes along the axon, the extent of spread being dependent on the space or length constant of the membrane. Also, the injection of a square pulse of charge causes a response in the membrane that lags behind the pulse by a time dependent on the time constant of the membrane. The time constant of the membrane is determined by the resistive and capacitive components of the membrane, and the space constant by these components and the resistance of the axoplasm to current flow.

These passive properties of the cell membrane are of extreme importance both for the integrative properties of neurons and for the propagation of nerve impulses. It will be seen (Chaps. 8 and 9) that neurons interact at synapses by generating synaptic potentials, and these potentials have durations that are determined by, among other factors, the time constant of the membrane. A neuron with a relatively long membrane time constant may be able to summate a series of synaptic responses, whereas one with a short time constant may not. Furthermore, synapses are located at widely separate points on the neuron's membrane and therefore the

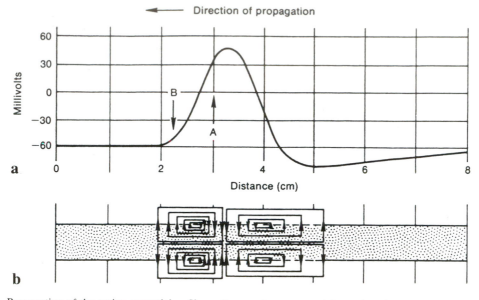

Fig. 4.1a,b. Propagation of the action potential. **a** Shows the membrane potential as a function of distance along the axon. **b** Shows the electric currents flowing across the membrane, inside the axon and in the external medium as a result of the potential differences. These currents (local circuits) depolarize the membrane ahead of the action potential, at *B* in **a**, and lead to greatly increased Na conductance at *A* in **a**. (Reproduced with permission from Keynes 1958.)

interaction of synaptic potentials is dependent on the membrane length constant, a larger length constant allowing summation over a longer length of membrane. The space constant affects the longitudinal spread of current in an axon and determines the rate of propagation of the nerve impulse.

Local Circuits

Once an action potential is generated by opening of the voltage-gated sodium channels, that part of the membrane where the potential exists is depolarized compared with adjacent parts. The local depolarization spreads, by means of the passive properties of the membrane, discharges the membrane capacitance and therefore depolarizes adjacent membrane (Fig. 4.1). Under physiological conditions where a nerve impulse is initiated at a particular point on a neuron and propagates in one direction only, it is the membrane in advance of the impulse that is depolarized by local current flow since the membrane behind the active region will be in a refractory state.

Evidence for the participation of local circuits in the propagation of the nerve impulse was provided by Hodgkin (Fig. 4.2). He used the frog's sciatic nerve and recorded the compound action potential which is made up of large num-

bers of individual action potentials in individual nerve fibres (for a discussion of compound action potentials see below). Hodgkin showed that when a small length of the nerve was blocked, by pressure or cooling, the impulses failed to pass the block, but passive current spreading through the blocked region produced a subthreshold depolarization. Further evidence was provided by Hodgkin, who showed that for axons in the crab the velocity of propagation of the impulse (conduction velocity) was affected, in the predicted manner, by altering the external resistance of the axons (Fig. 4.3).

Effect of Axon Diameter on Conduction Velocity

The conduction velocities of nerve impulses vary widely in different nerves. For non-myelinated axons (see below for myelinated ones) the velocity can vary over more than a hundred-fold range, from less than 0.1 m/s in some fine axons to about 70 m/s in some giant axons. The conduction velocity of the nerve impulse depends mainly on the rate at which the local circuits discharge the membrane capacitance ahead of the active region of membrane. This rate depends on the amount of current generated and on the passive properties of the membrane. Thus the larger the membrane capacitance then the greater the amount of current that has to be

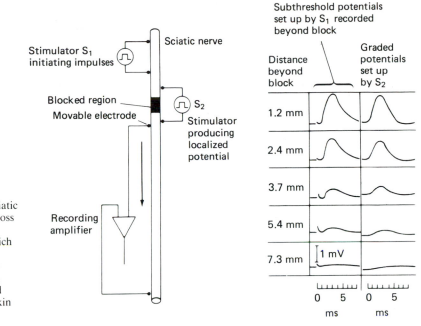

Fig. 4.2. Experimental evidence for local circuits. Impulses in the frog sciatic nerve generate currents that pass across a region of nerve block, where they produce subthreshold potentials, which decay with distance from the block. Subthreshold potentials set up in the same region by electrical stimulation decay in a similar manner. (Modified from Kuffler et al. 1984, after Hodgkin 1937.)

deposited on the membrane to change the membrane potential by a given amount. Also, the greater the axial resistance of the axoplasm, the smaller the current flow for a given potential change. The rate of passive spread of current varies as the product of axial resistance and the capacitance per unit length of axon. Axial resistance varies inversely with the square of axon diameter, and capacitance per unit length of axon varies directly with axon diameter. Thus the effect of an increase in diameter is to increase the product of resistance and capacitance and to increase the conduction velocity.

Myelination and Saltatory Conduction

There are physical limits to the diameters of axons, for example approaching 2 mm in giant axons, where the usual upper limit of conduction velocity is about 70 m/s in non-crustacean giant fibres at 20 °C. In vertebrate species another solution has been found to provide fast impulse propagation while keeping the axon diameter small. This solution involves the cooperation between axons and glial cells, the Schwann cells in the peripheral nervous system and oligodendroglia in the central nervous system. These satellite cells wrap themselves around the axon during development, and as they do so the cytoplasm of the cell is squeezed out so that the satellite cell's membrane forms a series of tightly packed lamellae, the myelin sheath (Fig. 4.4). Thus, because of the lipid nature of the membrane, there is formed around the axon a series of fatty membranes (between about 10 and 150 according to the number of times the satellite cell wraps itself around the axon) which, from an electrical point of view, are in series with the

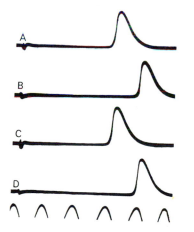

Fig. 4.3. The effect of altering external resistance on conduction velocity of a nerve impulse. A crab giant axon was stimulated at one end and the impulse recorded from the other, first in sea water (*A* and *C*), and again when the external resistance was increased by replacing the sea water with mineral oil, leaving only a thin film of sea water around the axon (*B* and *D*). (Reproduced with permission from Hodgkin 1939.)

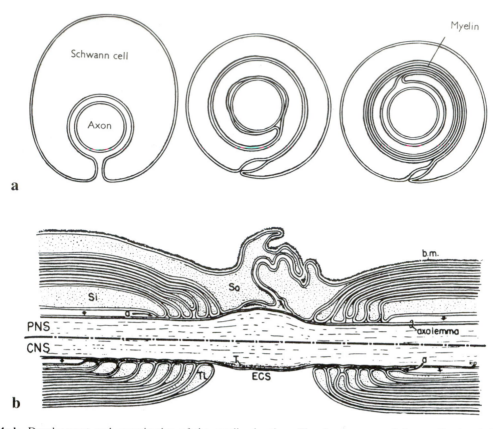

Fig. 4.4a,b. Development and organization of the myelin sheath. **a** The development of the myelin sheath by a glial cell (Schwann cell or oligodendroglial cell) wrapping around an axon. **b** A schematic diagram of the longitudinal arrangement of myelin at either side of a node of Ranvier. The *upper part* of **b** shows the arrangement in the peripheral nervous system (*PNS*), where a Schwann cell provides both an inner (*Si*) and an outer (*So*) collar of cytoplasm to the compact myelin, which comes into close apposition to the axon at the region near the node. The *lower part* shows the arrangement in the central nervous system (*CNS*), where the myelin ends similarly in terminal loops (*Tl*) near the node. At many CNS nodes there is considerable extracellular space (*ECS*). b.m., basement membrane; *T*, thickening of oxolemma. [Reproduced with permission from Robertson 1960 (**a**) and Bunge 1968 (**b**).]

axon's membrane. This mechanism greatly increases the resistance of the membrane and also decreases the membrane's capacitance. The overall diameter of a myelinated axon is made up of the axonal diameter and the thickness of the surrounding myelin, the two components making up some 60%–80% and 20%–40% respectively. For axons conducting at the same velocity, at the same temperature, there is about a hundred-fold saving in cross-sectional area in the myelinated axon.

The myelin is not continuous along the length of an axon but is interrupted periodically at the nodes of Ranvier, where bare axonal membrane is exposed. It is at the nodes where the inward movement of sodium ions occurs, the myelin effectively preventing this at the internodal regions. The nerve impulse therefore jumps along the myelinated axon from node to node, a pro-

cess called saltatory conduction. Experimental evidence for this mode of conduction was provided by Tasaki (1939), who showed that the inward current only occurred at the nodes, and by Huxley and Stämpfli (1949), who also showed that the impulse propagated in a saltatory fashion (Fig. 4.5).

The distance between nodes varies according to the axonal diameter from about 0.2 to 2.0 mm, the thinnest axons having the shortest internodal lengths. The internodal length is about 100 times the axon diameter, that is, about 1 mm for an axon 10 μm thick. The safety factor for conduction in myelinated axons is large, about 5. This means that the current produced at the next node by excitation at one node is about five times that necessary to reach threshold. Thus, even if a node is blocked the impulse can excite the axon at the next node further along the fibre.

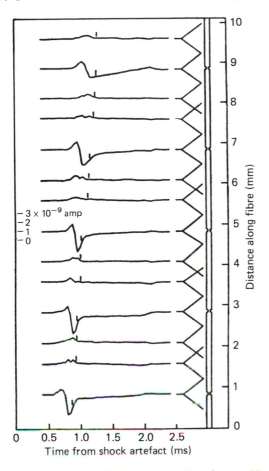

myelinated arrangement also has some metabolic benefits for the nerve cell. In myelinated axons less energy is expended by the sodium–potassium pump in restoring the internal sodium and potassium concentrations after impulse activity.

In rabbit myelinated nerves it has been observed by Ritchie and colleagues that there is only an inward current at the nodes. There is no later outward current, and it may be concluded that the voltage-gated potassium channels are absent. Repolarization presumably occurs as a result of a large leak current (non-gated).

The Length of Axon Involved in a Nerve Impulse

It is instructive to consider how much of the length of an axon is active during nerve impulse activity. A rough estimate may be made by considering the duration of the action potential and the conduction velocity of the impulse. Thus, for an action potential lasting 1 ms in an axon conducting at 100 m/s (that is, 100 mm/ms) the action potential occupies up to 100 mm of nerve length. Similarly, for an action potential lasting 2 ms and travelling at 2 mm/ms it would occupy about 4 mm of nerve. In axons that conduct quickly the impulse can take up an appreciable proportion of the overall length of the nerve fibre.

Fig. 4.5. Saltatory conduction in a myelinated axon. Membrane currents were measured along the length of a single frog myelinated axon at 0.75 mm intervals after stimulation at one end. Inward currents (*downwards deflections* in the current traces) were only recorded when a node occurred between the recording electrodes, whose positions are indicated along the nerve fibre. The *vertical ticks* show the time of peak membrane potential. Note that the latency of the peak membrane potentials jumps from node to node. (Reproduced with permission from Huxley and Stämpfli 1949.)

Voltage-Gated Channels and Impulse Propagation

In non-myelinated axons the voltage-gated sodium and potassium channels are evenly distributed in the membrane. In myelinated axons, however, ionic current only flows at the nodes, and it is at the nodes where the voltage-gated channels are found. There is a relatively high concentration of voltage-gated sodium channels at the nodes (for example, in frog about $2000/\mu m^2$ compared with about $330/\mu m^2$ for the squid giant axon), and this is the reason for the high safety factor for conduction. But even though there is a high concentration of sodium channels at the nodes the

Extracellular Field Potentials

It will be useful to consider some practical consequences of local circuits and their importance for the experimental recording of action potentials from both single axons and bundles of axons as they run, for example, in peripheral nerve. The local circuits allow such action potentials to be recorded by means of extracellular electrodes.

Extracellular Recording from a Single Axon

Extracellular electrodes do not record the potential change occurring across the membrane during a propagated impulse but record the potential change produced by the local currents along the outside of the active fibre. These local currents flow from resting regions in front of and from behind the active region of membrane (see Fig. 4.1).

As indicated in Fig. 4.1, the net current flow through any one cross section of the axon is zero, since at any point the currents along the inside (core) of the axon are of equal strength but of opposite direction to the currents along the external medium. The density of longitudinal current and longitudinal potential difference between two points are not necessarily the same inside and outside the axon, since current inside is concentrated within the fibre while that outside is distributed among the extracellular elements such as the interstitial fluid, other nerve fibres, connective tissue etc. The external current density will be very low if only a few axons are active in a peripheral nerve (Box 4.1).

BOX 4.1

POTENTIAL RECORDED EXTERNALLY FROM AN AXON (after Katz 1966)

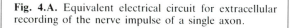

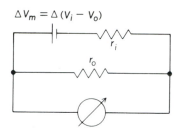

Fig. 4.A. Equivalent electrical circuit for extracellular recording of the nerve impulse of a single axon.

Consider the equivalent electrical circuit of Fig. 4.A for extracellular recording of an action potential from a single active nerve fibre. The external potential change (ΔV_o) produced by current flow along the external medium, which has a resistance (r_o), is only a fraction of the total displacement of membrane potential (ΔV_m). That is:

$$\Delta V_m = \Delta(V_i - V_o)$$

By Ohm's Law the current along the outside is given by:

$$i_o = -\frac{1}{r_o}\frac{dV_o}{dx} \qquad (1)$$

where V_o is the potential on the surface of the axon, dV_o/dx is the external potential gradient and r_o is the resistance of a unit length of outside medium (the minus sign is

_____ Continued

Continued _____

conventional: the direction of current is positive along a falling potential gradient).

Similarly, the current along the inside is given by:

$$i_i = -\frac{1}{r_i}\frac{dV_i}{dx} \qquad (2)$$

But the sum of the currents inside and outside is zero:

$$i_o + i_i = 0$$

Therefore:

from (1) $V_o = a - r_o \int i_o dx$ (3)

from (2) $V_i = b - r_i \int i_i dx$ (4)

and $V_i = b + r_i \int i_o dx$ (5)

since $i_o = -i_i$

a and b are the constant levels of potential outside and inside the fibre at rest. If we ignore these, then equations (3) and (5) give the change of potential produced by the flow of longitudinal current along the fibre core and along its surface.

But:

$$\Delta V_m \doteq \Delta(V_i - V_o)$$

therefore, from (3) and (5):

$$\Delta(V_i - V_o) = (r_o + r_i)\int i_o dx$$

and the recorded external potential change, ΔV_o, is given by:

$$\Delta V_o = -r_o \int i_o dx$$

Thus only a fraction of the total membrane potential change is observed, that is:

$$\frac{\Delta V_o}{\Delta(V_i - V_o)} = -\frac{r_o}{r_o + r_i}$$

External recording will monitor a fraction which depends on the ratio of the external resistance, r_o, and the sum of the total resistance, $(r_o + r_i)$.

Extracellular Recording from a Nerve Bundle – The Compound Action Potential

If a nerve bundle, such as a peripheral nerve, is placed on a pair of recording electrodes (silver or platinum wires) and the bundle is stimulated

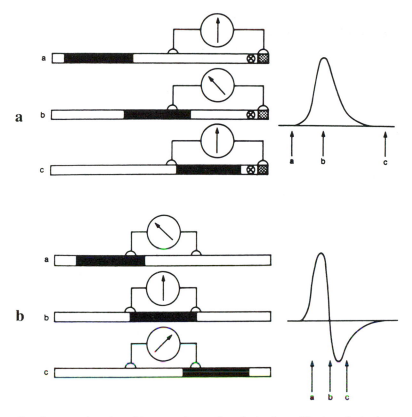

Fig. 4.6a,b. Recording the nerve impulse with external recording electrodes. **a** The two electrodes are placed on the axon and the potential difference between them is recorded. When the impulse reaches the first electrode it swings negative relative to the second, and when the impulse reaches the second electrode it, in turn, swings negative relative to the first. A biphasic potential change is recorded. **b** The nerve has been crushed between the two electrodes and the second is now effectively at earth potential. The nerve impulse never reaches the second electrode and a monophasic negatively going potential is recorded. (Reproduced with permission from Bullock et al. 1977.)

electrically through another pair of electrodes some distance away, then, if the stimulating current is large enough to excite a considerable number of individual axons, a compound action potential will be recorded, composed of individual action potentials in the active axons. With a pair of recording electrodes a biphasic compound potential will be recorded, since the potential difference between the two electrodes is what will be registered (Fig. 4.6a). It is usual to crush the nerve under the electrode furthest away from the site of stimulation so that the nerve impulses do not reach this electrode, which is now at earth potential. In this way a monophasic compound potential may be recorded (Fig. 4.6b).

The compound action potential recorded from a nerve trunk, e.g. the frog sciatic nerve, in response to a maximal stimulus consists of a series of elevations. As the conduction distance increases, the individual elevations become more spread out in time and the different elevations become more and more separated from each other (Fig. 4.7). These observations are due to the fact that different axons have different conduction velocities, and the individual action potentials become more temporally dispersed the further they travel. Another easily verified observation is that the faster components in the compound potential have the lowest electrical threshold for stimulation, and as the strength of stimulation is raised from threshold for the fastest fibres the compound action potential grows progressively (it is not an all-or-nothing phenomenon even though made up of all-or-nothing events) and the slower fibres are excited successively.

Mammalian nerve fibres may be classified according to the various elevations in the compound action potential. Thus A fibres are myelinated, somatic, afferent and efferent axons – myelinated fibres that run in peripheral nerve to muscle and joints and to skin and subcutaneous tissue to (afferent) and from (efferent) the central nervous system; B fibres are myelinated,

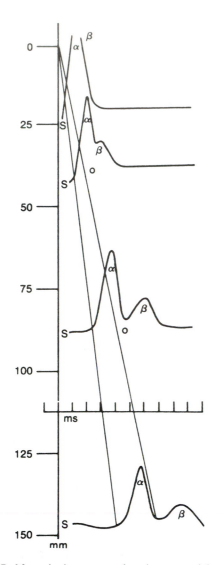

Fig. 4.7. Monophasic compound action potential recorded from the sciatic nerve of a frog. As the distance between stimulating and recording sites is increased (from the *top* to the *bottom* of the figure) there is an increasing delay between the time of stimulation and the start of the action potential, and the two peaks in the potential become more clearly defined. The relation between conduction time and latency for the two groups of fibres is linear, indicating a constant conduction velocity. (Reproduced with permission from Erlanger and Gasser 1937.)

efferent, preganglionic axons in autonomic nerves – myelinated fibres running from the central nervous system to ganglia in the autonomic nervous system; and C fibres are non-myelinated afferent and efferent axons. The A fibres may be further subdivided into α, β, γ and δ according to conduction velocity. Another classification much used by neuroscientists is that due to Lloyd and based on the fibre diameters of the axons (in the cat). Group I fibres have dia-

meters of 12–21 μm, Group II 6–12 μm and Group III 1–6 μm; all are myelinated. The conversion factor for conduction velocity is about 6; that is, a myelinated axon 10 μm in diameter conducts at about 60 m/s. The non-myelinated (C) fibres are called Group IV.

Summary

1.   Propagation of the nerve impulse depends on the passive membrane properties of the cell membrane – its resistance (conductance) and capacitance. Local depolarizations open voltage-gated sodium channels, and this active process depolarizes the membrane further. The depolarization spreads along a nerve or muscle fibre by current flow in local circuits, discharging the membrane capacitance and depolarizing adjacent membrane, thus opening voltage-gated channels ahead of the initially active region.

2.   The conduction velocity of a nerve impulse (or muscle action potential) depends on the diameter of the fibre, since the rate at which local circuits discharge the membrane capacitance depends on the amount of current generated and the passive properties of the membrane. The axial resistance of the axoplasm varies inversely as the axon diameter, and the membrane capacitance per unit length of axons varies directly as the axon diameter. Increasing the axonal diameter increases the product of resistance and capacitance and leads to an increase in conduction velocity.

3.   Myelination of axons in vertebrates greatly increases the resistance of the membrane and decreases the membrane capacitance. The myelin is not continuous but is interrupted periodically at the nodes of Ranvier, where voltage-gated sodium channels are concentrated. The impulse jumps from node to node – saltatory conduction. This speeds up conduction.

4.   External recording from a single axon monitors only a fraction of the membrane potential change that depends on the ration of the external resistance of the medium in which the axon is located to the sum of the total internal and external resistances.

5.   The compound action potential recorded extracellularly from a nerve trunk reflects the activity of all the active axons in the trunk. Axons conducting more slowly produce later elevations in the compound action potential than those conducting more quickly.

5 General Properties of Synaptic Transmission

As mentioned in Chapter 1, the prime function of nervous systems is one of communication: communication within the organism itself and with the external environment, including communication with other organisms. Furthermore, the individual nerve cells that make up the nervous system communicate with one another and with a variety of cells (effector cells) that carry out the nervous system's commands. These effector cells include muscle cells (striated, smooth and cardiac) and a variety of secretory (gland) cells. The nerve impulse is a mechanism whereby these commands may be sent quickly from one end of a nerve cell to the other. In general, there is no cytoplasmic continuity between individual nerve cells or between nerve cells and effector cells. This is the neuron doctrine of Ramon y Cajal, which, in turn, is the cell theory of Schleiden and Schwann applied to the nervous system. Neurons contact one another at synapses (a term coined by Sherrington) or they contact muscle cells at neuromuscular junctions and gland cells at neuroglandular junctions. It is a convenient shorthand, which has become common usage, to call all these contacts "synapses".

Synaptic transmission may be electrical or chemical in nature (or both). The effects of transmission between a pair of nerve cells or between a nerve cell and an effector cell may be excitatory or inhibitory (or both). These two bald statements summarize over 150 years of speculation and nearly 100 years of careful experimentation, during which time very lively controversies occurred. The story is not yet complete, and the increasing awareness of the sophistication of chemically transmitting synapses and of the mechanisms that control the effectiveness of synaptic transmission continues to provide very active fields of research. Not only is such research of great intrinsic interest to students of the nervous system, but it also has great practical applications, since many disorders of the nervous system, including psychiatric illnesses, are caused by alterations in the normal function of synaptic transmission.

The following three chapters will deal in some detail with chemical synaptic transmission and its control. In the rest of this chapter electrical transmission will be discussed, followed by a general outline of chemical transmission, which will act as an introduction to the following chapters.

Electrical Synaptic Transmission

Many examples of excitatory electrical synaptic transmission are now recognized, not only in invertebrate species (where it was first clearly established) but also in vertebrate species, including mammals. One fascinating example of an inhibitory electrical synapse has been described.

Excitatory Electrical Synaptic Transmission

The essence of excitatory electrical transmission is that current flow generated in one cell (the presynaptic cell), for example by an action potential, passes across a synapse and leads to a depolarization in the postsynaptic cell. In order for such electrical transmission to take place there

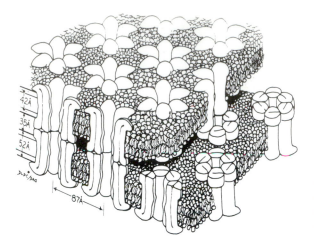

Fig. 5.1. Diagram of the structure of a gap junction. Two cell membranes are closely opposed and channels (connexons) are lined up with each other in the two membranes. Each connexon is made up of six protein subunits which span the membrane, providing channels for the interchange of low molecular weight substances and also for the passage of ionic current. (Reproduced with permission from Makowski et al. 1977.)

must be minimal interference with the passage of current between cells, and this is achieved by special synapses – the electrotonic synapse or bridged junction. Bridged junctions are gap junctions which are similar to the gap junctions

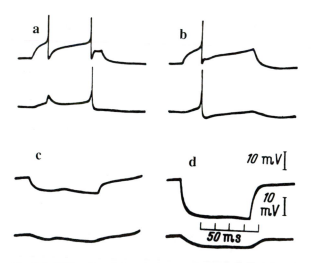

Fig. 5.2. Bidirectional electrical transmission in the segmental ganglion of the leech. Simultaneous intracellular microelectrode recordings from two giant cells. Rectangular current pulses were applied through one microelectrode (*upper traces*) and its effect on the other cell recorded (*lower traces*). Depolarizing currents were passed in A and B, and hyperpolarizing currents in C and D. Currents were larger in A than B and in D than C. (Reproduced with permission from Hagiwara and Morita 1962.)

found between many different types of cells, e.g. cells in the liver. At gap junctions (Fig. 5.1) there is an especially close apposition of the cell membranes of the two cells of about 2 nm (compared with about 20 nm at regions outside gap junctions). On each side of the junction there are aggregations of particles about 6–15 nm in diameter, and the particles are paired across the junction. Each pair of particles forms a channel (connexon) spanning the gap junction and these channels allow metabolic and electrical communication between the cells. The diameter of the channels imposes restrictions on the size of molecules that can pass from cell to cell, and the channels will also allow movement of ions during current flow.

There are two main types of excitatory electrical synapses. In one, the synapse transmits equally well in either direction, that is, either member of the pair may be the presynaptic "driving" cell. Examples of such bidirectional transmission are found, for example, between certain neurons in segmental ganglia of the leech (Fig. 5.2), electromotor neurons of Mormyrid fish, supramedullary neurons in puffer fish, in follower cells of the cardiac ganglia of lobster and in the inferior olivary nucleus of various mammalian species. In general, electrical synapses of this type transmit slow potential changes well, but not brief ones such as action potentials (except in the leech ganglia and the inferior olivary nucleus). In the other type of excitatory electrical transmission, exemplified by the synapse between the lateral giant fibre in the abdominal nerve cord of the crayfish and a motor nerve that innervates a fast-acting muscle that flexes the tail, the transmission is unidirectional (Fig. 5.3). Furshpan and Potter (1959) showed that depolarizing current passed easily from the presynaptic to the postsynaptic fibres but that there was almost no current flow in the opposite direction. Thus the synapse shows rectifying properties, allowing transmission in one direction only, like chemical synapses. Other examples of such rectifying electrical synapses have been found, e.g. in the rat's mesencephalic nucleus.

The gap junction provides a low resistance path for current flow between the two cells, and therefore there is little delay, since it is the speed of electronic transmission that matters. As we shall see, this contrasts with chemical transmission, where there is a marked synaptic delay. Thus electrical transmission is found, (1) in situations where even a small synaptic delay of a few tenths of a millisecond may be important; (2) in mechanisms underlying escape reactions (in the cray-

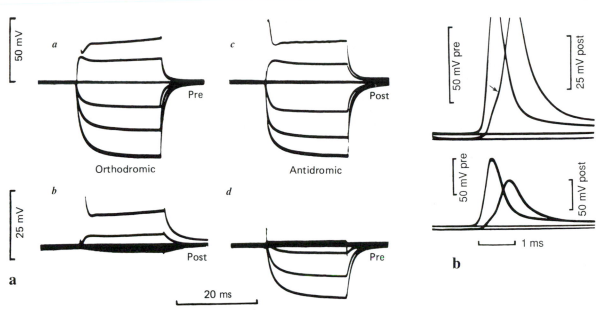

Fig. 5.3a,b. Unidirectional transmission at the crayfish giant motor synapse. Simultaneous intracellular microelectrode recordings from two electrically coupled giant fibres. **a** Records *a* and *b* show responses in the pre- and post-fibres to current pulses in the pre-fibre. Only depolarizing currents cross the synapse. Records *c* and *d* show responses in the fibres to current pulses in the post-fibre. Only hyperpolarizing currents cross the synapse. **b** Shows the pre- and postsynaptic action potentials at the synapse. Two pairs of records are shown at different amplifications. In each the *upper record* is the presynaptic response. The deflection in the postsynaptic action potential (*arrow*) shows the level at which the postsynaptic response crosses threshold. Note the very short latency between the times of onset of the two potentials. (Reproduced with permission from Furshpan and Potter 1959.)

fish example above), where it is important to synchronize activity in a group of cells (in leech ganglia where cells with similar functions on opposite sides of the organism are electrically coupled); (3) where constancy of action is required; (4) where very fine timing is important (mammalian inferior olivary nucleus); and (5) in systems where secondary cells are driven by a primary pacemaker cell, as in the cardiac ganglion of the lobster.

Inhibitory Electrical Transmission

A single example of electrical inhibition is known. This occurs in Mauthner cells in the medulla of bony fish. Mauthner cells are large neurons, and there is one on each side of the medulla. From the cell body arise two large dendrites, a lateral one and a ventral one, and an axon (Fig. 5.4). The axon arises from the axon hillock and it is at this point that the nerve impulse arises. The axon hillock is surrounded by a network of glial cells, the axon cap, and the neurons that are responsible for electrical inhibition of the Mauthner cell send their axons into the space between the glial cells and the axon hillock. Activation of

these inhibitory neurons leads to a large extracellular positive potential change in the space surrounding the axon hillock. This positivity is caused by the current flow in the fibres that penetrate the cap, these currents being spatially restricted by the connective tissue sheath of the axon cap. The inhibitory axons do not make synaptic contact with the axon hillock region of the Mauthner cell, and the extracellular positivity is a reflection of the intense intracellular positivity that occurs in the fibres during the action potential. The increased extracellular positivity at the axon hillock has the same effect as if an extracellular anode were placed in that position, that is, it raises the threshold for the initiation of an action potential at the axon hillock by hyperpolarization (Fig. 5.4). It is therefore more difficult to bring the Mauthner cell to threshold and the effect is inhibitory.

Chemical Synaptic Transmission

The essence of chemical transmission (Fig. 5.5) is that potential changes in the presynaptic cell

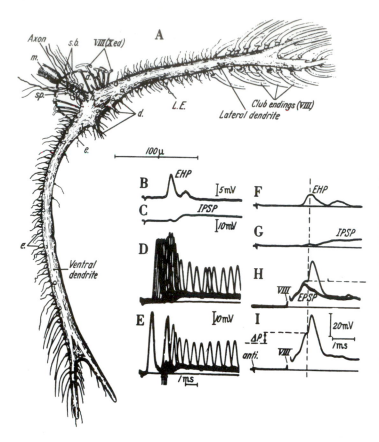

Fig. 5.4. Inhibitory synapse operating by electrical transmission. *A* is a drawing of the Mauthner cell in the goldfish. The axon cap is indicated by the *circle* and is shown containing a few of the inhibitory fibres spiralling (*sp.*) around the initial part of the axon near the axon hillock (*h*). Record *B* shows the extracellular hyperpolarizing potential (*EHP*) produced by activity in the spiral fibres, and record *C* shows the concomitant intracellular potential (*IPSP*). Records *D* and *E* are intracellular records from the Mauthner cell and show the depression or block of antidromic impulse invasion from the cell's axon. Records *F* and *G* are similar to records *B* and *C* but at a faster time base. Record *H* shows orthodromic excitation of the Mauthner cell (*EPSP*, excitatory postsynaptic potential), and in record *I* this has been preceded by a conditioning stimulus producing an EHP. The EHP increases the threshold necessary to fire the cell by a factor of *P*. (Reproduced with permission from Eccles 1964, after Furukawa and Furshpan 1963.)

lead to the secretion (exocytosis) of a chemical transmitter which crosses the synaptic cleft and combines with specific receptor molecules on the surface of the postsynaptic cell, and this combination leads to changes in the postsynaptic cell. There are strong similarities between the release of a neurotransmitter from a nerve cell and the release of a hormone from an endocrine cell; indeed, some nerve cells release hormones, for example cells of the supraoptic and paraventricular nuclei of the vertebrate hypothalamus that release vasopressin and oxytocin, and the modified nerve cells of the adrenal medullary gland that release adrenaline (epinephrine). The main differences between neurotransmission and hormonal transmission are in the location of the target cell – usually very close to the presynaptic cell in neurotransmission but at a considerable distance from the endocrine cell in hormonal transmission – and in the localization of action of the chemical messengers – usually very localized (to a particular part of the postsynaptic cell) in neurotransmission but widespread and on many target cells in hormonal transmission. A further difference is in the speed of action. Neurotrans-

mission is usually faster in onset and shorter in duration than hormonal transmission, but there are exceptions to these generalizations. Some consideration of neuroendocrine control mechanisms will be given in Chapter 16.

Recently it has been realized that some peptides released from nerve cells and which act as neurotransmitters or neuromodulators (see below) may be hormones. Thus, for example, the hormones oxytocin and vasopressin, released from nerve endings in the posterior pituitary, and the gastrointestinal hormones gastrin, secretin and cholecystokinin may also be found in neurons in many parts of the central nervous system and probably act as neurotransmitters or neuromodulators.

Neurotransmitters

The classical view of chemical transmission was that an individual nerve cell only released a single transmitter substance and that the effects of that substance depended on the particular receptor on the postsynaptic cell. Thus, postganglionic para-

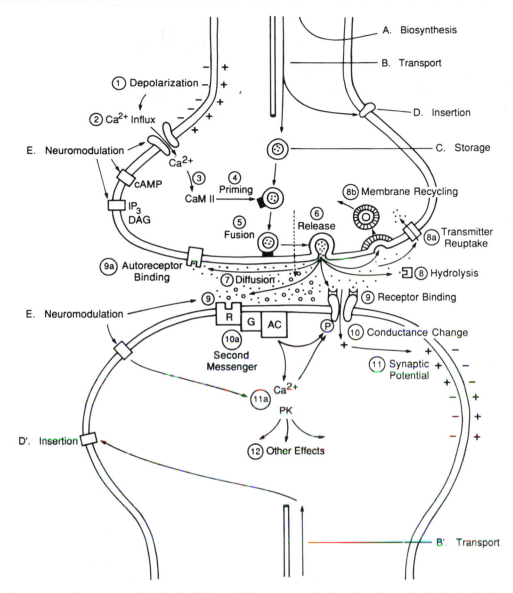

Fig. 5.5. The processes that can occur in chemically transmitting synapses. $A-E$ are long-term steps in the synthesis, transport and storage of transmitters and neuromodulators. $1-12$ summarize the more rapid steps involved in signalling at chemical synapses. *IP*, inositol triphosphate; *CaM II*, Ca/calmodulin-dependent protein kinase II; *DAG*, diacylglycerol; *PK*, protein kinase; *R*, receptor; *G*, G protein; *AC*, adenylate cyclase. (Reproduced with permission from Shepherd 1988.)

sympathetic neurons in the heart release acetylcholine, which has an inhibitory action, slowing the heart beat, whereas the motor nerves to skeletal muscle also release acetylcholine, but here the action is excitatory leading to contraction of the muscle. The two actions of acetylcholine may be differentiated by pharmacological means, the action on the heart being mimicked by the drug muscarine and the action on skeletal muscle being mimicked by nicotine. It is now known, however, that many (and perhaps a majority) of nerve cells

release more than one transmitter and that they may have quite different actions. However, any single neuron always releases the same transmitter or the same combination of transmitters (although perhaps in different ratios under different circumstances). In the presynaptic neuron the transmitter is stored in membrane-bound synaptic vesicles.

Neurotransmitters may be divided into two classes: substances of low molecular weight and neuroactive peptides (which have larger molecular weights). Eight low molecular weight trans-mitters have been generally accepted and all of them are amines. Seven are amino acids or are derived from amino acids and one, acetylcho-line, is not. The seven are either biogenic amines (noradrenaline, dopamine, serotonin or 5-hydro-xytryptamine, and histamine) or amino acids (glycine, glutamate and gamma-aminobutyric acid; GABA). There is a possibility that aspartate is also one of the amino acid transmitters. There is a long list of neuroactive peptides that are re-leased from neurons and act as transmitters or as neuromodulators. A neuromodulator may be de-fined as a substance released from a nerve cell that affects the response of its postsynaptic target cells to neurotransmitters. Some of these pepti-des, such as oxytocin, vasopressin, gastrin, secre-tin, vasoactive intestinal peptide, growth hormone releasing hormone, were previously recognized as hormones. Others, such as the enkephalins and nueropeptide Y, have been identified more recently. The vast array of chemical substances that have been identified as transmitters or neuromodulators or that are candidates for these roles will be considered in Chapter 7.

Release of Transmitter

Transmitter is released by exocytosis in which the membrane-bound synaptic vesicles fuse with the cell membrane of the presynaptic cell. This exocytosis is brought about by means of an influx of calcium ions. The membrane of the nerve terminal contains voltage-gated calcium channels. These channels are opened by depolarization, which may be due to an action potential or, in neurons that do not generate action potentials, by an excitatory depolarizing potential. Here, then, is another example of the specific localization of particular voltage-gated ion channels in neurons. Release of transmitter will be covered in Chapter 6.

Effects of Transmitter–Receptor Combination

Combination of transmitter with receptor, after the transmitter has diffused across the synaptic cleft, may lead to a variety of events. There may be opening of chemically gated ion channels that are closed at rest. Depending on which ions are allowed to move through the channels the result-ing conductance changes may have excitatory or

inhibitory actions on the postsynaptic cell. Some transmitter–receptor combinations may lead to the closure of chemically gated ion channels. In these latter situations a second intracellular mes-senger is needed, and again the ionic conductance changes produced may lead to either excitatory or inhibitory actions, usually with a rather slow time course. Finally, some transmitter–receptor com-binations do not lead to conductance changes but to metabolic changes in the postsynaptic cell. Again a second intracellular messenger is required. The effects of transmitter–receptor combination will be discussed in Chapter 8.

Presynaptic Control of Chemical Transmission

It will already be apparent to the reader that chemical transmission is a much more complex and sophisticated process than electrical trans-mission. It lends itself to a variety of controlling mechanisms, but, in addition, the release of trans-mitter from the presynaptic neuron can be control-led by chemical synaptic transmission. Consider Fig. 5.6, where a nerve cell (A) makes synaptic contact with another cell (B). The terminals of cell A themselves receive synaptic contacts from cell C. This anatomical organization, which is extremely common in both vertebrate and inver-tebrate nervous systems, forms a substrate for presynaptic control of neuron A. Cell C can re-lease a transmitter which will combine with re-ceptors on the membrane of the terminals of cell A and lead to conductance changes that may either reduce the amount of transmitter released by A (presynaptic inhibition) or increase the amount of transmitter released (presynaptic facilitation). Presynaptic inhibition is a well-recognized phenomenon in vertebrate nervous systems and both phenomena occur in inverte-brate systems. Mechanisms of presynaptic inhibi-

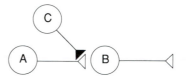

Fig. 5.6. Diagrammatic scheme of the anatomical basis for presynaptic effects. The axon of cell *A* makes a chemically transmitting synapse with cell *B*. The terminal bouton of A is itself postsynaptic to a terminal bouton from the axon of cell *C*. Activity in cell *C* can affect transmission between A and B.

tory control will be discussed in Chapter 8, and the organizational aspects will be considered at appropriate points in the later sections.

Summary

1. Synaptic transmission between nerve cells or between nerve and effector cells may be either electrical or chemical. Both electrical and chemical transmission may have either excitatory or inhibitory effects on the postsynaptic cell.

2. Excitatory electrical transmission takes place at electrotonic synapses where there is close apposition of pre-and postsynaptic cells. It may be bidirectional or unidirectional. It is found where very quick action is needed, where synchronization of action is required, where constancy of action is desirable and where fine timing is important.

3. One well-documented example of inhibitory electrical transmission is known.

4. In chemical synaptic transmission the presynaptic neuron releases a chemical or a mixture of two or even more chemicals. These transmitters diffuse across the synaptic gap to the postsynaptic cell, where they combine with specific receptor molecules. Combination of transmitter with receptor leads to changes in the postsynaptic cell that include the opening or closing of chemically gated ion channels and metabolic changes in the cell.

5. Neurotransmitters are either low molecular weight substances (amines or amino acids and acetylcholine) or larger molecular weight peptides. Many of the peptides are also classical hormones and may act as neuromodulators rather than as classical transmitters, that is, they may modify the response of the postsynaptic cell to classical transmitter.

6. Transmitters are contained within synaptic vesicles, and the contents of the vesicles are released by exocytosis brought about by an influx of calcium ions through voltage-gated calcium channels. These channels are opened by depolarization.

7. The release of transmitters may also be controlled by synaptic mechanisms (presynaptic inhibition or facilitation).

6 The Presynaptic Neuron I: Release and Storage of Transmitter

Two experimental preparations have been used extensively in unravelling the intricacies of neuro-transmitter release and the effects of transmitters on the postsynaptic neuron. These are the vertebrate neuromuscular junction, which has been especially useful for studying the actions of transmitter on the postsynaptic cell and the general properties of transmitter release, and the giant synapse in the stellate ganglion of the squid, which has been especially useful for studying the link between a neuronal action potential and the release (exocytosis) of transmitter from the presynaptic neuron.

Control of Transmitter Release

The giant fibre synapse in the stellate ganglion of the squid is a chemical excitatory synapse in which a single impulse in the presynaptic fibre leads to an impulse in the postsynaptic neuron. In this respect the synapse operates like the neuromuscular junction with one-to-one transmission. It should be stressed that this is a rather unusual situation, as will be seen later, but one that has advantages for study. Furthermore, the sizes of the pre- and postsynaptic elements are such that microelectrodes may be inserted into both of them to allow controlled intracellular stimulation and recording.

Since transmitter is normally released following an action potential in the presynaptic neuron it is instructive to ask whether the action potential (nerve impulse) is itself directly responsible for this release. Katz and Miledi (1967b) addressed this problem by ascertaining whether either the sodium influx or the potassium efflux that underly the action potential were necessary for release. Their results are shown in Figs. 6.1 and 6.2. First, they blocked the sodium channels selectively with tetrodotoxin (TTX). As Fig. 6.1a shows, before TTX application a single impulse in the presynaptic fibre led to a single impulse in the postsynaptic cell. Within a few minutes of TTX application the presynaptic action potential became smaller in amplitude and slightly longer in duration, and the postsynaptic impulse failed, leaving the underlying excitatory postsynaptic potential (EPSP). Then the presynaptic impulse failed progressively and there was a corresponding reduction in amplitude of the EPSP until, about 15 min after TTX application the presynaptic action potential had fallen to 45 mV in amplitude and there was no discernible EPSP. There is, therefore, a steep relationship between presynaptic action potential amplitude and the size of the EPSP (Fig. 6.1b) and it might be concluded that the influx of sodium was indeed necessary for transmitter release. But once all the sodium channels were blocked by TTX, Katz and Miledi showed that direct depolarization of the presynaptic axon, by intracellular injection of current, led to the appearance of a postsynaptic potential once the terminal had been depolarized beyond about 25–40 mV and that the relation between depolarization and postsynaptic potential amplitude was exponential with, above threshold, a 10 mV presynaptic depolarization producing a ten-fold increase in trans-

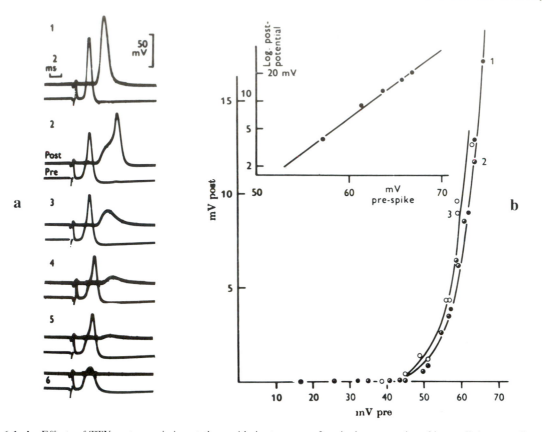

Fig. 6.1a,b. Effects of TTX on transmission at the squid giant synapse. In **a** is shown a series of intracellular recordings taken simultaneously from the pre- and postsynaptic neurons close to the synapse. Note the failure of the post-synaptic impulse (between records 2 and 3) and then the failure of the EPSP as the presynaptic impulse becomes smaller. In **b** is plotted the relationship between the pre- and postsynaptic potential changes. Presynaptic action potentials are shown as *filled circles*. After complete TTX paralysis curves 2 (*half-filled circles*) and 3 (open circles) were obtained by applying direct depolarizing pulses through the micro-electrode in the presynaptic fibre, showing that transmitter release is not dependent on Na influx. (Reproduced with permission from Katz and Miledi 1967b.)

mitter release (as assessed by postsynaptic potential amplitude). Thus, transmitter can still be released even though there is no influx of sodium through the voltage-gated sodium channels.

Katz and Miledi then investigated whether or not the efflux of potassium through voltage-gated channels was a necessary prerequisite for transmitter release. In this experiment the sodium channels were blocked, as before, by the application of TTX externally and in addition the voltage-gated potassium channels were blocked by the injection of tetraethylammonium (TEA) into the presynaptic fibre. Again presynaptic depolarization produced by intracellular current pulses led to postsynaptic depolarizing potentials and it was concluded that neither sodium influx nor potassium efflux was required for transmitter release (Fig. 6.2).

If neither sodium nor potassium were involved in transmitter release and yet depolarization of

the presynaptic terminal produced release, what are the likely mechanisms? A depolarization might be caused by the influx of some other positively charged ions or by the efflux of negatively charged ions. A likely candidate was calcium, since it had been known for some time that neuromuscular transmission fails in low calcium solutions. Katz and Miledi returned to the frog neuromuscular junction as their experimental preparation and showed that in a bathing solution containing no calcium neuromuscular transmission was abolished, but that it could be restored by releasing a very small pulse of calcium from a microelectrode in close proximity to the terminal region if the calcium application occurred just before invasion of the terminal by the nerve impulse (Fig. 6.3).

Direct evidence for the entry of calcium into the presynaptic terminals was provided by Llínas and his co-workers (see Llínas, 1982) who in-

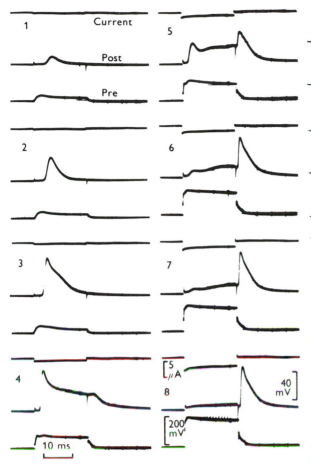

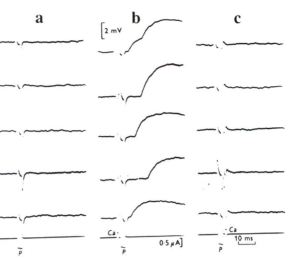

Fig. 6.3. Effect of an iontophoretic pulse of Ca^{2+} on the end-plate response at the frog neuromuscular junction. The preparation was devoid of Ca^{2+}. Depolarizing pulses (P) and Ca^{2+} were applied from a twin-barrel miropipette and intracellular recordings were made from the end-plate. Column A shows depolarizing pulses alone, column B shows the Ca^{2+} pulse preceding the depolarizing pulse, and column C shows depolarization preceding the Ca^{2+} pulse. Only when Ca^{2+} had been injected around the nerve before depolarization was there any end-plate response. (Reproduced with permission from Katz and Miledi 1976a.)

Fig. 6.2. Effects of TTX and TEA on transmission at the squid giant synapse. Long current pulses were applied through the microelectrode in the presynaptic axon producing potential changes. Note the responses in the postsynaptic neuron showing that neither Na^+ influx nor K^+ efflux is required for transmitter release. (Reproduced with permission from Katz and Miledi 1967b.)

jected the dye aequorin into the giant fibre. Aequorin luminesces in the presence of ionized calcium. These workers also voltage clamped the presynaptic terminals in the presence of both TTX and TEA and showed that graded depolarizations led to activation of an inward calcium current in a graded manner. Thus there is a voltage-gated calcium current in the nerve terminals which is due to the presence of voltage-gated calcium channels in this part of the axonal membrane. The influx of calcium produces a secretory potential which is a regenerative calcium action potential (Fig. 6.4) The calcium channels do not inactivate readily but remain open whilst the depolarization lasts. Normally, the duration of the secretory potential is determined by the duration of the sodium–potassium

action potential. (See Fig. 5.5 for a summary of the events occurring in the presynaptic axon that lead to transmitter release and its subsequent effects.)

Release of Transmitter in Packets or Quanta

The experiments described above show that presynaptic depolarization leads to activation of voltage-gated calcium channels and the influx of calcium. The calcium entry, in turn, leads to transmitter release. How is the transmitter released, or secreted, from the nerve terminals? In fact it has been known since the 1950s that transmitter is released in multimolecular packets which were called "quanta" by Fatt and Katz. A quantum is the smallest amount (unit) of transmitter that is normally released. The evidence for the quantal release came from work on the frog neuromuscular junction.

Fatt and Katz (1952) observed that at the neuromuscular end-plate region small spontaneous depolarizations could be recorded. These were

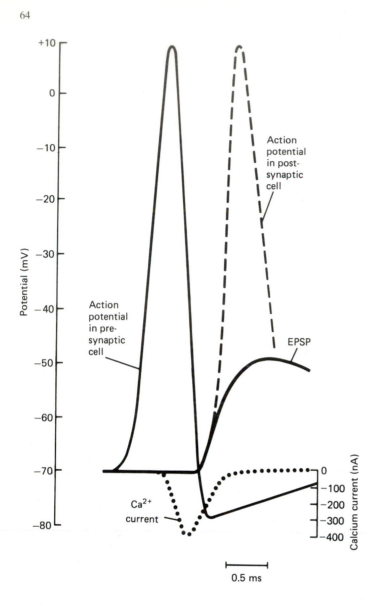

Fig. 6.4 The time courses of events during synaptic transmission. The presynaptic action potential causes voltage-gated Ca^{2+} channels to open leading to a Ca^{2+} current. The Ca^{2+} current causes transmitter release and this, in turn, leads to a postsynaptic potential (EPSP) that can cause a postsynaptic impulse (spike). (After Llínas 1982.)

about 0.5–1 mV in amplitude and had the same time course, and were affected by drugs in the same way, as the end-plate potential elicited by an impulse in the motor axon innervating the muscle (Fig. 6.5). The transmitter at the neuromuscular junction is acetylcholine (ACh), and these spontaneous depolarizations – miniature end-plate potentials – were decreased in amplitude and then abolished as curare was added to the bathing solution, and were increased in amplitude and duration by the addition of the drug prostigmine, which inhibits the breakdown of ACh by the enzyme acetylcholinesterase. These drugs have similar actions on the impulse-evoked end-plate potential.

The miniature end-plate potentials occur in a random fashion, indicating that they are independent events. Their frequency of occurrence, but not their amplitude, can be increased by depolarizing the presynaptic terminal region. They disappear if the motor axon is cut or crushed and allowed to degenerate distal to the lesion and they reappear if the nerve regenerates.

All of the above observations show that miniature end-plate potentials are produced by the spontaneous release of ACh from the presynaptic terminal. Do the miniature end-plate potentials represent the response of some receptor molecule to the release of single molecules of Ach? The answer to this question is "No". Del Castillo and Katz (1954) showed that if ACh was released from a microelectrode at the end-plate the response was graded and not quantized.

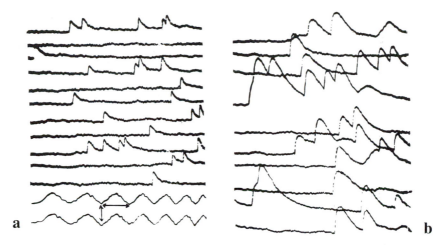

Fig. 6.5a,b. Spontaneous miniature end-plate potentials at the frog neuromuscular junction and the effects of neostigmine. **a** These records are control responses in normal frog (Ringer's solution). **b** These responses are recorded after addition of neostigmine – the miniature end-plate potentials are larger and longer. The *arrows* in **a** indicate 1 mV and 20 ms. (Reproduced with permission from Fatt and Katz 1952.)

Del Castillo and Katz also noted that the end-plate potential that was evoked by an action potential in the motor nerve became smaller and smaller as the external calcium concentration was reduced or the external magnesium concen-

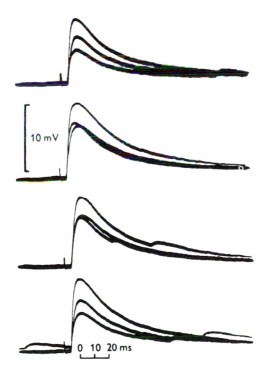

Fig. 6.6. Fluctuation of the end-plate potential in raised Mg^{2+} solution. The responses were evoked by stimulating the nerve. Note the scattered spontaneous miniature end-plate potentials. (Reproduced with permission from del Castillo and Katz 1954a.)

tration was increased (Fig. 6.6). Ultimately, at very low levels of calcium the end-plate potential itself began to fluctuate in a step-like fashion. The smallest steps were about 0.5–1 mV in amplitude and other potentials had amplitudes in multiples of these smallest steps. Del Castillo and Katz proposed that normally the end-plate potential was made up of a number of these individual quantal events due to the almost simultaneous release of a number of packets of ACh. Calculations suggested that at the frog neuromuscular junction the end-plate potential was generated by the release of about 200 quanta.

Further analysis of the fluctuations in the amplitude of impulse-evoked end-plate potentials that occur in low calcium solutions were made for the frog and also the mammalian neuromuscular junction. It was shown (Fig. 6.7) that the fluctuations occurred in multiples of the smallest potential (equivalent to the size of the miniature end-plate potential). Furthermore, the amplitude distribution was remarkably well-described by the Poisson distribution, indicating that the quanta were released independently. The alterations in external calcium concentration, therefore, did not affect the size of the quanta (that is, did not affect the number of molecules of ACh in each package) but did alter the number of quanta released by affecting the probability that a given quantum was released. This explanation, due to del Castillo and Katz, is the quantum hypothesis of transmitter release.

Quantal release has been demonstrated at all chemically transmitting synapses studied. The release of as many as 200 quanta by a single

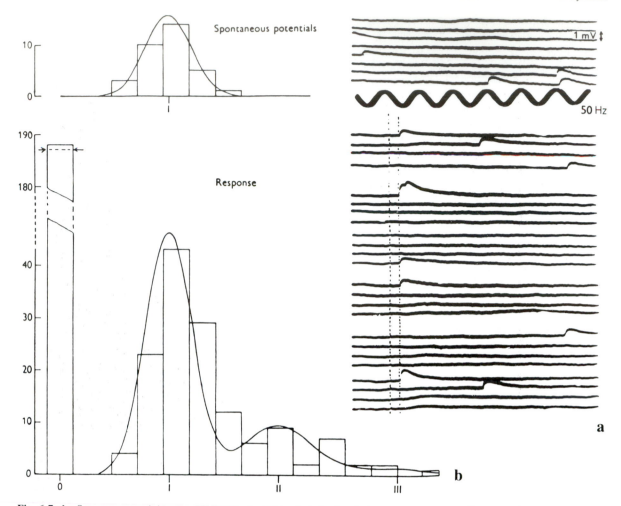

Fig. 6.7a,b. Spontaneous miniature end-plate potentials and evoked end-plate potentials in a Ca^{2+}-deficient medium. **a** These records show, at the *top*, a few spontaneous potentials and, at the *bottom*, responses evoked by single nerve impulses. (The stimulus artefact and response latency are shown by the *dotted lines*.) Note the high proportion of times the impulse failed to evoke a response and the similarity between the amplitudes of the spontaneous and evoked potentials. **b** The *upper histogram* shows the amplitudes of spontaneous miniature end-plate potentials and the *lower histogram* shows the amplitudes of potentials evoked in a Ca^{2+}-deficient medium. The continuous curve in the lower histogram was calculated on the hypothesis that the responses were built up statistically of units with a mean size and amplitude distribution similar to those of the spontaneous potentials. The *arrows* indicate the expected number of failures. (Reproduced with permission from del Castillo and Katz 1954a.)

presynaptic action potential, as occurs at the neuromuscular junction, is not the standard pattern in transmission between pairs of nerve cells. The very high safety factor for transmission at the neuromuscular junction, where a single nerve impulse always leads to a muscle action potential, and therefore to muscle contraction, would be inappropriate in the nervous system. Generally any individual nerve cell receives excitatory, and inhibitory, inputs from very many neurons (tens or hundreds of thousands), and whether or not the postsynaptic neuron fires depends on the balance between the various inputs. The number of quanta

released by a presynaptic neuron under these conditions is much less than 200, and, as we shall see, often of the order of 1–10.

As discussed above, the number of quanta released is affected by the size of the calcium current in the terminals. Anything that affects the calcium current under physiological conditions might therefore alter the efficacy of transmission at a particular synapse. Changes in the membrane potential of the presynaptic terminal will alter the number of quanta released – a depolarization leading to opening of voltage-gated Ca^{2+} channels and an increase in calcium influx and therefore to an increase in the number of quanta released, and a hyperpolarization having the opposite effect. These changes are brought about by changes in the steady calcium current that is present even at the resting level of membrane potential. The reader will probably have had a mental hiccup at this point: if depolarization leads to opening of the voltage-gated Ca^{2+} channels how does presynaptic inhibition (which depolarizes the presynaptic terminal) work? Presynaptic inhibition, which involves synaptic transmission at axo-axonic synapses and the control of chemically gated channels on the presynaptic membrane, probably acts by depressing the voltage-gated Ca^{2+} channel or by short-circuiting the membrane by increasing Cl^- conductance. Furthermore, activity in the presynaptic neuron can have effects on the efficacy of synaptic transmission. A second impulse reaching the terminal shortly after the first may arrive at a time when there is still a raised calcium level in the terminal due to the first impulse, and a train of impulses may lead to a build-up of calcium in the terminal. Under these conditions the succeeding impulse or impulses will cause a larger number of quanta to be released than the first impulse, if there is sufficient readily available transmitter. The facilitation at excitatory synapses produced by a train of impulses is known as post-tetanic potentiation and provides a simple example of synaptic plasticity and may even be considered as a form of learning.

Quantal Content

The experiments of Katz and his colleagues showed clearly that quanta represented the effects of multimolecular packages of transmitter. Various estimates were made of the number of transmitter molecules (ACh, for example, at the neuromuscular junction) that were contained in a single quantum package. The most accurate estimates were made by Kuffler and his co-workers in some beautifully designed experiments (see Kuffler and Yoshikami 1975a, b). Using a snake muscle preparation, Kuffler and Yoshikami (1975a) ejected ACh from a microelectrode onto the postsynaptic membrane after having stripped off the nerve terminals. By careful placement of the ACh-containing microelectrode and by careful adjustment of the pulse of current used to eject the ACh, they were able to mimic spontaneous miniature end-plate potentials (Fig. 6.8).

The next problem was to determine how many molecules of ACh had been released. For this purpose they ejected ACh into a droplet of oil

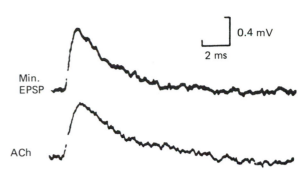

Fig. 6.8. Synaptic responses to nerve-released and iontophoresed ACh in the cutaneus pectoris muscle of the frog. The *upper trace* is a spontaneous miniature end-plate potential and the *lower trace* was obtained by the application of a 0.5 ms pulse of ACh from a micropipette placed close to the subsynaptic membrane. The rise time of the artificial ACh potential is slightly slower due to the pipette being slightly further away from the subsynaptic membrane than the nerve terminal. (Reproduced with permission from Kuffler and Yoshikami 1975a.)

by repeatedly passing pulses of current similar to those that had produced the response mimicking the miniature end-plate potential. The droplet was then applied to the end-plate of a snake muscle fibre and the potential produced was recorded. Following this, droplets of the same size containing known concentrations of ACh were applied to the end-plate and a stimulus–response curve was derived. It was therefore possible to determine the concentration of ACh in the droplet into which ACh had been ejected from the microelectrode, and from this figure the number of ACh molecules ejected per pulse was calculated. It turned out that each pulse contained rather less than 10000 molecules of ACh. It was concluded that this figure would be the upper limit for the number of ACh molecules in a quantum, since, under the conditions of the experiment, the location of the microelectrode used for ejecting ACh would not be as favourable as the location of the terminals from which ACh is released physiologically.

Storage of Transmitter

The Vesical Hypothesis

At the time that del Castillo and Katz were putting forward their quantal hypothesis of chemical transmission, electron microscopists had begun to provide high-magnification images of the neuromuscular juction. It was shown that the presynap-

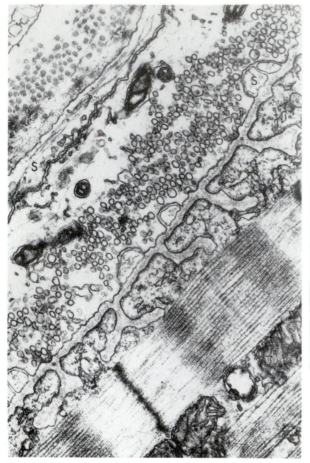

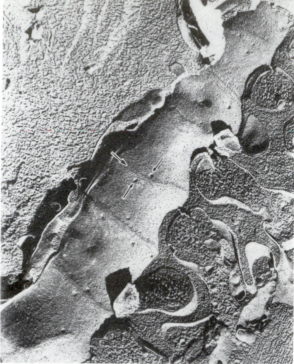

Fig. 6.10. Freeze-fracture replica of a motor nerve terminal. The nerve was stimulated before and during fixation. The view is of the cytoplasmic half of the axon terminal as seen from outside the terminal. Small dimples (*smaller arrows*) are seen beside the active zones only in stimulated junctions. They probably represent vesicles fusing with the cell membrane during transmitter discharge. The *larger arrows* point to ridges on the surface of the nerve terminal which face folds (*F*) in the surface of the muscle. (Reproduced with permission from Heuser et al. 1974.)

Fig. 6.9. Synaptic vesicles at a frog neuromuscular junction. This is a transmission electron micrograph of a longitudinal section of a junction. Many vesicles may be seen in the axon terminal and they appear to cluster around "active zones" (*asterisks*) opposite subneural folds. *S*, Schwann cell processes. (Reproduced with permission from Heuser and Reese 1977.)

tic nerve terminal contained an accumulation of membrane-bound vesicles (Fig. 6.9), and del Castillo and Katz suggested that the vesicles contained the transmitter and were the structural units underlying the quantal release of transmitter. Since that time all chemically transmitting synapses have been shown to contain synaptic vesicles, and although there is quite a wide variation in the size and appearance of these vesicles they are a constant feature of the system of chemical transmission.

Direct evidence that vesicles contain transmitter was provided by Whittaker and his colleagues (Whittaker et al. 1972), who showed that by homogenizing and fractionating preparations like the electric organ of the electric fish *Torpedo*, in which the transmitter is ACh, that some fractions contain large concentrations of membrane-bound synaptosomes containing ACh. The ACh content of the synaptosomal fraction could be changed by stimulating the nerves before fractionation. In intact nerve terminals depletion of vesicles may be observed after repeated stimulation or the application of black widow spider venom, which causes a massive release of transmitter. Finally, Heuser and Reese and their colleagues (see Heuser and Reese 1977) have studied the fine structure of chemically transmitting synapses by electron microscopy after fracturing the tissue along natural planes of cleavage by very rapid freezing (freeze-fracturing) and have observed vesicles apparently in the process of exocytosis (Fig. 6.10).

The vesicles are not randomly distributed in the presynaptic terminal, but are concentrated over certain parts of the presynaptic membrane – the active zones – where the pre- and postsynaptic membranes seem thicker and appear more

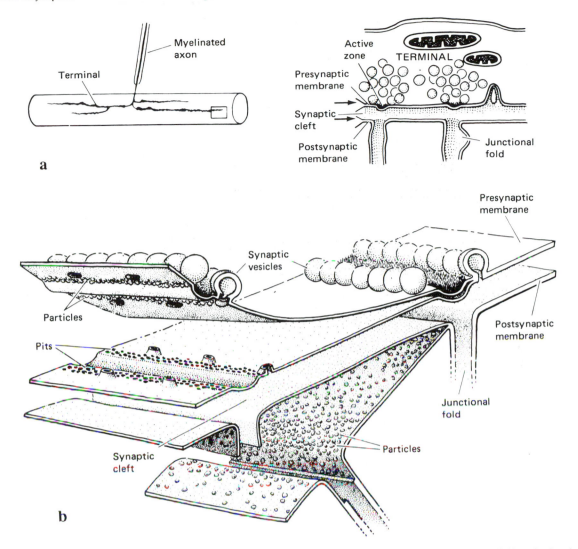

Fig. 6.11a,b. Diagrams of synaptic membrane structure. **a** Shows the entire frog neuromuscular junction (*left*) and a longitudinal section through the nerve terminal (*right*). The *arrows* indicate the plane of cleavage in freeze-fracture. **b** Shows a three-dimensional view of the junction. (Reproduced with permission from Kuffler et al. 1984.)

dense. The apparent thickenings have now been resolved at high magnification and shown to be a series of dense bars attached to the inside of the presynaptic membrane (Fig. 6.11). It is at these active zones that transmitter is released.

Heuser and Reese and their colleagues have developed the freeze-fracture technique to the point where they have been able to provide direct anatomical evidence to support the view that quanta are indeed the result of the release of the contents of individual synaptic vesicles. They have observed vesicles undergoing exocytosis and analysed their distribution statistically. The distribution of such exocytosing vesicles at the active zones indicates that individual vesicles fuse with the presynaptic membrane in an independent manner, and the results also indicate that a single vesicle undergoes exocytosis for every quantum that is released.

Obviously, if vesicles fuse with the presynaptic cell membrane in order to release their content of transmitter, then this fusion should produce an increased surface area of the presynaptic terminals. Repeated vesicle release should therefore lead to continued enlargement of the terminal surface area. This does not occur, so it must be assumed that there is recycling of vesicle membrane. Quantitative studies have indicated that the total amount of membrane (plasma membrane, vesicles and the cisternal membrane

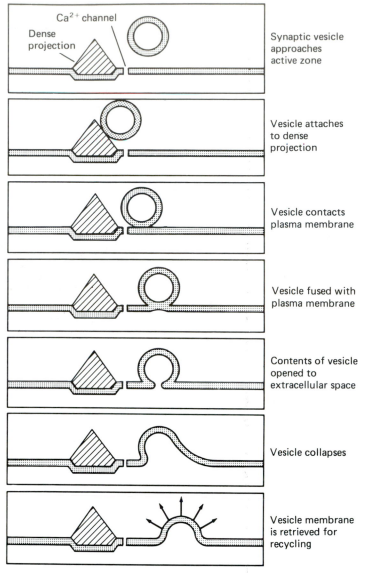

Fig. 6.12. Exocytosis and recycling of vesicular membrane at the neuromuscular junction. (Modified from Kandel and Schwartz 1985, after Llínas and Heuser 1977.)

in the terminal) remains constant. Also, if the enzyme horseradish peroxidase (which can be reacted histochemically to produce an electron-dense reaction product) is placed in the solution bathing the neuromuscular junction it is taken up into stimulated axons and first appears in membrane-coated vesicles, then in cisternae and finally in synaptic vesicles. It may be released from the vesicles upon nerve stimulation. Evidence suggests that the only membrane retrieved from the plasma membrane in this way is vesicle membrane, indicating a highly specific process that recognizes vesicle membrane. According to

Heuser and Reese there are the following steps in exocytosis and recycling of vesicle membrane (Fig. 6.12): (1) the approach of a vesicle to the active zone; (2) the attachment of the vesicle to the dense projections; (3) contact of the vesicle to, and (4) fusion with, the presynaptic plasma membrane, leading to (5) opening (fission) of the vesicle and the ejection of the vesicular contents; (6) the collapse of the vesicular membrane and (7) its coalescence into the plasma membrane; and, finally, (8) retrieval of the vesicular membrane for re-use or for degradation and return to the cell body by retrograde axonal transport.

Transmitter Stores

It is convenient to consider that transmitter is held in several different stores in the nerve terminal. The immediately available store is the transmitter held in vesicles, which is available for release by a presynaptic impulse. Evidence for such a store comes from experiments (neuromuscular junction) in which the second of a pair of closely spaced (in time) presynaptic impulses leads to a smaller postsynaptic response than the first impulse. In many situations, however, (especially when many impulses are passed along the presynaptic nerve – see post-tetanic potentiation, above) a second impulse will lead to a greater postsynaptic effect. In this case it is as if transmitter has been mobilized into the immediately available store, and this leads to the concept of a mobilization store from which this mobilization can take place. Obviously, the role of Ca^{2+} ions are of possible importance here, since the amount of transmitter released has been shown to depend on the amount of Ca^{2+} available. Finally, the main presynaptic store of transmitter is presumably determined by the rate at which transmitter arrives at the presynaptic terminal and packaged in vesicles, either after re-uptake (ACh) or from the cell body and transport to the terminals. Although these various stores may be no more than conceptual aids and have little real existence as separate entities, such concepts are useful in thinking about transmitter storage and release.

Summary

1. Release of transmitter is controlled by the influx of Ca^{2+} into the presynaptic nerve terminal through voltage-gated Ca^{2+} channels controlled by the membrane potential of the terminals. Normally the nerve impulse is responsible for opening these voltage-gated Ca^{2+} channels.

2. The transmitter is released in packets, or quanta, and it is the frequency of release of these quanta that is controlled by the influx of Ca^{2+}, not the size of the quanta.

3. The transmitter is stored in the presynaptic nerve terminal in synaptic vesicles. The contents of a single vesicle are responsible for a single quantum of postsynaptic activity. Release of transmitter is by exocytosis of synaptic vesicles.

4. After vesicular exocytosis the vesicular membrane is retrieved by the presynaptic terminal for re-use.

5. Various phenomena of synaptic plasticity, such as depression and facilitation of synaptic transmission, are explicable in terms of the role of Ca^{2+} and the storage of transmitter in various compartments in the presynaptic terminal.

7 The Presynaptic Neuron II: Neurotransmitters

In the previous chapter the squid giant fibre synapse and the vertebrate neuromuscular junction were considered as the archetypal chemical synapse. The transmitter at both of these synapses is acetylcholine (ACh). In the present chapter transmitters in general will be considered, in particular the criteria needed to identify a transmitter, the way in which different transmitters can be classified, the metabolic pathways for synthesis of some transmitters, the ways in which neurons synthesize transmitters and package them for release at their terminals, and the locations in the nervous system of neurons utilizing particular transmitters. In the next chapter the actions that follow from combination of the transmitter with its specific receptor molecules on the postsynaptic cell will be discussed.

Transmitters – Definition and Identification

A neurotransmitter is a chemical substance that is released from a neuron (at a synapse, a neuromuscular or neuroglandular junction or by terminals of a neurosecretory neuron) and affects a postsynaptic cell. In general the transmitter is released in packets from vesicles in the presynaptic cell and combines with specific receptors on the postsynaptic cell. The postsynaptic cell may be another neuron or an effector cell innervated by the presynaptic neuron (such as a muscle or gland cell), or it may be an effector cell that

responds to a neurotransmitter released into the blood stream by the presynaptic neuron. In the latter case it is common to call the process neurosecretion, and the transmitter in this situation is, by definition, a hormone (neurohormone). Indeed, one and the same substance can be a neurotransmitter between a pre- and postsynaptic neuron and a hormone between a neurosecretory cell and various target cells (e.g. vasopressin, somatostatin).

In order to be identified as a transmitter at a particular set of synapses, a chemical should, theoretically, satisfy a number of criteria. These criteria are:

1. The substance should be synthesized by the presynaptic neuron.
2. The substance should be present in the presynaptic nerve terminals (in the synaptic vesicles).
3. The substance should be released from the nerve terminals by activity in the neuron.
4. The substance should have the same action on the postsynaptic cells as the natural transmitter released by presynaptic activity.
5. The substance should be removed from the synaptic cleft by a specific mechanism.

As a corollary of criterion 4 the putative transmitter should combine specifically with the same receptor molecules on the postsynaptic membrane as the transmitter does, and therefore agonist and antagonist chemicals should affect the actions of the natural transmitter and the putative transmitter in the same way.

The above criteria were established in the early days of pharmacological research on chemical transmission. ACh satisfies these criteria at the various peripheral junctions where it is the transmitter. It is very difficult to apply these criteria at central synapses, and many substances that are almost certainly transmitters in the vertebrate brain and spinal cord have still not satisfied all the criteria. Furthermore, transmission is now known to be a more complicated process than was previously thought. For example, it was at one time believed that a single neuron only used a single transmitter at all of its terminals. This generalization does not hold for many, perhaps the majority, of neurons, which may synthesize, store and release more than one substance – co-synthesis, co-storage and co-release. It is now necessary to reformulate the generalization to the following: a single neuron releases the same transmitters at all of its terminals. It is of interest to realize that all neurons have the genetic machinery necessary to allow the manufacture of any transmitter and embryonic neurons often contain a large number of different transmitters (as do neurons in culture). Once the nervous system has differentiated, however, the number of transmitters manufactured is severely restricted.

Criterion 5 – removal from the synaptic cleft by a specific mechanism – may not be satisfied by a number of transmitters. It is possible that some peptide transmitters are not removed by a specific mechanism but simply diffuse away.

A Classification of Transmitters

It is convenient to divide transmitters into two groups: low molecular weight transmitters and neuroactive peptides (which have larger molecular weights).

Low Molecular Weight Transmitters

Eight low molecular weight transmitters are recognized and all are amines. Seven of the eight are amino acids or their derivatives and the other is acetylcholine.

Acetylcholine

Although the first transmitter to be identified, ACh is in fact the odd one out among the low molecular weight transmitters in that it is not derived directly from an amino acid. ACh is formed by the acetylation of choline, a reaction catalysed by the enzyme choline acetyltransferase (Fig. 7.1). It is the transmitter used by all motoneurons that innervate skeletal muscle (including the gamma-motoneurons that innervate the muscle fibres contained within the muscle spindles – see Chap. 13) and is also used by preganglionic neurons in the autonomic nervous system and by postganglionic neurons of the parasympathetic division of the autonomic nervous system, as well as by some postganglionic sympathetic neurons. In addition to these roles as a transmitter of output systems from the central nervous system it is also used by many neurons in the brain, notable among which are neurons in the basal forebrain, including those of the nucleus basalis which project widely to other areas, the large Betz cells in the cerebral cortex which provide one of the origins of an important descending pathway – the corticospinal tract, and many short-axoned neurons in the neostriatum (caudate nucleus, putamen and nucleus accumbens) (Fig. 7.2). As will be discussed in the next chapter, ACh may combine with either nicotinic or muscarinic receptors on the postsynaptic cell and transmitter–receptor combination may lead to a variety of responses. Nicotinic actions of ACh are rapid in onset and short in duration.

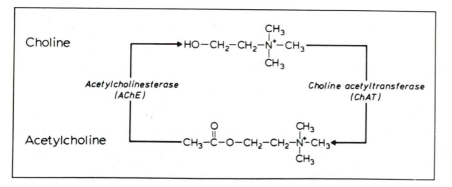

Fig. 7.1. The synthesis and breakdown of acetylcholine.

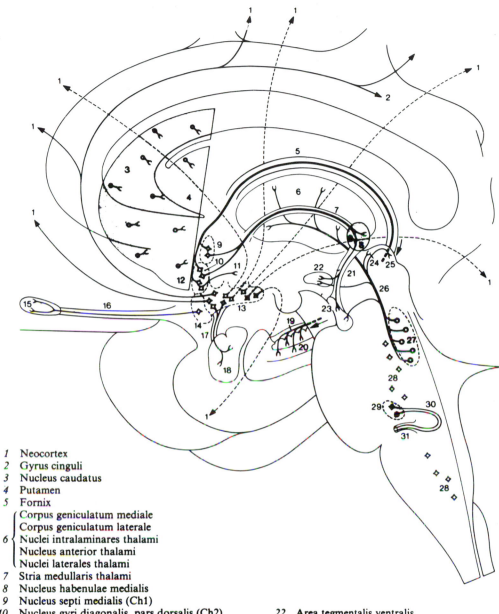

1   Neocortex
2   Gyrus cinguli
3   Nucleus caudatus
4   Putamen
5   Fornix
⎧ Corpus geniculatum mediale
⎪ Corpus geniculatum laterale
6 ⎨ Nuclei intralaminares thalami
⎪ Nucleus anterior thalami
⎩ Nuclei laterales thalami
7   Stria medullaris thalami
8   Nucleus habenulae medialis
9   Nucleus septi medialis (Ch1)
10 Nucleus gyri diagonalis, pars dorsalis (Ch2)
11 Area lateralis hypothalami
12 Nucleus accumbens
13 Nucleus basalis of Meynert (Ch4)
14 Nucleus gyri diagonalis, pars ventralis (Ch3)
15 Bulbus olfactorius
16 Tractus olfactorius
17 Fibrae amygdalofugales ventrales
18 Nucleus basalis amygdalae
19 Fimbria hippocampi
20 Hippocampus
21 Tractus habenulointerpeduncularis

22 Area tegmentalis ventralis
23 Nucleus interpeduncularis
24 Area pretectalis
25 Colliculus superior
26 Fasciculus tegmentalis dorsalis (Shute and Lewis)
27 Area tegmentalis dorsolateralis (including nuclei parabrachiales) plus adjacent central grey (Ch5 + Ch6)
28 Formatio reticularis medialis
29 Nuclei periolivares
30 Fasciculus olivocochlearis (Rasmussen)
31 Nervus vestibulocochlearis

Fig. 7.2. Cholinergic cell groups and pathways. This figure, and similar figures in this chapter, are based on a medial view of the bisected human brain. The various nuclei and pathways etc. have been projected onto the median plane. Several diagrammatic schemes have been included, for example the hippocampus has been unrolled and the globus pallidus turned through 90°. In this diagram the skeletal alpha and gamma motoneurons and the preganglionic autonomic neurons in the brain stem and spinal cord (which are, of course, cholinergic) have been omitted. (Reproduced from Nieuwenhuys 1985.)

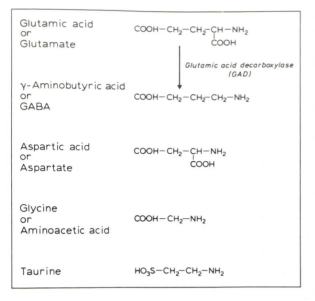

Fig. 7.3. Amino acid neurotransmitters.

The ACh is rapidly hydrolysed and removed from the synaptic cleft by the enzyme acetylcholinesterase (see Fig. 7.1). The hydrolysis releases choline, which is taken up by the nerve terminals and acetylated to form more ACh, which is then packaged into vesicles formed from recycled vesicular membrane (see Chap. 6). This ability of cholinergic nerve terminals to take up choline and to manufacture ACh is unusual; most transmitters are made in the neuron's cell body and transported to the terminals or, in addition, the transmitter is taken up by the nerve terminals from the synaptic cleft (biogenic amines). Choline itself cannot be synthesized by nerve cells but needs to be supplied to them, ultimately from food intake.

Amino Acids

Three, and possibly four, amino acids have been identified as strong candidates for transmitters. These are glycine, gamma-aminobutyric acid (GABA) and glutamate, and possibly aspartate (Fig. 7.3). Because amino acids take part in general metabolic activities in the cell there was considerable resistance to the idea that they might also act as specific transmitters. It is likely that the amino acid used as transmitter is separated from that used in general metabolic pathways, perhaps by its localization in vesicles. Glycine is now recognized as a major transmitter involved in postsynaptic inhibitory mechanisms,

especially in the spinal cord and lower brain stem. It appears to be released, in general, from short-axoned local circuit neurons. Glutamate (and possibly aspartate) is certainly involved in transmission between the large primary afferent fibres from cutaneous and muscle receptors and their target neurons in the central nervous system, and glutamate has been identified as a transmitter in the cerebellum and other parts of the brain (Fig. 7.4). GABA is synthesized from glutamate and has been identified as an inhibitory transmitter in invertebrate nervous systems. It is also highly concentrated in certain parts of the vertebrate central nervous system. It is almost certainly responsible for presynaptic inhibition in the mammalian spinal cord, and Maxwell and his colleagues have identified GABA-containing terminals presynaptic to the terminals of identified cutaneous afferent fibres (see Fig. 8.10). GABA is thought to act as the transmitter in granule cells of the olfactory bulb (see Chap. 10), in amacrine cells of the retina, in Purkinje and basket cells of the cerebellum and in basket cells of the hippocampus (Fig. 7.5). At all these sites GABA acts as an inhibitory transmitter.

Biogenic Amines

The biogenic amines consist of the catecholamines – adrenaline (or epinephrine), noradrenaline (or norepinephrine) and dopamine – and certain other amines such as serotonin (5-hydroxytryptamine; 5-HT), histamine and possibly tyramine and octopamine (Fig. 7.6). Adrenaline is the hormone released from the adrenal medulla. Noradrenaline is the transmitter of neurons with cell bodies in the locus coeruleus and whose processes project to many parts of the central nervous system including the cerebral cortex, the cerebellum and the spinal cord (Fig. 7.7). Noradrenaline is also the transmitter of cells in other areas of the brain stem (Fig. 7.8) and also of many postganglionic sympathetic neurons. Serotonin is found in neurons in the midline raphe nuclei of the brain stem and adjacent areas which project to wide areas of the brain and spinal cord (Fig. 7.9). Histamine is present in high concentration in the hypothalamus and is also found in certain dorsal root ganglion cells; it is also possibly a transmitter in vertebrates.

Neuroactive Peptides

In recent years it has been demonstrated that a large number of short peptides that are pre-

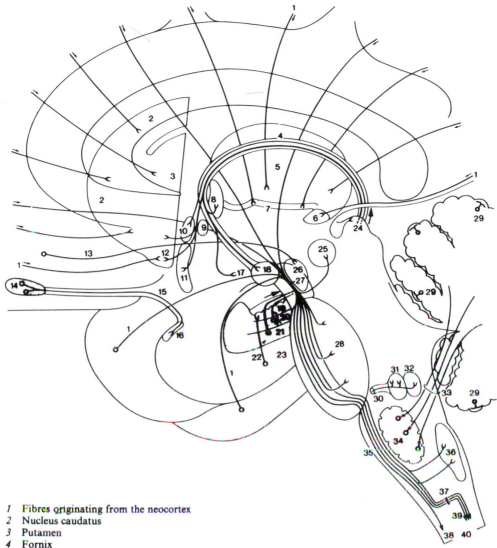

Fig. 7.4. Glutamate-containing cell groups and pathways in the central nervous system. Large-diameter primary afferent fibres also contain glutamate. (Reproduced from Nieuwenhuys 1985.)

1   Fibres originating from the neocortex
2   Nucleus caudatus
3   Putamen
4   Fornix
5   Thalamus
6   Corpus geniculatum laterale
7   Nucleus reticularis thalami
8   Nucleus interstitialis striae terminalis
9   Commissura anterior
10 Nucleus septi lateralis
11 Area diagonalis
12 Nucleus accumbens
13 Fibres from the rostral and medial parts of the pre-
     frontal cortex, passing to the substantia nigra
14 Bulbus olfactorius
15 Stria olfactoria lateralis
16 Cortex prepiriformis
17 Mediobasal hypothalamus
18 Corpus mamillare
19 Fascia dentata
20 Cornu Ammonis
21 Subiculum
22 'Perforant path'
23 Gyrus parahippocampalis

24 Colliculus superior
25 Nucleus ruber
26 Substantia nigra
27 Pedunculus cerebri
28 Pons
29 Granule cells, giving rise to parallel fibres
30 Nervus cochlearis (VIII)
31 Nucleus cochlearis ventralis
32 Nucleus cochlearis dorsalis
33 Tractus olivocerebellaris
34 Nucleus olivaris inferior
35 Pyramis
36 Nucleus cuneatus medialis (+ nucleus gracilis)
37 Decussatio pyramidum
38 Tractus pyramidalis anterior
39 Tractus pyramidalis lateralis
40 Medulla spinalis

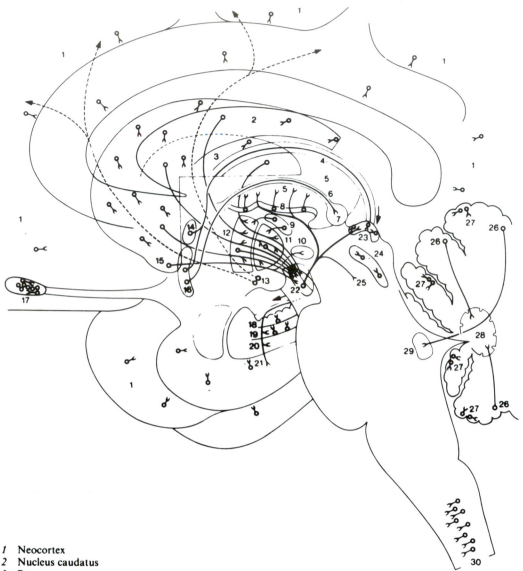

1   Neocortex
2   Nucleus caudatus
3   Putamen
4   Fornix
5   Thalamus
6   Stria medullaris thalami
7   Nucleus habenulae medialis
8   Nucleus reticularis thalami
9   Nucleus subthalamicus
10 Area tegmentalis ventralis
11 Globus pallidus, pars medialis
12 Globus pallidus, pars lateralis
13 GABA-containing cell groups in
    caudal hypothalamus
14 Nucleus septi medialis
15 Nucleus accumbens
16 Nucleus gyri diagonalis
17 Bulbus olfactorius
18 Fascia dentata
19 Cornu Ammonis
20 Subiculum

21 Cortex entorhinalis
22 Substantia nigra
23 Colliculus superior
24 Nucleus raphes dorsalis
25 Tegmentum mesencephali
26 Purkinje cells
27 Golgi, stellate and basket cells
28 Nuclei centrales cerebelli
29 Nucleus vestibularis lateralis
30 Medulla spinalis

Fig. 7.5. GABA-containing cell groups and pathways. (Reproduced from Nieuwenhuys 1985.)

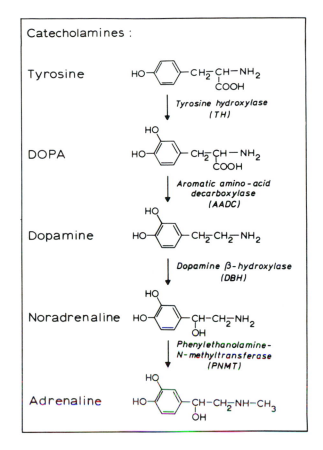

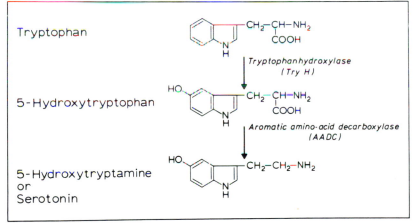

Fig. 7.6. Monoamine transmitters.

ferentially localized in high concentrations in certain neurons have very active pharmacological actions on neurons, causing excitation or inhibition. Some of these peptides have been known for a long time as hormones, such as gastrin, vasoactive intestinal peptide (VIP) and secretin. Others were known as substances secreted by neurons (neurosecretion) of the hypothalamo-hypophyseal system, such as vasopressin, oxytocin, luteinizing hormone, somatostatin etc. (see Chap. 16).

The known list of neuroactive peptides now recognized is very long. However, it is possible to classify them into several groups with members of each group having structural similarities. There are at least seven families – the opioids,

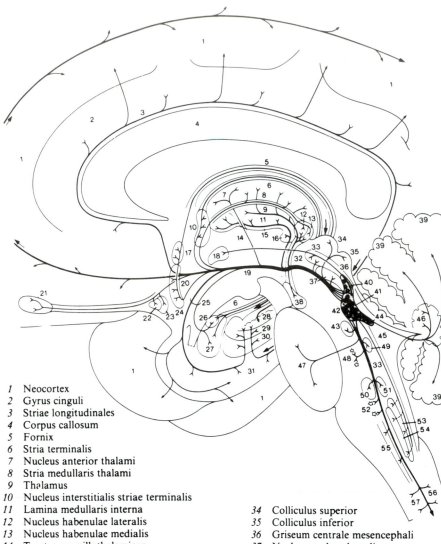

1	Neocortex
2	Gyrus cinguli
3	Striae longitudinales
4	Corpus callosum
5	Fornix
6	Stria terminalis
7	Nucleus anterior thalami
8	Stria medullaris thalami
9	Thalamus
10	Nucleus interstitialis striae terminalis
11	Lamina medullaris interna
12	Nucleus habenulae lateralis
13	Nucleus habenulae medialis
14	Tractus mamillothalamicus
15	Lamina medullaris externa
16	Corpus geniculatum mediale + laterale
17	Nucleus septi medialis
18	Nucleus paraventricularis, pars parvocellularis
19	Fasciculus telencephalicus medialis
20	Bandeletta diagonalis
21	Bulbus olfactorius
22	Nucleus olfactorius anterior
23	Substantia perforata anterior
24	Nucleus gyri diagonalis
25	Ansa peduncularis + fibrae amygdalofugales ventrales
26	Nucleus centralis amygdalae
27	Nucleus basalis amygdalae
28	Gyrus dentatus
29	Cornu Ammonis
30	Subiculum
31	Gyrus parahippocampalis
32	Tractus habenulointerpeduncularis
33	Fasciculus longitudinalis dorsalis

34	Colliculus superior
35	Colliculus inferior
36	Griseum centrale mesencephali
37	Nucleus raphes dorsalis
38	Nucleus interpeduncularis
39	Cortex cerebelli
40	Locus coeruleus, rostral extension (A6cg)
41	Locus coeruleus (A6)
42	Area subcoerulea (A6sc)
43	Nuclei lemnisci lateralis
44	Locus coeruleus, caudal extension (A4)
45	Brachium conjunctivum
46	Nuclei centrales cerebelli
47	Nuclei pontis
48	Formatio reticularis metencephali
49	Nucleus sensorius principalis nervi trigemini
50	Nucleus cochlearis ventralis
51	Nucleus cochlearis dorsalis
52	Formatio reticularis myelencephali
53	Nucleus solitarius
54	Nucleus dorsalis nervi vagi
55	Nucleus spinalis nervi trigemini
56	Cornu posterius (Laminae IV, V, VI)
57	Cornu anterius

Fig. 7.7. Noradrenaline-containing cell groups and pathways. I. The locus coeruleus complex. (Reproduced from Nieuwenhuys 1985.)

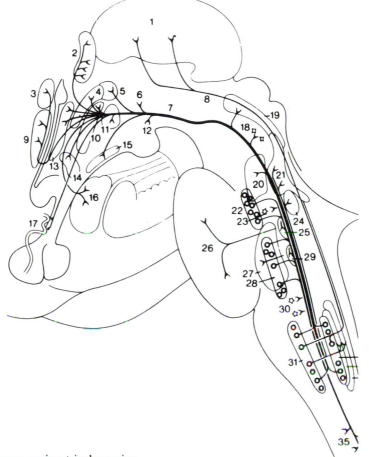

Fig. 7.8. Noradrenaline-containing cell groups and pathways. II. Remaining cell groups. (Reproduced from Nieuwenhuys 1985.)

1 Thalamus, periventricular region	
2 Nucleus interstitialis striae terminalis	
3 Nucleus septi lateralis	
4 Nucleus paraventricularis, pars magnocellularis	
5 Nucleus paraventricularis, pars parvocellularis	
6 Area lateralis hypothalami	
7 Fasciculus telencephalicus medialis	
8 Fasciculus longitudinalis dorsalis	
9 Nucleus gyri diagonalis	
10 Nucleus anterior hypothalami	
11 Nucleus dorsomedialis	
12 Area caudalis hypothalami	
13 Nucleus praeopticus medialis	
14 Nucleus supraopticus	*26* Nuclei pontis
15 Nucleus infundibularis	*27* Nucleus raphes magnus
16 Corpus amygdaloideum	*28* Cell group A5
17 Eminentia mediana	*29* Nucleus nervi facialis
18 Formatio reticularis mesencephali	*30* Formatio reticularis myelencephali
19 Griseum centrale mesencephali	*31* Cell group A1
20 Nucleus centralis superior	*32* Cell group A2
21 Locus coeruleus	*33* Nucleus dorsalis nervi vagi
22 Cell group A7	*34* Nucleus solitarius
23 Formatio reticularis metencephali	*35* Substantia grisea centralis
24 Nuclei parabrachiales	*36* Substantia gelatinosa
25 Nucleus motorius nervi trigemini	*37* Nucleus intermediola

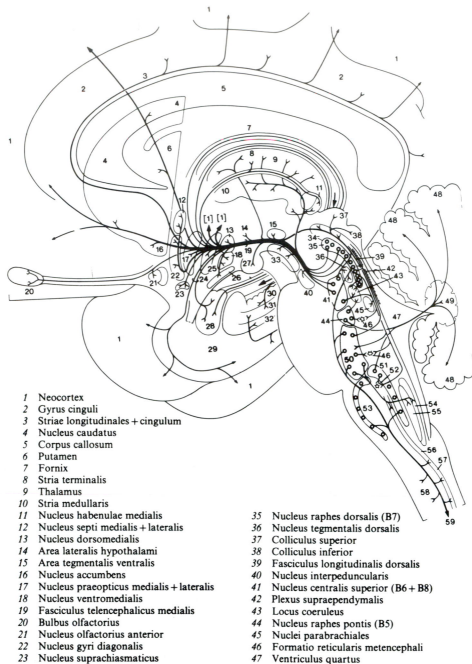

1   Neocortex
2   Gyrus cinguli
3   Striae longitudinales + cingulum
4   Nucleus caudatus
5   Corpus callosum
6   Putamen
7   Fornix
8   Stria terminalis
9   Thalamus
10 Stria medullaris
11 Nucleus habenulae medialis
12 Nucleus septi medialis + lateralis
13 Nucleus dorsomedialis
14 Area lateralis hypothalami
15 Area tegmentalis ventralis
16 Nucleus accumbens
17 Nucleus praeopticus medialis + lateralis
18 Nucleus ventromedialis
19 Fasciculus telencephalicus medialis
20 Bulbus olfactorius
21 Nucleus olfactorius anterior
22 Nucleus gyri diagonalis
23 Nucleus suprachiasmaticus
24 Ansa peduncularis + fibrae amygdalofugales
    ventrales
25 Nucleus anterior hypothalami
26 Nucleus infundibularis
27 Corpus mamillare
28 Corpus amygdaloideum
29 Gyrus parahippocampalis
30 Gyrus dentatus
31 Cornu Ammonis
32 Subiculum
33 Substantia nigra
34 Griseum centrale mesencephali

35 Nucleus raphes dorsalis (B7)
36 Nucleus tegmentalis dorsalis
37 Colliculus superior
38 Colliculus inferior
39 Fasciculus longitudinalis dorsalis
40 Nucleus interpeduncularis
41 Nucleus centralis superior (B6 + B8)
42 Plexus supraependymalis
43 Locus coeruleus
44 Nucleus raphes pontis (B5)
45 Nuclei parabrachiales
46 Formatio reticularis metencephali
47 Ventriculus quartus
48 Cortex cerebelli
49 Nuclei centrales cerebelli
50 Nucleus raphes magnus (B3)
51 Nucleus raphes obscurus (B2)
52 Formatio reticularis myelencephali
53 Nucleus raphes pallidus (B1)
54 Nucleus solitarius
55 Nucleus dorsalis nervi vagi
56 Nucleus spinalis nervi trigemini
57 Substantia gelatinosa
58 Cornu anterius
59 Nucleus intermediolateralis

Fig. 7.9. Serotonin (5-HT)–containing cell groups and pathways. (Reproduced from Nieuwenhuys 1985.)

neurohypophyseal peptides, tachykinins, secretins, insulins, somatostatins and the gastrins. It is beyond the scope of this introductory text to detail what is known in this rapidly expanding area. The localization of a few neuroactive peptides (Substance P, VIP, cholecystokinin, somatostatin and the enkephalins) are shown in Fig. 7.10. A few generalizations are noted here:

1. The peptides are produced only by a restricted group of cells, neurons and gland cells that are derived from embryological precursors of nervous tissue.

2. Within the nervous system only certain neurons appear to express the genes for neuroactive peptides in the adult animal (although in the embryo or in tissue culture the genes may be expressed by neurons that do not express them in the adult).

3. Neuroactive peptides are synthesized in the cell bodies of those neurons expressing the gene.

4. Peptides and the "classical" neurotransmitters often co-exist in the same neuron. This may be the more usual situation and raises questions about the role of the peptides (see below). Furthermore, more than one peptide may be present in a particular neuron.

5. Neuroactive peptides often have long-lasting actions on their target cells and an important role for them may be to modulate the action of "classical" transmitters.

6. The long-lasting action may be largely due to a lack of specific re-uptake or enzymatic breakdown mechanisms at the synaptic cleft.

Some General Principles About Transmitters

Some Transmitters Appear To Be Either Excitatory or Inhibitory but Not Both

Glycine has inhibitory actions on its postsynaptic target neurons and may be classed as an inhibitory transmitter. GABA also is thought to have exclusively inhibitory actions. By contrast, glutamate (and aspartate) have excitatory actions. These transmitters (glycine, GABA and glutamate) have their appropriate actions on the postsynaptic cells in spite of the fact that there is more than a single type of receptor molecule for each.

Some Transmitters May Have Either Excitatory or Inhibitory Actions

The classical transmitter with both excitatory and inhibitory actions is ACh. The mode of operation depends on the postsynaptic receptors; two major ones – the nicotinic and the muscarinic – are recognized (see Chap. 8).

Many Neurons Contain Both a Classical Small Molecule Transmitter and a Neuroactive Peptide

Many nerve cells synthesize and store more than one transmitter substance, usually a small molecule "classical" transmitter such as noradrenaline together with a peptide such as somatostatin. These phenomena are known as co-synthesis, co-localization (in same nerve terminal) and co-storage (in same vesicle).

A Single Neuron May Release More Than One Transmitter

Not only do neurons often synthesize and store more than one transmitter but they may also release more than one – a phenomenon known as co-release. Indeed, co-release is the logical outcome of co-synthesis and co-storage. Evidence for co-release in the central nervous system is weak, but there is good evidence in the periphery. Thus the parasympathetic nerves that innervate the sweat glands contain both ACh and VIP. The ACh mainly causes secretion by the gland, whereas VIP mainly causes vasodilatation. Hökfelt and Lundberg and their colleagues have shown that ACh and VIP can be co-released and also that a single impulse in the parasympathetic nerves preferentially liberates ACh, whereas a train of high-frequency impulses preferentially liberates VIP (see Hökfelt et al. 1980). If this latter observation can be generalized it would allow a subtle degree of presynaptic control over the release of particular transmitters (or modulators).

Some Neuronal Systems Containing Particular Transmitters Appear To Have Very Wide-ranging Actions in the Brain

In the mammalian brain the biogenic amines serotonin (5-HT), noradrenaline or dopamine

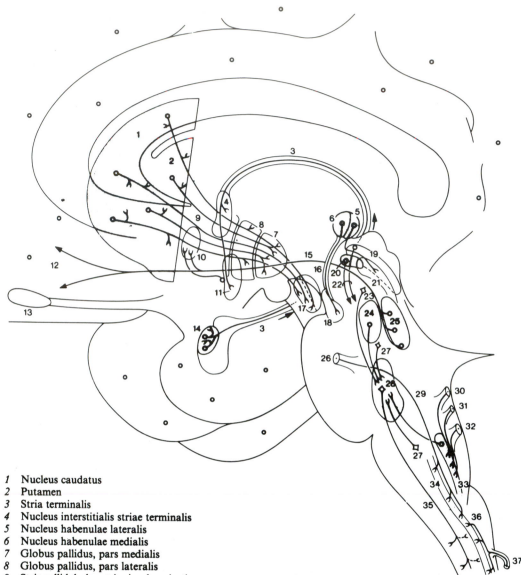

1 Nucleus caudatus	
2 Putamen	
3 Stria terminalis	
4 Nucleus interstitialis striae terminalis	
5 Nucleus habenulae lateralis	
6 Nucleus habenulae medialis	
7 Globus pallidus, pars medialis	
8 Globus pallidus, pars lateralis	
9 Striopallidal plus strionigral projections	
10 Nucleus septi lateralis	
11 Nucleus anterior hypothalami	
12 Cortex frontalis	
13 Bulbus olfactorius	
14 Corpus amygdaloideum, pars medialis	
15 Fasciculus telencephalicus medialis	*26* Radix sensoria nervi trigemini
16 Tractus habenulointerpeduncularis	*27* Formatio reticularis rhombencephali
17 Substantia nigra, pars reticulata	*28* Nucleus raphes magnus
18 Nucleus interpeduncularis	*29* Tractus spinalis nervi trigemini
19 Griseum centrale mesencephali	*30* Nervus facialis
20 Nucleus accessorius nervi oculomotorii (Edinger-Westphal)	*31* Nervus glossopharyngeus
	32 Nervus vagus
21 Nucleus raphes dorsalis	*33* Nucleus solitarius
22 Spinal projections originating from 19 and 20	*34* Nucleus spinalis nervi trigemini, pars caudalis
23 Nucleus cuneiformis	*35* Raphespinal projection
24 Nucleus centralis superior	*36* Substantia gelatinosa
a *25* Area tegmentalis dorsolateralis	*37* Radix dorsalis nervi spinalis

Fig. 7.10a–e. Some peptide-containing cell groups and pathways. **a** Substance P. **b** Vasoactive intestinal peptide. **c** Cholecystokinin. **d** Somatostatin. **e** Enkephalin. (Reproduced from Nieuwenhuys 1985.)

Fig. 7.10. (continued)

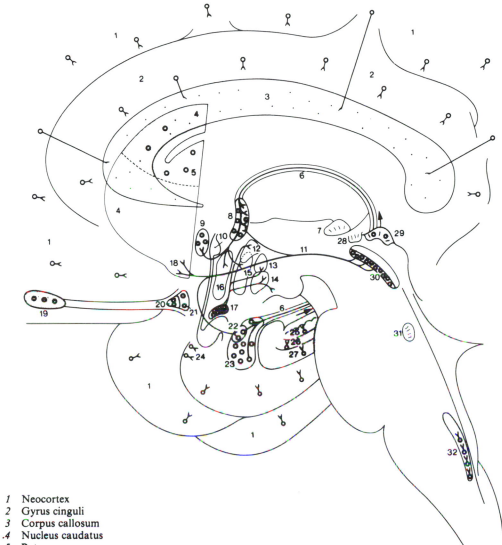

1	Neocortex		
2	Gyrus cinguli		
3	Corpus callosum		
.4	Nucleus caudatus		
5	Putamen		
6	Stria terminalis		
7	Corpus geniculatum laterale		
8	Nucleus interstitialis striae terminalis		
9	Nucleus septi lateralis		
10	Commissura anterior		
11	Fasciculus telencephalicus medialis		
12	Nucleus paraventricularis		
13	Nucleus dorsomedialis		
14	Nucleus ventromedialis		
15	Nucleus anterior hypothalami	*24*	Cortex praepiriformis
16	Regio preoptica	*25*	Gyrus dentatus
17	Nucleus suprachiasmaticus	*26*	Cornu Ammonis
18	Nucleus accumbens	*27*	Subiculum
19	Bulbus olfactorius	*28*	Area pretectalis
20	Nucleus olfactorius anterior	*29*	Colliculus superior
21	Tuberculum olfactorium	*30*	Griseum centrale mesencephali
22	Nucleus centralis amygdalae	*31*	Nucleus parabrachialis lateralis
23	Corpus amygdaloideum	*32*	Nucleus solitarius

b

Fig. 7.10. (continued)

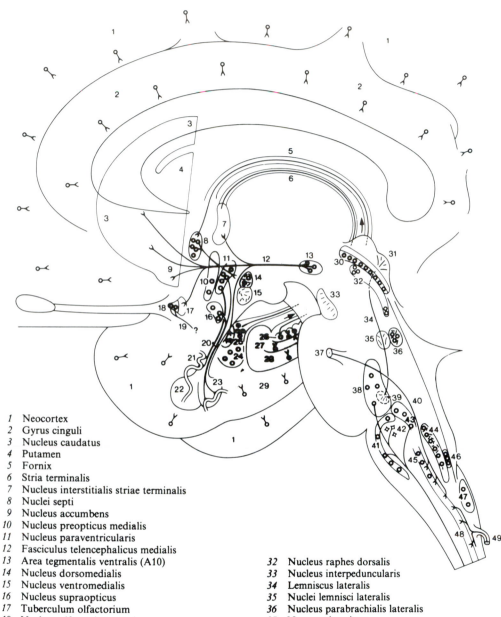

1	Neocortex	32	Nucleus raphes dorsalis
2	Gyrus cinguli	33	Nucleus interpeduncularis
3	Nucleus caudatus	34	Lemniscus lateralis
4	Putamen	35	Nuclei lemnisci lateralis
5	Fornix	36	Nucleus parabrachialis lateralis
6	Stria terminalis	37	Nervus trigeminus
7	Nucleus interstitialis striae terminalis	38	Nucleus raphes magnus
8	Nuclei septi	39	Oliva superior
9	Nucleus accumbens	40	Tractus spinalis nervi trigemini
10	Nucleus preopticus medialis	41	Nucleus raphes pallidus
11	Nucleus paraventricularis	42	Nucleus reticularis gigantocellularis
12	Fasciculus telencephalicus medialis	43	Nucleus raphes obscurus
13	Area tegmentalis ventralis (A10)	44	Nucleus solitarius
14	Nucleus dorsomedialis	45	Substantia gelatinosa nuclei spinalis nervi trigemini
15	Nucleus ventromedialis		pars caudalis
16	Nucleus supraopticus	46	Area postrema
17	Tuberculum olfactorium	47	Nucleus cuneatus medialis
18	Nucleus olfactorius anterior	48	Substantia gelatinosa spinalis
19	Stria olfactoria lateralis	49	Radix dorsalis nervi spinalis
20	Tractus paraventriculo-supraoptico-hypophyseos		
21	Eminentia mediana		
22	Lobus anterior hypophyseos		
23	Lobus posterior hypophyseos		
24	Corpus amygdaloideum		
25	Nucleus corticalis amygdalae		
26	Fascia dentata		
27	Cornu Ammonis		
28	Subiculum		
29	Gyrus parahippocampalis		
30	Griseum centrale mesencephali		
31	Colliculus inferior		

c

Fig. 7.10. (continued)

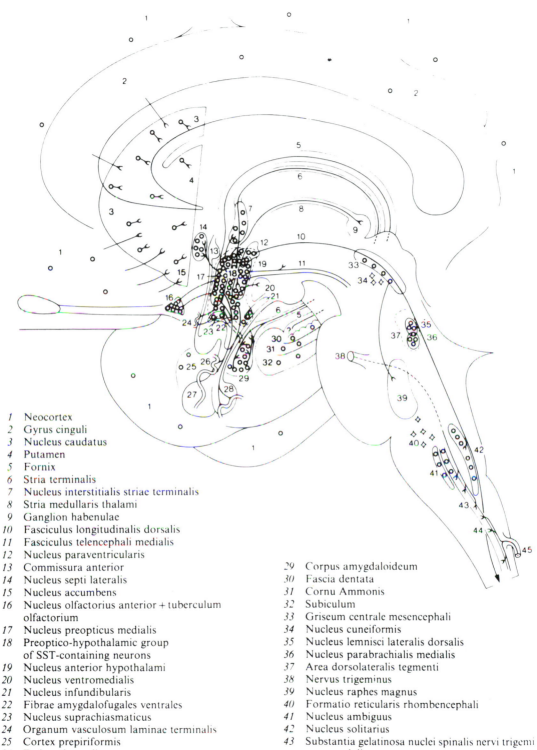

1 Neocortex
2 Gyrus cinguli
3 Nucleus caudatus
4 Putamen
5 Fornix
6 Stria terminalis
7 Nucleus interstitialis striae terminalis
8 Stria medullaris thalami
9 Ganglion habenulae
10 Fasciculus longitudinalis dorsalis
11 Fasciculus telencephali medialis
12 Nucleus paraventricularis
13 Commissura anterior
14 Nucleus septi lateralis
15 Nucleus accumbens
16 Nucleus olfactorius anterior + tuberculum
    olfactorium
17 Nucleus preopticus medialis
18 Preoptico-hypothalamic group
    of SST-containing neurons
19 Nucleus anterior hypothalami
20 Nucleus ventromedialis
21 Nucleus infundibularis
22 Fibrae amygdalofugales ventrales
23 Nucleus suprachiasmaticus
24 Organum vasculosum laminae terminalis
25 Cortex prepiriformis
26 Eminentia mediana
27 Lobus anterior hypophyseos
28 Lobus posterior hypophyseos

29 Corpus amygdaloideum
30 Fascia dentata
31 Cornu Ammonis
32 Subiculum
33 Griseum centrale mesencephali
34 Nucleus cuneiformis
35 Nucleus lemnisci lateralis dorsalis
36 Nucleus parabrachialis medialis
37 Area dorsolateralis tegmenti
38 Nervus trigeminus
39 Nucleus raphes magnus
40 Formatio reticularis rhombencephali
41 Nucleus ambiguus
42 Nucleus solitarius
43 Substantia gelatinosa nuclei spinalis nervi trigemi
    pars caudalis
44 Substantia gelatinosa spinalis
45 Radix dorsalis nervi spinalis

d

Fig. 7.10. (continued)

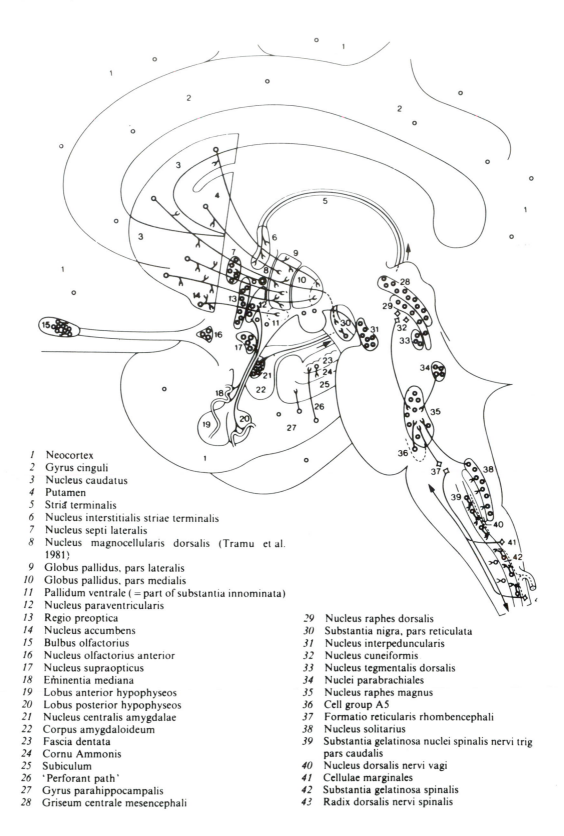

1 Neocortex
2 Gyrus cinguli
3 Nucleus caudatus
4 Putamen
5 Stria terminalis
6 Nucleus interstitialis striae terminalis
7 Nucleus septi lateralis
8 Nucleus magnocellularis dorsalis (Tramu et al. 1981)
9 Globus pallidus, pars lateralis
10 Globus pallidus, pars medialis
11 Pallidum ventrale (= part of substantia innominata)
12 Nucleus paraventricularis
13 Regio preoptica
14 Nucleus accumbens
15 Bulbus olfactorius
16 Nucleus olfactorius anterior
17 Nucleus supraopticus
18 Eminentia mediana
19 Lobus anterior hypophyseos
20 Lobus posterior hypophyseos
21 Nucleus centralis amygdalae
22 Corpus amygdaloideum
23 Fascia dentata
24 Cornu Ammonis
25 Subiculum
26 'Perforant path'
27 Gyrus parahippocampalis
28 Griseum centrale mesencephali

29 Nucleus raphes dorsalis
30 Substantia nigra, pars reticulata
31 Nucleus interpeduncularis
32 Nucleus cuneiformis
33 Nucleus tegmentalis dorsalis
34 Nuclei parabrachiales
35 Nucleus raphes magnus
36 Cell group A5
37 Formatio reticularis rhombencephali
38 Nucleus solitarius
39 Substantia gelatinosa nuclei spinalis nervi trig pars caudalis
40 Nucleus dorsalis nervi vagi
41 Cellulae marginales
42 Substantia gelatinosa spinalis
43 Radix dorsalis nervi spinalis

e

are contained in relatively few neurons. These neurons are grouped together in restricted regions of the brain, mainly the raphe nuclei, the locus coeruleus and the substantia nigra, respectively. Furthermore, these neurons project to virtually all regions of the central nervous system. Damage to the cells of origin of these widely divergent projections leads to crippling behavioural, motor or sensory disorders. For example, damage to the serotoninergic system may affect the level of wakefulness and responses to noxious stimuli; damage to the locus coeruleus can affect the developing sensory cortex in kittens; and damage to the dopaminergic pathways may lead to disorders of movement like Parkinsonism, and also dopaminergic neurons are strongly implicated in schizophrenia.

It has been suggested that these systems with their wide-ranging projections do not make highly specific connexions with target neurons. Rather, it is suggested that they liberate their transmitters in a diffuse way (perhaps from axonal varicosities rather than from synapses between pre- and postsynaptic neurons), and these transmitters then act to modulate the function of more specifically wired sets of neurons.

Axonal Transport

As described above, many neurotransmitters are synthesized in the neuronal cell body. Yet they are released from nerve terminals that may be a long way away from the cell body (up to 2 or 3

m or more in large mammals). The neurotransmitters are transported to the nerve terminals by active processes of axonal transport. Not only are the neurotransmitters transported in this way but various other subcellular components necessary for the process of neurotransmission – such as the specialized cell membrane at the nerve terminal, the synaptic vesicular membrane and various enzymes – are too, since they are manufactured by the Golgi apparatus and endoplasmic reticulum of the cell body. In fact, all newly synthesized membranous organelles are made in the cell body and transported to their appropriate locations. Furthermore, the systems necessary for the recycling of transmitter at the nerve terminals and the re-uptake of synaptic vesicular membrane are also transported from the cell body to the terminals. Finally, there is a retrograde transport of substances from the terminals back to the cell body.

There are both slow and fast transport mechanisms that move substances and subcellular organelles etc. along axons in both the anterograde and retrograde direction. Fast transport can move organelles, such as membrane-bound vesicles, as fast as about 400 mm per day (Fig. 7.11). Slow transport, or slow axoplasmic flow, moves the cytosolic components such as soluble proteins at rates of a few millimetres per day.

Fast transport mechanisms seem to use microtubules in some way involving an ATPase enzyme in order to move organelles. Evidence for this comes from the observation that various substances such as colchicine and vinblastine, which disrupt microtubules, block fast transport processes.

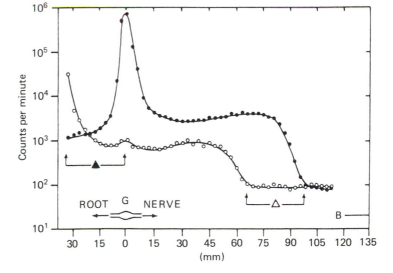

Fig. 7.11. Fast axonal transport in sensory and motor fibres in the cat. The motoneuronal region of the seventh lumbar segment (*open circles*) and the seventh lumbar ganglion (*filled circles*) were injected with tritiated leucine. After 6h the nerves were removed and the radioactivity sampled. The displacement of the fronts of the crests of activity (*open triangle*) is comparable to the displacement of the locations of the spinal cord segment and the ganglion (*filled triangle*). After 6 h the rate of transport was similar in sensory and motor nerves at about 100 mm, corresponding with a rate of about 400 mm per day. (Reproduced with permission from Ochs and Ranish 1969.)

The transport of various substances in both the anterograde and retrograde directions by fast transport mechanisms have been used to very good effect by experimental anatomists. Thus the enzyme horseradish peroxidase (HRP) is taken up by nerve terminals, packaged in membrane-bound vesicles and retrogradely transported to the cell body. By injecting the enzyme around nerve terminals, allowing subsequent take-up and retrograde transport, the locations of the neuronal cell bodies having axonal projections to the injection site can be determined since the HRP can be easily visualized (for both light and electron microscopy) by straightforward histochemical techniques. Various other substances, including HRP conjugates, plant lectins and fluorescent dyes may also be used for both anterograde and retrograde neuronal pathway tracing.

Summary

1.   A neurotransmitter is a chemical substance that is released from a neuron and has a specific action on a target cell (either on another neuron or an effector cell – muscle or gland cells).

2.   Neurotransmitters are contained within and released from synaptic vesicles in the presynaptic cell.

3.   Many neurons manufacture and store more than one transmitter (co-synthesis and co-storage) and also release more than one transmitter (co-release).

4.   There are two major groups of transmitters: low molecular weight transmitters and neuropeptides.

5.   Low molecular weight transmitters are amines and include acetylcholine, various amino acids (glycine, gamma-aminobutyric acid, glutamate and possibly aspartate) and the biogenic amines (adrenaline, noradrenaline, serotonin or 5-hydroxytryptamine, and dopamine).

6.   There are numerous neuropeptides that act as neurotransmitters or neuromodulators. They include substances that can also act as hormones, e.g. gastrin, secretin, oxytocin, vasopressin, cholecystokinin, somatostatin, luteinizing hormone and members of the opioid group.

7.   Some transmitters have either excitatory actions or inhibitory actions but not both. Thus glycine appears always to act as an inhibitory transmitter and glutamate as an excitatory one.

8.   Some transmitters may have either excitatory or inhibitory actions e.g. ACh. The response depends on the postsynaptic receptor.

9.   Substances such as membrane components, enzymes and subcellular organelles are transported from the cell body to the nerve terminals and from the nerve terminals to the cell body by axoplasmic transport mechanisms at speeds ranging from a few millimetres per day to 400 mm per day.

8 The Postsynaptic Neuron I: Actions of Transmitters

Transmitter released from the presynaptic neuron diffuses across the synaptic gap and combines with specific receptor molecules located in the membrane of the postsynaptic cell. The combination of transmitter with receptor leads to changes in the postsynaptic cell that can be of two general types, either affecting chemically gated ion channels or affecting the metabolism of the cell. Once the appropriate postsynaptic response has occurred it is obviously important that the system should be reset to allow further actions to take place. The transmitter is therefore released from its combination with the receptor and, furthermore, removed from the synaptic cleft. Removal of transmitter may be achieved by re-uptake into the terminals of the presynaptic neuron, by enzymatic degradation (which may be combined with re-uptake) or by diffusion away from the cleft.

Postsynaptic Receptors

The effects of a particular transmitter on its postsynaptic target cell are not specific for the transmitter but rather are the result of the combination of the transmitter with a specific receptor. Thus, the transmitter acetylcholine (ACh) may lead to excitation at some synapses (such as the vertebrate skeletal neuromuscular junction) but to inhibition at others (such as the synapses between the postganglionic parasympathetic neurons and muscle cells in the heart), and may even have both actions at some synapses. It is the receptor that determines the postsynaptic response. Receptor molecules that have been described so far are protein molecules that form an integral part of the postsynaptic cell membrane. The active component of the molecule that binds with the transmitter is on the outer surface of the membrane, where it is easily reached by the transmitter diffusing from the presynaptic terminals.

The two main types of postsynaptic responses – ionic conductance changes produced by actions on chemically gated ion channels and metabolic changes by actions that work through the mediation of intracellular second messengers – are produced by two main types of receptors.

Receptors That Control Ionic Channels

More is known about this type of receptor than about those that mediate responses through metabolic changes. This is largely due to the fact that the electric organ of electric fish contains a great concentration of a particular receptor, the nicotinic ACh receptor. ACh receptors are of two main types: the nicotinic variety which combines with the drug nicotine, and the muscarinic variety which combines with the drug muscarine. In both cases combination with the appropriate drug leads to postsynaptic actions similar to those that occur upon ACh-receptor combination in the appropriate cells. The nicotinic ACh receptor has been isolated from the electric organ and characterized as a glycoprotein, with a molecular weight of

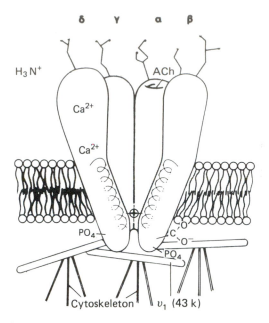

Fig. 8.1. Model of the ion channel of the nicotinic acetylcholine receptor in longitudinal section. α, β, γ and δ are amino acid residues with largely hydrophilic side chains. (Reproduced with permission from Guy and Hucho 1987.)

about 275 000, consisting of five subunits which surround a central channel that passes through the membrane (Fig. 8.1). Combination of ACh with the receptor appears to involve two molecules of transmitter, each binding to one of the two alpha subunits on the receptor. Transmitter–receptor combination leads to a configurational change in the receptor molecule that alters the diameter of the channel and thereby allows ions to flow through it (see below). The receptor itself is, therefore, the chemically gated ion channel since it is chemically sensitive (combines specifically with the appropriate receptor) and forms the channel through which ions pass.

A considerable amount is now known about the molecular biology of the ACh receptor. Each of the different types of sub-units is translated from its own messenger RNA, which, in turn, is transcribed from its own gene. The DNA molecules corresponding to the messenger RNA have now all been sequenced. Once the sub-units have

been made they are somehow brought together and inserted into the cell membrane at the appropriate place, where they have a half-life of about 1 week.

Much less is known about other chemically gated ion channels. It is generally assumed that they all are integral membrane proteins that form a cylindrical structure running through the membrane. Some, such as the gamma-aminobutyric acid (GABA) receptors (there are more than one), appear more complex than the nicotinic ACh receptor in that the receptors appear to have subunits that control the receptor activity and indeed appear to have several receptor sites. For example, the $GABA_A$ receptor has receptor sites for GABA itself, for barbiturates and for benzodiazepines, the latter two being powerful hypnotic (and anaesthetic) drugs and tranquillizing drugs, respectively.

Receptors That Act Through Intracellular Second Messengers

Combination of transmitter with some receptors does not lead to ionic conductance changes directly but to metabolic changes in the cell mediated by intracellular second messenger molecules such as cyclic adenine monophosphate (cAMP) or some lipid molecules. As described below, transmitter–receptor combination of this type may lead indirectly to changes in ionic conductance or to changes in the cell's metabolism by phosphorylation of proteins. In general, activation of these receptors lasts longer than that of chemically gated ion channels (minutes rather than milliseconds or seconds). Examples of receptors that act through intracellular messengers include the serotonin (5-hydroxytryptamine; 5-HT) receptor, the muscarinic ACh receptor, the alpha-adrenergic receptor and some peptide receptors.

Consequences of Transmitter–Receptor Combination

Combination of transmitter with receptor may either affect chemically gated ion channels or influence the metabolism of the postsynaptic cell.

Actions at Chemically Gated Ion Channels

Chemically gated ion channels may be either opened or closed as a consequence of transmitter–receptor combination.

Opening of Ion Channels That Are Normally Closed

The Vertebrate Neuromuscular Junction. The vertebrate neuromuscular junction has provided an important preparation for understanding the mode of action of chemically gated ion channels. As described in Chapter 6, ACh is released by the motoneuronal terminals at the neuromuscular junction. Here it combines with nicotinic ACh receptor molecules to produce the end-plate potential (EPP), which, as we have seen is composed of a large number of quantal miniature end-plate potentials each due to the release of a single package of ACh from a single vesicle. Now it is time to discuss the ionic mechanisms underlying the end-plate potential. Similar mechanisms also underly the excitatory postsynaptic potential (EPSP) seen at central nervous synapses.

Del Castillo and Katz (1954b) determined the reversal potential for the EPP in an ingenious experiment by causing an EPP to occur at various times during the occurrence of a directly evoked muscle action potential (Fig. 8.2). They then observed how the action potential was affected by the underlying EPP. Thus, the peak of the action potential was reduced if the EPP occurred during the peak. If the EPP occurred as the action potential was rising or falling, then depolarization occurred when the membrane potential was more negative than about -15 mV, and hyperpolarization occurred if the potential was less negative than about -15 mV. In other words, del Castillo and Katz had shown that the EPP reverses at a membrane potential of about -15 mV. A reversal potential of this magnitude does not coincide with the equilibrium potential for any single ion species available (sodium $+55$ mV; potassium -90 mV, chloride about -90 mV). It was concluded that the EPP was due to an unselective increase in membrane permeability to all ion species with a small size. In fact, it is now known that the EPP (and the EPSP in nerve cells) is due to a selective increase in permeability to small cations, of which sodium and potassium are by far the most important (see below).

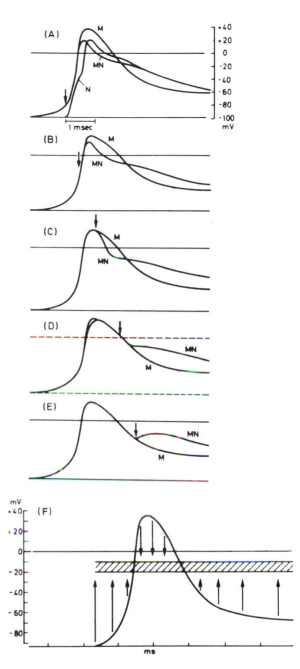

Fig. 8.2. The reversal potential of the end-plate potential. Records *A–E* show the effect on control muscle action potentials (*M* in each record) of transmitter-evoked responses at the frog neuromuscular junction following nerve stimulation at the *arrows*. *MN* in each set of records is the modification of the control muscle action potential. In record *A*, *N* is the action potential, arising from an end-plate potential, set up by nerve stimulation alone. Record *F* summarizes the results. The *arrows* indicate the direction and relative magnitude of the changes caused by transmitter. The *cross-hatched area* shows the approximate level at which the effect of transmitter on membrane potential reverses in direction. (Reproduced with permission from del Castillo and Katz 1954b.)

The EPP is produced by an underlying end-plate current due to the flow of ions down their electrochemical gradients. The end-plate current was demonstrated by Takeuchi and Takeuchi (1959), who were able to voltage clamp the end-plate region by injecting current through one intracellular microelectrode and recording the voltage changes produced by ACh (released either naturally or from an extracellular microelectrode) through another intracellular microelectrode. End-plate current was the current necessary to hold the membrane potential at the desired level in the face of ACh action. As shown in Fig. 8.3, the end-plate current has a faster rise time and shorter time course than the EPP. This is due to the fact that the EPP properties are determined in part by the passive membrane properties of the muscle membrane.

Takeuchi and Takeuchi, and later workers, showed that the end-plate current reversed at a membrane potential at, or very close to, 0 mV and that it was influenced by changes in extra-

cellular concentrations of sodium, potassium (and calcium) ions but not by chloride. Normally calcium plays little or no part in generating the EPP, and only sodium and potassium are involved. The movements of sodium and potassium through the chemically gated ion channel are simultaneous, unlike the movements of the same ions through the voltage-gated ion channels that open during the action potential where the movements are sequential. This is an important difference. The voltage-gated ion channels for sodium and potassium are two independent channels, whereas the chemically gated channels activated by the combination of transmitter with receptor allow both sodium and potassium to pass through the same channel. Furthermore, the opening of the voltage-dependent sodium channel leads to a regenerative increase in sodium influx: as the membrane is more and more depolarized more and more sodium enters. In contrast, the chemically gated channel openings are dependent on the concentration of the transmitter available for combination with the receptor: the level of the membrane potential does not affect the channel openings and the total synaptic conductance is not affected (although the time course of the current is).

The patch clamp technique may be used to examine the ionic current that flows through single ACh-gated channels in the muscle. Small patches of muscle membrane from the end-plate region are attached to the polished tips of the patch electrode by suction and form a tight electrical seal with the electrode. Such patches may contain one or a few channels, and in the presence of ACh these channels open (and close) in an all-or-nothing way (Fig. 8.4). The openings occur randomly in time and the channels remain open for about 1 ms on the average. When open, a single channel has a conductance of about 30 pS and contributes a current pulse of about 2 pA of current to the total end-plate current. It has been calculated that during the period that a single channel is open about $20\,000$ Na^+ ions flow into the cell and a similar (but smaller) number of K^+ ions flow out. Analysis of single channel currents by Neher and Sackmann and their colleagues has shown that the currents have the same reversal potential as the macroscopic end-plate current – about 0 mV (Fig. 8.4).

Under physiological conditions a miniature end-plate potential, which results from the release of ACh from a single synaptic vesicle, produces a potential change in the muscle cell of 0.5–1.0 mV, and the underlying miniature end-plate current has a peak amplitude of about 3

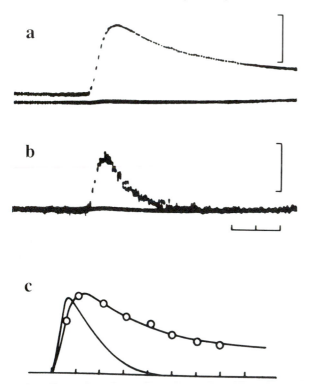

Fig. 8.3a–c. Voltage clamp of the end-plate potential. **a** Shows the end-plate potential at a frog sartorius neuromuscular junction recorded in a curarized preparation. **b** Shows the end-plate current (*upper trace*) when the voltage change had been prevented by the clamp (*lower trace*). **c** Shows the end-plate potential and current superimposed. The *circles* on the potential trace indicate the values of potential calculated from the end-plate current. (Reproduced with permission from Takeuchi and Takeuchi 1959.)

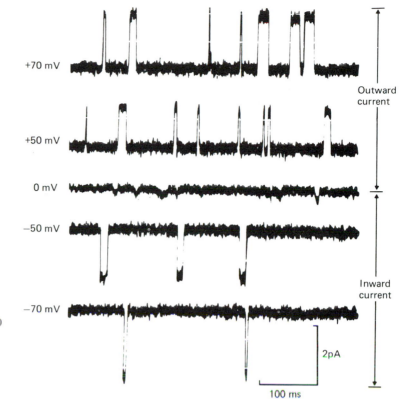

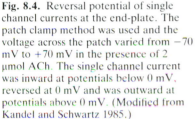

Fig. 8.4. Reversal potential of single channel currents at the end-plate. The patch clamp method was used and the voltage across the patch varied from −70 mV to +70 mV in the presence of 2 μmol ACh. The single channel current was inward at potentials below 0 mV, reversed at 0 mV and was outward at potentials above 0 mV. (Modified from Kandel and Schwartz 1985.)

nA. If each ACh-gated channel contributes 2 pA of current, then each miniature EPP is caused by the almost simultaneous opening of 1500 individual channels. Since it is believed that two molecules of ACh are required to open each channel, then each vesicle should contain at least 3000 molecules of the transmitter. The experiments of Kuffler and Yoshikami (see Chap. 6) had indicated that a single vesicle in the motoneurons in the snake contained an upper limit of rather less than 10 000 molecules of ACh. These figures are in remarkably good agreement as it is not known whether all the ACh molecules released from a single vesicle actually manage to combine with the receptor molecules on the muscle membrane; some may diffuse away or be broken down before they can reach the receptor sites.

Central Excitatory Synapses – The Ia-motoneuron Synapse. At the vertebrate neuromuscular junction a single nerve impulse in the axon of a single motoneuron leads (in twitch muscle) to the release of enough transmitter to cause a sufficiently large end-plate potential to evoke a muscle action potential. The muscle action potential is conducted throughout the length of the muscle fibre and in turn leads to contraction of the

muscle. In other words, a single nerve action potential, in the presynaptic neuron, leads to a single muscle action potential, in the postsynaptic cell. This simple one-to-one relay is obviously adapted to the work of the muscle, but such simple relay between neurons in the nervous system is the exception. In the nervous system it is rare for a single presynaptic impulse to lead to the setting up of a single postsynaptic impulse. A single neuron in the nervous system receives many synaptic contacts, often several hundred thousand, from very many individual neurons. The synapses may have either excitatory or inhibitory actions, and whether or not the neuron is caused to fire impulses depends on the balance of the various excitatory and inhibitory actions. Activity in a considerable proportion of the excitatory inputs is usually necessary to cause neuronal firing.

The pioneering work of Eccles and his colleagues (see, for example, Eccles 1964) established the foundations of our knowledge of the basic workings of excitatory postsynaptic synaptic transmission in the vertebrate central nervous system by mechanisms that were later shown to be due to the opening of chemically gated ion channels. The preparation used was the cat spinal

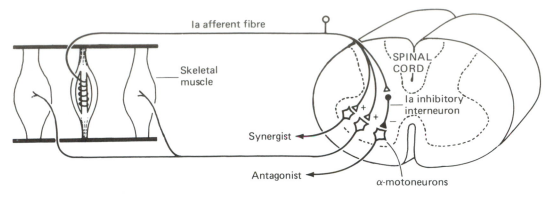

Fig. 8.5. Diagrammatic representation of the monosynaptic reflex arc between Ia afferent fibres from muscle spindles and alpha-motoneurons in the spinal cord. The spinal cord is represented as a transverse section. (Modified from Kandel and Schwartz 1985.)

cord, and in particular the monosynaptic connexions between the large (Ia) afferent fibres from the annulospiral endings in the muscle spindle and the large alpha-motoneurons that innervate the muscles containing the same spindles (and also muscles having similar actions – the synergists). In Chapter 11, more detailed consideration will be made of transmission at these synapses, and in Chapter 13 we shall consider the role of the system in reflex action and in posture and movement control. For the time being it is necessary to realize that there is a direct synaptic contact between the Ia fibres and the motoneurons and that almost every one of the Ia fibres from every muscle spindle in a particular muscle makes a small number (one to probably less than ten) of excitatory synapses with every motoneuron that innervates the muscle containing the spindles. The system is illustrated in Fig. 8.5.

The Ia afferent fibres from muscle spindles are the largest in a peripheral nerve. They therefore have the lowest electrical threshold for excitation and may be caused to fire impulses selectively by electrical stimulation at and near threshold for the peripheral nerve under study. Such near-threshold stimulation leads to a short-lasting wave of depolarization (the excitatory postsynaptic potential; EPSP) in the appropriate motoneurons and this EPSP is a graded phenomenon, its amplitude depending on the size of the current used to stimulate the afferent nerve and therefore depending on the number of nerve fibres activated by the stimulus (Fig. 8.6). Only when the EPSP reaches an amplitude of about 15 mV does the motoneuron generate an impulse. In other words, simultaneous activity of several (probably at least ten) Ia afferent fibres is needed to lift the motoneuron's membrane potential from its resting

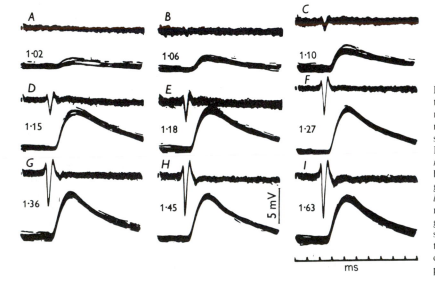

Fig. 8.6. The relationship between the size of the intracellularly recorded EPSP in alpha-motoneurons and the strength of stimulation of muscle afferent fibres. In each pair of traces the *upper record* is the afferent volley produced by stimulating the medial gastrocnemius nerve (cat) and the *lower record* the intracellular recording from a medial gastrocnemius motoneuron. The stimulus strengths, relative to a threshold value of 1.0, are indicated on the records. (Reproduced with permission from Eccles et al. 1957.)

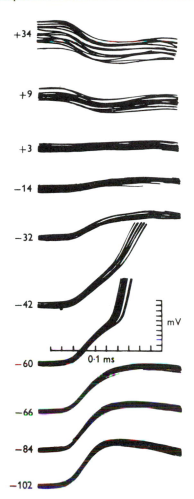

Fig. 8.7. The effect of membrane polarization on the EPSP. The EPSPs were recorded, via one barrel of a double-barrelled microelectrode, from a cat biceps-semitendinosus motoneuron in response to electrical stimulation of the afferent fibres from the muscle, and the membrane potential of the motoneuron was varied by passing current through the other barrel. Note the reversal of the EPSP at about 0 mV. Each record consists of about 20 superposed individual traces. (Reproduced with permission from Coombs et al. 1955c.)

level of −70 mV to its firing level of about −55 mV. This EPSP is known as the composite EPSP since it is produced by impulses arriving more or less synchronously along several afferent nerve fibres. The composite EPSP is very similar to the end-plate potential, having a rise time of about 2 ms and a total duration of 10–15 ms. The similarities extend beyond these two characteristics – the EPSP changes in amplitude and in polarity as the membrane potential of the motoneuron is changed by passing current through an intracellular microelectrode (Fig. 8.7). As the membrane potential is increased (made more negative)

the amplitude of the EPSP increases, whereas as the membrane potential is decreased the EPSP amplitude decreases until, at about 0 mV, it reverses. That is, the reversal potential for the EPSP in mammalian alpha-motoneurons is at about 0 mV. It has, in fact, proved difficult to reverse Ia EPSPs in motoneurons, but relatively recently Finkel and Redman (1983) have been able satisfactorily to voltage clamp motoneurons and determine the reversal potential for the synaptic current underlying the EPSP. Earlier, Eccles and co-workers had shown, by injecting various ions into motoneurons through an intracellular microelectrode, that the membrane became permeable to both Na^+ and K^+ ions during the EPSP, but not to larger cations nor to anions.

Thus, the EPSP evoked in mammalian motoneurons by activity in the Ia afferent fibres from muscle spindles has an underlying mechanism similar to that of the EPP. The transmitter released from primary afferent fibres is not yet identified with certainty, but, for Ia fibres, is probably glutamate or aspartate. Combination of transmitter with receptor leads to the opening of chemically gated channels that are permeable to small cations – Na^+ and K^+ under physiological conditions. Many other excitatory actions at central neurons, especially where the excitatory action is short-lived, have the same underlying mechanism.

Postsynaptic Inhibition at the Mammalian Motoneuron. In addition to determining the basis of excitatory processes in the motoneuron, Eccles and his co-workers were also instrumental in establishing our understanding of inhibitory mechanisms. As mentioned above, whether or not a central neuron fires is determined by the balance of excitatory and inhibitory inputs. Eccles and his collaborators examined the inhibitory actions of Ia muscle spindle afferent fibres on motoneurons of antagonist muscles. Stimulation of Ia fibres leads to a hyperpolarizing potential (the inhibitory postsynaptic potential; IPSP) in antagonist motoneurons which has a slightly longer central latency than the Ia-evoked EPSP and also a similar, though slightly shorter, time course (Fig. 8.8). Altering the membrane potential of the motoneuron from its resting potential of about −70 mV showed that the IPSP grew in amplitude as the membrane was depolarized and that it became smaller as the membrane was hyperpolarized. At about −80 mV the IPSP reversed and beyond this level it became a depolarizing potential (Fig. 8.9), i.e.

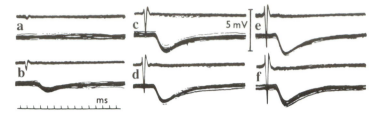

Fig. 8.8. Inhibitory postsynaptic potentials (IPSPs) in a mammalian motoneuron. The *lower records* give the intracellular responses of a biceps-semitendinosus motoneuron to afferent volleys of increasing size (*upper records*) evoked by electrical stimulation of the nerve from the antagonist muscle, quadriceps. All records were formed by the superposition of a number of traces. (Reproduced with permission from Coombs et al. 1955d.)

the reversal potential for the Ia-evoked IPSP in mammalian motoneurons is −80 mV.

For a potential to reverse at −80 mV the underlying ionic mechanism must involve either

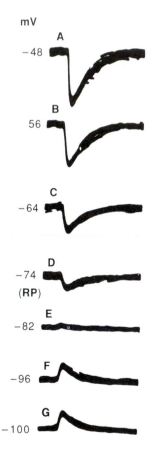

Fig. 8.9. The effect of membrane potential on the IPSP. The IPSPs were recorded from a biceps-semitendinosus motoneuron (cat) in response to electrical excitation of Group Ia afferent fibres in the quadriceps nerve. The membrane potential of the motoneuron was changed by passing current through one barrel of the intracellular electrode (values of membrane potential given to the *left*). The resting potential (*RP*) of the neuron was −74 mV and the IPSP reversed in sign at about 82 mV. (Reproduced with permission from Coombs et al. 1955b.)

an influx of anions or an efflux of cations (or both). A reversal potential of −80 mV is close to the equilibrium potentials of both potassium and chloride, and it was originally thought that the inhibitory transmitter opened chemically gated channels permeable to both of these ions. However, careful studies involving intracellular injection of various ion species have shown that changing the intracellular potassium has little effect, and it is now thought that the IPSP in mammalian motoneurons is due to a selective increase in membrane permeability to chloride ions alone. Injection of chloride ions into the neuron leads to a reversal of the IPSP to a depolarizing potential, and it is generally accepted that the concentration of chloride ions inside the motoneuron is held at below its passive distribution level by an active process. Channel activation thus leads to an entry of chloride ions.

As mentioned above, the IPSP produced in mammalian motoneurons by Ia afferent fibres from antagonistic muscles has a slightly longer central delay in onset compared with the EPSP from synergistic muscles (after differences in conduction path length are taken into account). This longer latency is due to the interpolation of an extra inhibitory interneuron in the system. As far as is known at present, all primary afferent neurons that innervate sensory receptors and are the only neurons to enter the central nervous system from the periphery have excitatory actions on their target cells (even though their transmitters are certainly not all the same). In order for inhibitory action to occur there must be an extra interpolated inhibitory interneuron between the primary afferent neuron and the neuron that is to be inhibited (see Fig. 8.5).

It is useful to ask how the inhibition is brought about. One obvious mechanism is that the IPSP moves the membrane potential of the neuron away from its firing threshold, thereby making it more difficult for excitatory inputs to fire the cell. But this is not the only way inhibition works.

By opening chloride channels in the membrane the transmitter also increases the conductance of the membrane of the postsynaptic cell. This increased conductance has the effect of short-circuiting any concurrent EPSP activity and thus reducing the amplitude of the EPSP. In fact, this short-circuiting action is of paramount importance. An inhibitory action on a neuron need not produce a hyperpolarizing IPSP – an increase in membrane conductance is all that is required, and the associated potential change may be hyperpolarizing or depolarizing (or zero). As long as any potential change does not reach impulse firing threshold (the reversal potential is greater than the firing threshold), then the short-circuiting action will reduce concurrent EPSPs and the effect will be inhibitory. In some neurons postsynaptic inhibition is due to a selective increase in potassium permeability.

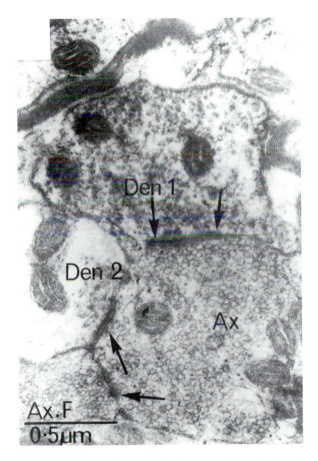

Fig. 8.10. Axo-axonic synapse in the mammalian spinal cord. This electron micrograph shows a synaptic bouton (*Ax*) which makes axodendritic contacts with two dendrites (*Den 1* and *Den 2*) and is itself postsynaptic to another axon terminal (*Ax.F*). (Reproduced with permission from Maxwell et al. 1983.)

The inhibitory transmitter responsible for the Ia-evoked IPSP in mammalian motoneurons is the amino acid glycine. Another amino acid transmitter responsible for many postsynaptic inhibitory actions is gamma-aminobutyric acid (GABA). Chemically gated channels opened by both of these transmitters have been studied using the patch clamp technique. In spinal cord neurons both transmitters open channels selectively permeable to chloride ions – in the case of GABA via the $GABA_A$ channel.

Presynaptic Inhibition in the Mammalian Spinal Cord. Many of the synaptic boutons of primary afferent fibres in the mammalian spinal cord are themselves postsynaptic to other boutons. The synapses thus formed (axo-axonic synapses) have all the ultrastructural requirements for chemically transmitting synapses (Fig. 8.10). These axo-axonic synapses are the anatomical basis for presynaptic inhibition, the basic operational effects of which were delineated by Eccles and his colleagues (see Eccles 1964) and Schmidt and his co-workers (Schmidt 1971, 1973). Although presynaptic inhibition occurs at many sites in the vertebrate central nervous system, it is certainly easiest to study it at spinal cord level, and, more precisely, to study its control of transmission between primary afferent fibres and their target cells. The terminals of large-diameter cutaneous afferent fibres (from receptors in the skin) are under presynaptic inhibitory control from a variety of sources, including other cutaneous afferent fibres. If a microelectrode is placed inside a cutaneous axon within the spinal cord near its terminals and other cutaneous axons stimulated electrically as they run in a peripheral nerve, a depolarizing potential is recorded from the single cutaneous axon (Fig. 8.11). This potential change is called primary afferent depolarization (PAD) when it occurs in primary afferent fibres. This PAD has a central latency of a few milliseconds, a time to peak of about 15–20 ms and a total duration of the order of 200 ms. It is thus a longer lasting potential change than either the EPSP or the IPSP.

A clue to the function of PAD is given by studying the changes in transmission characteristics between the primary afferent fibres known to receive axo-axonic synapses and their various target cells. One such system consists of cutaneous afferent fibres and spinal neurons belonging to the spinocervical tract, part of a somatosensory pathway. Transmission through this system may be affected by activity in cutaneous nerves that do not themselves excite the spinocervical tract

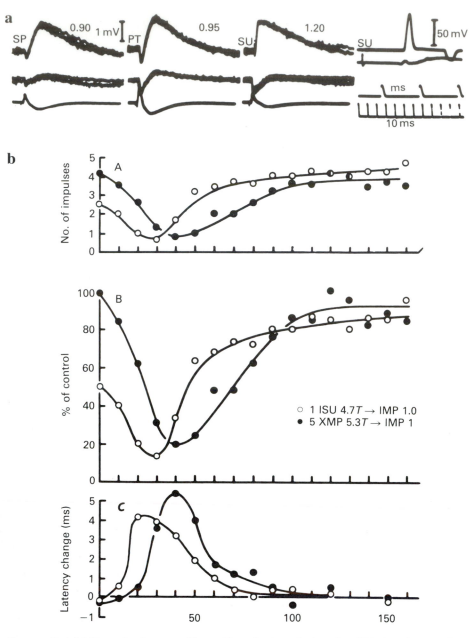

Fig. 8.11a,b. Presynaptic inhibition of cutaneous afferent fibres in the spinal cord. **a** This set of traces shows intra-axonal recordings from a sural nerve fibre (*uppermost*), the corresponding extracellular records (*middle*) and the afferent volleys producing the responses (*lowermost*). In response to electrical stimulation of the superficial peroneal (*SP*), posterior tibial (*PT*) and sural (*SU*) nerves at the indicated strengths, the sural axon is depolarized (primary afferent depolarization). To the *right* is a record of the action potential recorded from the sural axon. **b** This set of curves shows the effects of presynaptic inhibition on transmission through the spinocervical tract of the cat. The spinocervical tract cell was caused to fire by electrical stimulation of the ipsilateral medial plantar nerve at 1.06 times threshold, and this response was conditioned by previous activity in either the ipsilateral sural nerve (*ISU*) or contralateral medial plantar (*XMP*) nerves at the indicated strengths. The inhibition peaks at 30–50 ms and lasts for at least 150 ms. (Reproduced with permission from Eccles et al. 1963 (**a**) and from Brown et al. 1973 (**b**).)

neuron under study and this effect is a reduction in transmission efficacy with a time to maximum and total time course similar to that of PAD (Fig. 8.11). More evidence comes from studies of

the conditioning effects of stimulating peripheral nerves on the monosynaptic EPSP produced in motoneurons (see Eccles 1964). Such conditioning reduces the amplitude of the EPSP with a

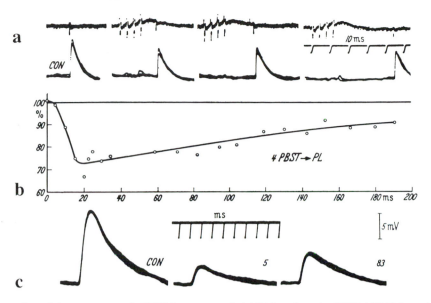

Fig. 8.12a–c. Depression of the monosynaptic EPSP by presynaptic inhibition. In **a** the EPSP (*CON*) in a plantaris motoneuron (cat) is depressed by four conditioning volleys in Group I muscle afferents. **b** Shows the time course of the EPSP depression. *PBST*, posterior biceps semitendinosus nerve; *PL*, plantaris nerve. In **c** the control EPSP (*CON*) of another experiment is depressed at 5 and 83 ms after a conditioning tetanus of 22 Group I volleys. (Reproduced with permission from Eccles et al. 1961.)

time course similar to that of the associated PAD (Fig. 8.12). At the same time there are no obvious conductance changes in the motoneuronal membrane, and so an involvement of postsynaptic inhibitory actions is ruled out.

Presynaptic inhibition works by reducing the amount of transmitter released by the presynaptic neuron and therefore leads to a reduction in EPSP amplitude. These inhibitory actions may be blocked by certain convulsant poisons such as bicuculline and picrotoxin, especially the former, which seems more selective. Both of these substances are competitive antagonists of GABA at sites where GABA is known to be the transmitter. Furthermore, recent work has established that the presynaptic component in spinal axo-axonic contacts onto identified cutaneous afferent fibres contain GABA. How does GABA act at this synapse? It would appear to act (at $GABA_A$ receptor sites) by increasing the conductance of the primary afferent terminal to chloride ions and thus producing a short-circuiting of the nerve action potential and reducing its height. Such a reduction would, by producing less depolarization, lead to activation of fewer voltage-gated calcium channels in the terminal and a consequential reduction in the amount of transmitter released. GABA also appears to act at $GABA_B$ receptor sites by reducing the influx of Ca^{2+}. A reduction in the amount of transmitter released

has the operational effect of inhibiting transmission at the synapse between the primary afferent fibre and its target neurons. Presynaptic inhibition controls the input to a neuron, whereas postsynaptic inhibition controls the output of a neuron.

Voltage-Dependent Chemically Gated Channels: The NMDA Receptor. Excitatory amino acid transmitters may combine with a variety of postsynaptic receptors. The receptors are defined according to which agonists they bind to as kainate, quisqualate and *N*-methyl-D-aspartate (NMDA) receptors. NMDA receptor actions have elicited great interest recently because of their unusual properties. Activation of NMDA receptors leads to relatively slow EPSPs lasting 200–300 ms, but most interestingly the NMDA receptor channel is blocked by Mg^{2+} ions in a voltage-dependent manner (Fig. 8.13). At membrane potentials of -60 to -70 mV the block is pronounced and progressive depolarization leads to a voltage-dependent removal of the block, opening the channel (which is permeable to Ca^{2+} ions in addition to Na^+ and K^+ ions. Thus any synaptic activity which leads to depolarization of the postsynaptic neuron will remove the Mg^{2+} block and allow the amino acid/NMDA receptor mediated channel to open. Here we have a

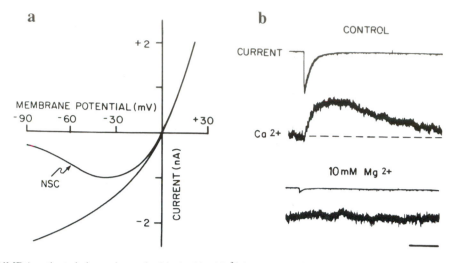

Fig. 8.13a,b. NMDA-activated channels can be blocked by Mg^{2+} ions at negative membrane potentials and are permeable to Ca^{2+}. In **a** NMDA-evoked currents are recorded under voltage-clamp conditions in cultured cells, in the presence (*NSC*) or absence of Mg^{2+} ions. **b** Shows that when NMDA is applied to a cell (voltage clamped at -60 mV) in the absence of added Mg^{2+} an inward current is evoked and the amount of free Ca^{2+} in the cell increases, but in the presence of 2 mM Mg^{2+} there is almost a total suppression of the current and no change in the intracellular Ca^{2+} concentration. (Reproduced with permission from MacDermott and Dale 1987.)

possible example of "synaptic plasticity", where activity via one input to a neuron can influence the potency of another input to the same neuron (see Chap. 18).

Closing of Ion Channels That Are Normally Open

The combination of transmitter with receptor may lead to the closing of ion channels as well as to the opening of ion channels. In recent years it has become obvious that such channel closure is not uncommon. The mechanism was first described for transmitter actions at various peripheral synapses, especially in the autonomic nervous system, but is now known to occur at many sites in the central nervous system too.

Channels that are closed by transmitter–receptor combination are open in the resting state. For example, potassium channels that contribute to the resting potential and are normally open in some sympathetic neurons (and also various neurons in the hippocampus and cerebral cortex) may be closed by combination of ACh with the muscarinic receptor. Such closure brings about a slow EPSP. In fact, in sympathetic ganglion cells (B cells) in the bullfrog ACh causes three types of responses (Fig. 8.14): a fast depolarization produced by combination with a nicotinic receptor, a slow depolarization produced by combination with a muscarinic receptor and a hyperpolarization which is, like the slow de-

polarization, blocked by atropine and is muscarinic in nature. Transmission between the preganglionic cholinergic neurons and the B cells is not the only transmission occurring at this site. In addition, there are other preganglionic neurons that release a peptide, luteinizing hormone releasing hormone (LHRH), which causes a late, slow EPSP that lasts for about 5 min (Fig. 8.14).

How can the closing of normally open channels bring about excitatory actions? Closure of potassium channels that are normally open leads to a depolarization – this is the slow EPSP – and thus brings the neuron closer to its firing threshold. In addition, because open channels are closed, there is a concomitant decrease in the cell's membrane conductance, and therefore any other excitatory input that leads to an EPSP (such as the fast EPSP produced by ACh at the nicotinic receptor) will produce a larger EPSP and have a greater chance of causing the cell to fire. Such actions in decreasing the conductance of a neuron modulate the actions of other transmitters that act directly to open channels and which are said to mediate an action.

Neurotransmitter actions that lead to closure of normally open channels have a longer latency of onset and a much longer duration than most transmitter actions that open channels by direct combination with receptor molecules. These actions are highly temperature dependent and the long-lasting actions are therefore not due to some sort of delayed diffusion of transmitter. The precise mode of action of many of these

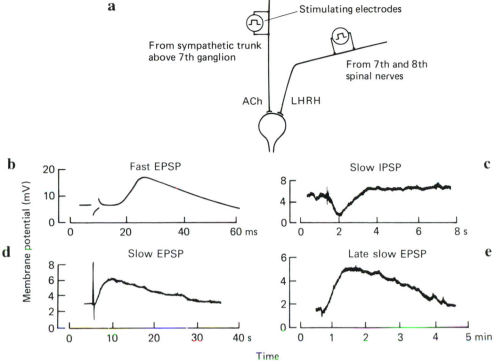

Fig. 8.14a–e. Synaptic response in sympathetic ganglion cells of the frog. **a** Shows the separation of the cholinergic and non-cholinergic innervation of a ganglion cell in the ninth ganglion of the paravertebral chain. **b–e** Four types of synaptic response: **b** A single presynaptic impulse produces a fast EPSP. **c** After blocking the fast EPSP with a nicotinic blocking agent, repetitive stimulation produces a slow IPSP. **d** Repetitive stimulation also produces a slow EPSP that occurs later than the responses in **b** and **c**. **e** The late slow EPSP evoked by activity in the LHRH-containing fibres. (Modified from Kuffler et al. 1984.)

transmitter–receptor combinations is not known. But it is known that some transmitters can lead to channel closure through biochemical processes involving a second messenger system. One such transmitter is 5-hydroxytryptamine (5-HT) or serotonin.

In the marine snail *Aplysia* serotonin produces an EPSP in certain sensory neurons. The EPSP is caused by the closure of normally open potassium channels (the so-called S channels). In this example, serotonin binds to receptor molecules on the neuronal membrane but these receptor molecules do not themselves partake in the formation of the S channels. The latter are located in different parts of the membrane. Combination of serotonin with the receptor leads to a protein (the G protein) in the membrane activating another membrane protein – adenylate cyclase. Adenylate cyclase is an enzyme that catalyses the synthesis of cyclic adenosine monophosphate (cyclic AMP) from adenosine triphosphate (ATP). Cyclic AMP is the second messenger. Increased levels of cyclic AMP in the neuron

lead to activation of another enzyme, a protein kinase, which catalyses the phosphorylation of a protein (which may be the S channel protein itself) and, somehow, causes the S channel to close. These steps are summarized in Fig. 8.15.

Such channel closures involving second messenger molecules are not limited to invertebrate synapses. It is now known that noradrenaline (norepinephrine) acts similarly on cells of the vertebrate cerebral cortex to close potassium channels. Both serotonin and noradrenaline are important transmitters in the human brain and have been implicated in various affective disorders such as depression.

Actions That Affect the Metabolism of the Postsynaptic Cell

Combination of transmitter with receptor does not necessarily lead to changes in the ionic conductance of the postsynaptic cell. It may lead to changes in the cell's metabolism. We have already

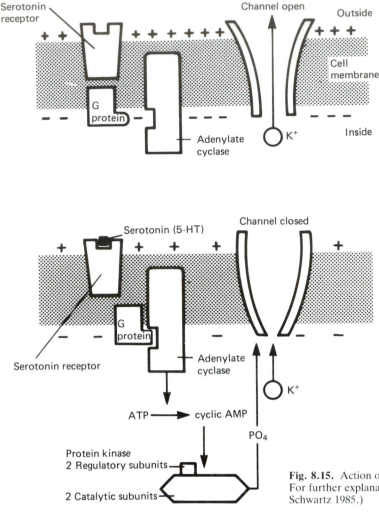

Fig. 8.15. Action of serotonin (5-HT) in closing ion channels. For further explanation see the text. (Modified from Kandel and Schwartz 1985.)

seen that some slow conductance changes may be brought about by a variety of transmitters by means of second messenger systems. Similar second messenger systems may bring about changes in the cell's metabolism. In this case, however, there is a more complex series of biochemical reactions.

The best known system of this type is that of the beta-adrenergic receptor which exists on a wide variety of cells, e.g. cardiac muscle, smooth muscle of arterioles. Combination of adrenaline (or noradrenaline) with the beta-adrenergic receptor sets in train a series of enzymically catalysed reactions – an enzyme cascade (Fig. 8.16) – via a G protein which phosphorylates guanosine diphosphate (GDP) to guanosine triphosphate (GTP). The G protein–GTP complex then activates adenylate cyclase which catalyses the conversion of ATP to cyclic AMP. The cyclic AMP in turn activates cyclic AMP-dependent protein kinases which catalyse the phosphorylation of various proteins.

In addition to cyclic AMP there are other important second messengers. Thus some receptors (muscarinic ACh receptors, alpha-adrenergic receptors as well as some peptide receptors) act by stimulating the hydrolysis of phosphatidylinositol to diacylglycerol and inositol tris phosphate. The diacyltryglycerol then activates a protein kinase. In some systems calcium ions act as a second messenger. Calcium brings about protein phosphorylation by calcium-dependent protein kinases or, by forming a complex with the protein calmodulin, activates a range of enzymes.

An example of how such changes in a cell's metabolism might affect its performance is given by considering the synthesis of transmitter,

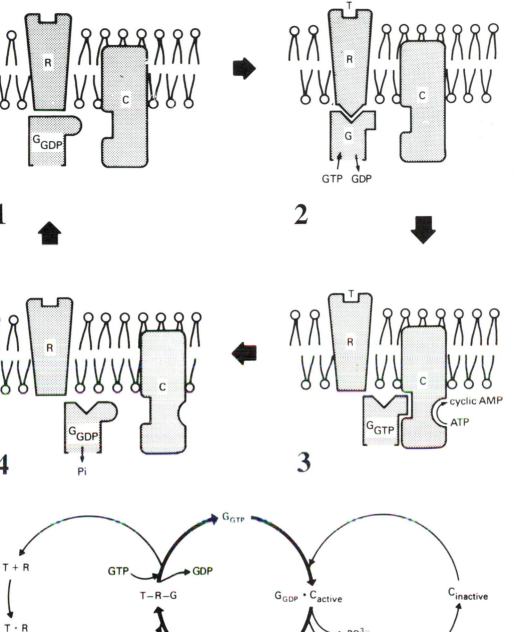

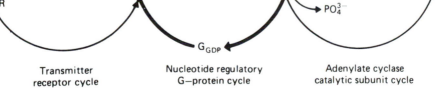

Fig. 8.16. Effects of transmitter combination with the β-adrenergic receptor. The synthesis of cyclic AMP that follows combination of transmitter (*T*) with the β-adrenergic receptor (*R*) is mediated through a G protein (*G*). The GDP of the G protein is replaced by GTP when transmitter and receptor combine (*2*). The G protein associates with adenylate cyclase (*C*), which catalyzes the conversion of ATP to cyclic AMP (*3*). The latter step also results in the hydrolysis of GTP to GDP and the G protein dissociates from the adenylate cyclase (*4*) and AMP synthesis stops. (Modified from Kandel and Schwartz 1985.)

e.g. noradrenaline. Noradrenaline is formed from the amino acid tyrosine by oxidation to L-dihydroxyphenylalanine (L-DOPA), by decarboxylation of L-DOPA to dopamine, which is in turn hydroxylated to noradrenaline (see Fig. 7.6). The first step is catalysed by the enzyme tyrosine hydroxylase and this is the rate-limiting step for the synthesis. Tyrosine hydroxylase is dependent on the presence of a pteridene cofactor. Phosphorylation of tyrosine hydroxylase by cyclic AMP (the second messenger) increases its affinity for both its substrate (tyrosine) and the cofactor and therefore enhances its action, thus increasing the rate of noradrenaline synthesis.

Summary

1. The action of a particular neurotransmitter at its postsynaptic target neuron depends on the particular specific receptor molecules with which it combines.

2. Combination of transmitter with receptor can lead to the opening of ion channels that are closed at rest. Such channel openings can lead to selective permeability increases to either single ion species, e.g. Cl^-, or to permeability increases

to more than one ion, e.g. Na^+ and K^+. Depending on the species of ion involved the ionic current may lead to a depolarization or a hyperpolarization of the membrane or may clamp the membrane potential at resting level. The receptor molecules themselves may be the ion channels. Some of these chemically gated ion channels, such as the NMDA-receptor channel, are also voltage-dependent and their state of opening depends on the membrane potential of the postsynaptic neuron.

3. Combination of transmitter with receptor may also lead to the closing of ion channels that are open at rest. Second messenger molecules may be involved in these channel closings.

4. Combination of transmitter with receptor may also lead to changes in the metabolic activity of the postsynaptic cell. Here the combination may lead to a series of enzymatically catalysed reactions (an enzyme cascade).

5. At this stage it will be useful to compare the properties of non-gated channels (see Chap. 2), voltage-gated channels (see Chaps. 3 and 6), chemically gated channels (see this chapter) and also channels gated by sensory stimuli such as light and mechanical displacement etc. (see Chap. 12). Table 8.1 summarizes the properties of these various channels.

Table 8.1. Common features of signalling potentials

Potentials	Channel specificity	Gating mechanism	Properties
Resting potential	Mostly non-gated K^+ and Cl^- channels	Usually non-gated	Usually steady, ranging in different cells from -35 to -70 mV
Action potential	Independently gated Na^+ and K^+ channels	Voltage	All or nothing; about 100 mV in amplitude; 1–10 ms in duration
Receptor potential	Modality-specific gated Na^+ and K^+ channels	Sensory (adequate) stimulus	Graded; fast, several milliseconds in duration; several millivolts in amplitude
Electrical PSP	None	None	Passive propagation of presynaptic potential change
Increased-conductance EPSP	Simultaneous gating of single class of non-voltage-gated channels for Na^+ and K^+	Chemical (extracellular messenger)	Graded; fast, several milliseconds to seconds in duration; several millivolts in amplitude
Increased-conductance IPSP	Non-voltage-gated K^+ or Cl^- channels	Chemical (extracellular messenger)	Graded; fast, several milliseconds to seconds in duration; several millivolts in amplitude
Decreased-conductance EPSP	Closure of K^+ channels	Chemical (intracellular messenger)	Graded; slow, seconds to minutes in duration; 1 to several millivolts in amplitude
Decreased-conductance EPSP	Closure of channels for Na^+ or Ca^{2+}	Chemical (? intracellular messenger)	Graded, slow, seconds to minutes in duration, 1 to several millivolts in amplitude

Modified from Kandel and Schwartz 1985.

9 The Postsynaptic Neuron II: The Initiation of Impulses

In Chapter 3 the nerve impulse was discussed from the point of view of its ionic mechanism and in Chapter 4 its propagation was described. In experimental work on the nerve impulse, electrical stimulation of axons is the usual means of eliciting action potentials. In nature, however, impulses are initiated either by the transduction of energy by sense organs (such as the muscle spindle, mechano- or thermoreceptors in the skin, photoreceptors etc.) or by the excitatory action of one neuron on another, that is, through excitatory transmission and excitatory postsynaptic potentials (EPSPs). In this chapter the natural initiation of impulses in central neurons will be considered, but the student should be aware of the fact that many neurons operate without impulses and cannot generate impulses (see Chap. 10).

Before describing the initiation of impulses by sensory receptors (see Chap. 12), the initiation of impulses in central neurons will be discussed, and it is of some interest to ask whether impulses may be initiated in any part of the neuronal membrane or only in localized parts, and even if impulse initiation is limited to a single site. In general, those parts of a neuron's membrane that are chemically sensitive (to transmitters) are often described as electrically inexcitable and incapable of generating an action potential. In a vertebrate neuron such as a motoneuron, where synapses are located on the dendrites, the soma and also the axon hillock and initial part of the axon, it might be thought that only the part of the axon free of synaptic contacts could generate impulses. The situation is not as simple as this, and we shall see that the sites of impulse initiation depend not only on the ability of the membrane to generate action potentials (that is, on those parts of the membrane containing voltage-gated channels) but also on the relative thresholds at different sites for the generation of action potentials.

Generation of Single Impulses in Motoneurons

The initiation of impulses in alpha-motoneurons was investigated by Eccles and his collaborators in the 1950s. The action potential in cat lumbosacral alpha-motoneurons has a different shape from, for example, the potential recorded from axons. Thus, whether set up by direct intracellular injection of current (Fig. 9.1c), by activation of excitatory inputs (orthodromic excitation, Fig. 9.1b) or whether recorded from within the motoneuron upon electrical excitation of the cell's axon with invasion of the impulse "from the wrong direction", i.e. the action potential travelling in a direction opposite to that which it would do normally (antidromic excitation, Fig. 9.1a), the action potential has an inflexion on its rising phase.

An analysis of the antidromic action potential in the motoneuron showed that the rising phase is made up of three distinctive components. These three components were all of the all-or-nothing character diagnostic of regenerative action potentials but had different thresholds. Thus, as shown

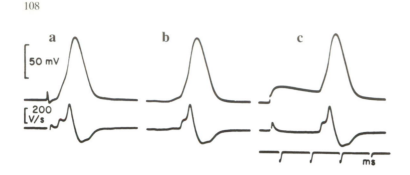

Fig. 9.1. Action potentials produced in a motoneuron when activated **a** by antidromic excitation, **b** by orthodromic excitation, and **c** by directly applied current. The *lower traces* are the electrically differentiated records of the upper traces. Note the inflexion, at approximately the same level, on the rising phases of the three potentials. (Reproduced with permission from Fatt 1957.)

in Fig. 9.2, if the membrane potential of a motoneuron was altered by passing current through one barrel of a double-barrelled intracellular microelectrode, the other barrel being used to record the responses, it was possible to isolate the components. At hyperpolarized levels of membrane potential (−87 mV) the antidromic action potential was reduced to a very small all-or-nothing component (the M spike) of about 5 mV amplitude. At −82 mV (still below the initial

resting potential of −80 mV) an additional and larger (40 mV) component was recorded. This was called the IS spike. At a membrane potential of −77 to −78 mV a third and larger component that completed the full-sized action potential was elicited. This was called the SD spike.

A consideration of these results, along with an analysis of the extracellular field potentials generated around motoneurons by antidromic activation of their axons, led to the following interpretation. It was assumed that the most likely location for the intracellular microelectrode was in the soma (or a large dendrite close to the soma). The largest component of the antidromic impulse (the SD spike) was most likely to have arisen from the part of the neuronal membrane closest to the electrode, that is, in the soma or in the soma plus the most proximal dendrites – hence SD spike. The IS spike was assigned to the initial segment, that is, the axon hillock plus the initial part of the axon before it acquires a myelin sheath. The reasoning behind this was that the region of surface membrane area expansion from axon to cell body was a likely place for the antidromic impulse to fail to invade the soma. The relatively large size (about 40 mV), however, of the IS spike suggested that it also arose close to the recording microelectrode and invasion of the axon hillock was assumed. The smallest (M spike) component was assigned to the myelinated axon since it was of small size, had a short refractory period and was capable of following high rates of stimulation.

This analysis of the antidromic action potential allowed the site of origin of the orthodromic and directly evoked impulses to be considered. Thus, as shown in Fig. 9.1, the inflexion on the rising phase of motoneuronal impulses, whatever the means by which they were evoked, always occurred at the same level of membrane potential, and this level coincided with the origin of the SD spike from the IS spike. Thus it was suggested that with all three types of initiation the IS spike precedes the SD spike, and in all cases the soma-

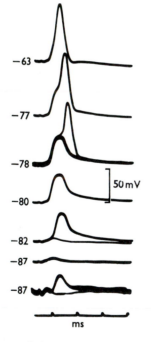

Fig. 9.2. Effects of changing the membrane potential of a motoneuron on the antidromic action potential. At −87 mV the potential is reduced to a small all-or-nothing component (M spike); at −82 mV a larger component (IS-spike) appears; and above −77 mV a third component (the SD-spike) appears. (Reproduced with permission from Coombs et al. 1955a.)

dendritic membrane is invaded by the action potential after a regenerative component has occurred in the initial segment. Furthermore, the antidromic invasion experiments had shown that the IS spike has a lower threshold than the SD spike, and this threshold is therefore the threshold for eliciting an impulse in the neuron (about 6–15 mV worth of depolarization from resting levels). The threshold for the generation of an impulse in the soma-dendritic membrane is about three times that of the IS segment (about 20–40 mV of depolarization is required). These differences are presumably due to a relative, but not absolute, lack of voltage-gated Na channels in the soma-dendritic membrane compared with the membrane of the initial segment. The chemically sensitive soma-dendritic and initial segment membranes are capable, therefore, of generating all-or-nothing responses. Under physiological conditions, however, the dendrites of spinal motoneurons (other than those parts nearest to the soma) are not capable of generating action potentials.

The above interpretation has been generally accepted for the spinal motoneuron and, by extrapolation, for many other types of nerve cells. What does such a mechanism mean for the operation of a neuron? Most importantly, the localization of the impulse-initiating zone to a particular part of the membrane (initial segment) implies that control over the membrane potential at that part is of prime significance in the control of neuronal firing. Put another way, the membrane at the initial segment may be considered to be integrating the total input (both excitatory and inhibitory) to the neuron, and if the excitatory input is such that the ionic currents depolarize the initial segment sufficiently then the neuron will fire. A further consequence of this mechanism is that the location of individual synapses becomes of supreme importance. This point will be taken up later (see Chap. 10), but it is worth pointing out now that, because of the cable properties of the (non-excitable) dendritic membrane, those synapses located far out on the dendrites will produce postsynaptic potentials at the initial segment that rise more slowly and decay over a longer time than those located near the initial segment, which will rise abruptly and decay quickly. Furthermore, inhibitory synapses located at or close to the initial segment will be very efficacious in preventing neuronal firing.

The observation that impulses arise at the initial segment and yet the soma and proximal dendrites also carry the all-or-nothing action potential also calls for comment. In this situation the impulse invades the soma and proximal dendrites after it has arisen in the initial segment and will interact with any postsynaptic currents present in the soma-dendritic membrane and will essentially wipe the soma-dendritic component clean of any remaining postsynaptic potentials. The soma-dendritic membrane is therefore reset and awaits further synaptic input.

It has recently been shown (Gogan et al. 1983) that in motoneurons of the abducens nerve (the abducens nerve is the sixth cranial nerve) that innervate the retractor bulbi muscle in the orbit of the eye impulse initiation may take place not at the initial segment but at the first or even the second node of Ranvier in the axon. Such activation was seen when the motoneurons were firing at relatively high frequencies. In these neurons invasion of the soma-dendritic membrane and even the initial segment did not necessarily take place, and thus EPSPs could influence the trigger zone for much longer periods than if the soma-dendritic membrane had been invaded.

Initiation of Trains of Impulses

Motoneurons

The initiation of a single impulse in a motoneuron is a relatively rare event. Under physiological conditions motoneurons, and most other neurons that can generate impulses, fire trains of impulses at varying frequencies. These impulse trains are elicited by incoming trains of impulses from the neurons afferent to the motoneuron. The initiation of trains of impulses in spinal alpha-motoneurons was investigated by Granit and Kernell and their colleagues.

When maintained excitatory synaptic activity is mimicked by passing long-duration depolarizing current pulses through an intracellular electrode many motoneurons show the following pattern of impulse activity (Fig. 9.3). After an initial fairly high-frequency burst of impulses the neuronal firing settles down, and ultimately a regular discharge occurs in which the firing rate is linearly related to the intensity of the injected current. This initial linear part of the current–frequency relation was called the primary range of firing. Further increase of depolarizing current leads, in many motoneurons, to an abrupt shift of firing frequency to another linear range with a greatly increased slope compared with the primary range – this is the secondary range (Fig. 9.3). Granit and his colleagues also made the important

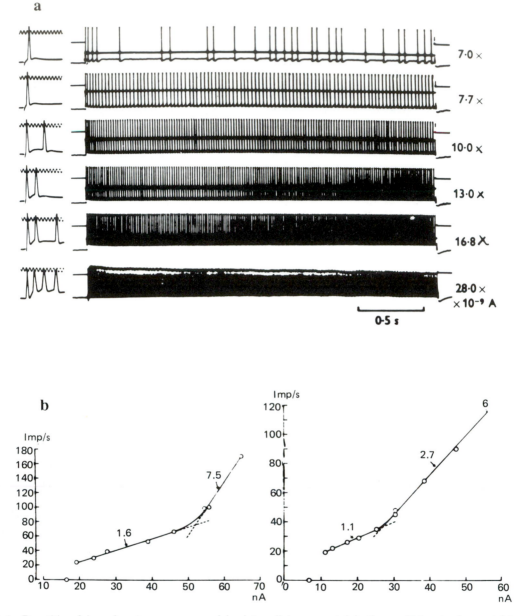

Fig. 9.3a,b. Repetitive firing of motoneurons caused by intracellular current injection. **a** This set of records´shows the responses recorded from rat motoneurons upon intracellular current injections at the strengths indicated on the *right*. The records on the *left* show the initial impulses to the injected current at a fast time-base (1000 Hz calibration). **b** These graphs show the relationship between frequency of impulse discharge and current strength for two cat motoneurons. The slopes of the curves are indicated (in impulses per second per nA) at the *arrows*. (Reproduced with permission from Granit et al. 1963b (**a**) and from Kernell 1965 (**b**).)

observation that, within the primary range, naturally evoked excitatory and inhibitory post-synaptic potentials (EPSPs and IPSPs) – elicited by muscle stretch – would interact with the de-polarizing pulses such that there was linear summation between them, EPSPs adding to the depolarization to increase the firing rate of the cell and IPSPs subtracting from the depolarizing pulses to decrease cell firing (Fig. 9.4).

The primary range varies from motoneuron to motoneuron but the lower limits of sustained firing are about 10–20 Hz and the point of transition to the secondary range is at about 30–50 Hz. Synaptically evoked firing in many moto-

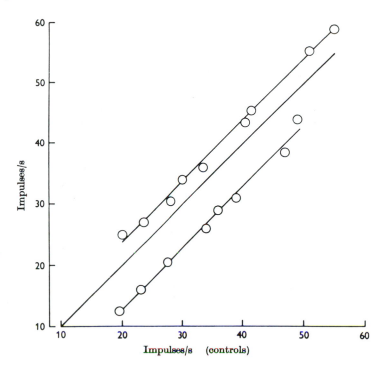

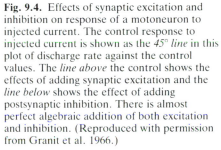

Fig. 9.4. Effects of synaptic excitation and inhibition on response of a motoneuron to injected current. The control response to injected current is shown as the *45° line* in this plot of discharge rate against the control values. The *line above* the control shows the effects of adding synaptic excitation and the *line below* shows the effect of adding postsynaptic inhibition. There is almost perfect algebraic addition of both excitation and inhibition. (Reproduced with permission from Granit et al. 1966.)

neurons causes discharges within the primary range, and this level of firing is responsible for about 85% of total steady tension in muscle. The remaining 15% of steady tension is supplied by firing within the secondary range, but this range is more important for fast contractions at the initiation of movement. Not all motoneurons can maintain firing in the face of long-duration depolarization. Thus, some motoneurons innervating fast-twitch muscle fibres are generally incapable of generating long trains of impulses. During stepping, the firing rates of motoneurons are generally within the primary range. During scratching, however, although flexor motoneurons fire within this range, extensor motoneurons tend to fire at 100–300 Hz.

When a motoneuron is firing within its primary range, the full SD spike is followed by an after-hyperpolarization (AHP) that lasts some 30–100 ms (the longer duration AHPs being found in motoneurons innervating slow twitch muscles). This AHP follows the SD spike but not the IS spike (Fig. 9.5) and is therefore produced by the soma-dendritic membrane. The AHP is increased

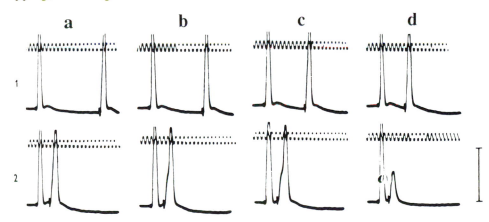

Fig. 9.5. After-hyperpolarization of motoneurons occurs only after a full SD spike. The records show pairs of antidromic action potentials at successively shorter intervals between the two. The first antidromic impulse in record *1a* can be seen to be followed by a short delayed depolarization which, in turn, is followed by an after-hyperpolarization. As the interval between the impulses becomes smaller the after-hyperpolarization increases. But when the SD spike fails, leaving only an IS spike (record *2d*) there is no after-hyperpolarization. (Reproduced with permission from Granit et al. 1963a.)

by depolarization of the motoneuron and reverses at a membrane potential of about -90 mV. It is due to an increased conductance to potassium ions. When two or more impulses occur at close intervals the AHPs show facilitation of both their voltage and conductance components and this has the effect of reducing the probability of further impulse discharge within a short time, i.e. the AHPs are responsible for controlling the frequency of discharge within the primary firing range. When a motoneuron is firing within its secondary range there is no, or very little, AHP. This observation has been interpreted to mean that in the secondary range there is a shrinking of the amount of soma-dendritic membrane involved towards the intitial segment. The analysis, however, is not complete, but the observations on abducens motoneurons referred to above indicate that a moving impulse initiation site is certainly a strong possibility.

The observations of algebraic summation between various combinations of firing produced by direct current injection, EPSPs and IPSPs have also not received a satisfactory explanation as to mechanism. What is important is that it is the steady levels of depolarization (or current) that summate and influence the firing rate. Thus any interaction between synaptic currents (shunting) that leads to non-linear addition of individual postsynaptic potentials is not of importance in this context. This is somewhat surprising as a powerful excitatory input would be expected to increase the input conductance of the cell and shunt the injected current. Likewise, shunting effects of IPSPs on injected current would also be expected. These shunting effects should alter the slopes of the current–frequency relation; however, as shown in Fig. 9.4, the slopes remain the same but move to the left or right.

Other Neurons

Neurons giving rise to long axons that form part of ascending tracts carrying sensory messages tend to behave somewhat differently from motoneurons. The neurons of the dorsal spinocerebellar tract (DSCT) have been carefully examined. This tract arises from cells in the spinal cord (in Clarke's column at the medial edge of the base of the dorsal horn in thoracic and upper lumbar segments) and projects, via the ipsilateral dorsolateral funiculus, to the cerebellar cortex, where the axons terminate as mossy fibres. These cells respond to injected current pulses with a high initial rate of firing that, like that of moto-

neurons, settles down (adapts) to a steady level with the rate linearly related to the strength of injected current. Unlike motoneurons, however, DSCT cells show only a primary range of firing and this extends up to firing rates of several hundred impulses a second (Fig. 9.6). DSCT cells have impulses with an IS-SD inflexion on their rising phase and also an AHP, but this AHP is much smaller and shorter-lasting than that of motoneurons. Thus, in contrast to motoneurons whose firing rates are held down to levels necessary for efficient muscle contraction, DSCT cells are capable of transmitting trains of impulses at high frequencies. There is a high safety factor for transmission between them and their monosynaptic excitatory input from primary afferent fibres of muscle spindles and cutaneous receptors.

Impulses in Dendrites

The ideas about impulse initiation in the spinal motoneuron, involving a single impulse-initiating zone and a passive dendritic tree, have been very influential. They have certainly provided a strong basis for further experimentation and also a largely satisfactory conceptual foundation for considering the individual neuron as an integrating device. But motoneurons, and neurons that behave like them, do not have an exclusive hold on mechanism. There is now a great deal of evidence showing that some neurons have more than one site for impulse initiation and have dendrites that contain electroresponsive membrane capable of generating all-or-nothing action potentials. In vertebrate species these cells include hippocampal pyramidal cells, cerebellar Purkinje cells and inferior olivary neurons. These three types of cells have certain advantages for experimental work (for the first two types the advantages include a most useful orientation and structure of their dendritic trees), but it should be assumed that many other types of neurons also can probably generate dendritic impulses. For the purposes of the present discussion the cerebellar Purkinje cell will be considered.

The vertebrate cerebellar cortex is a highly ordered structure with a modular design (see Chap. 13). The basic anatomical plan of the cerebellar cortex and the actions of the various neurons is described in Box 13.1. The Purkinje cell, which provides the sole output from the cerebellar cortex is, itself, an inhibitory neuron that projects to the cerebellar nuclei. The Purkinje cell dendritic tree is elaborately developed

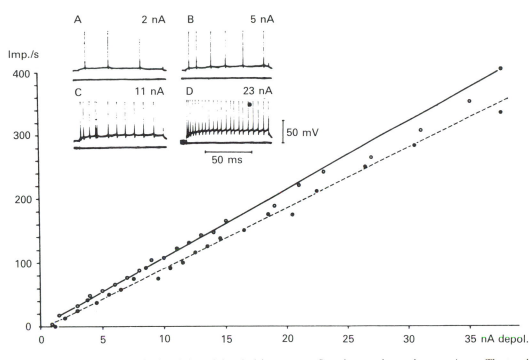

Fig. 9.6. Firing of a DSCT neuron (cat) to injected depolarizing current. Sample records are shown as *insets*. The two lines on the graph are plots of the mean frequencies during the entire current pulse (*open circles*) and for the period following the first 30 ms (*filled circles*). (Reproduced with permission from Eide et al. 1969.)

dorsal to the cell soma and is essentially restricted to a single plane, at right angles to which run the numerous parallel fibres that form excitatory synapses on the Purkinje cell dendrites. The other major excitatory input to the Purkinje cells is the climbing fibre input from the inferior olive. Each climbing fibre supplies a number of Purkinje cells (often a considerable distance apart) and winds around the dendritic tree making numerous contacts. Each Purkinje cell receives excitation from only one climbing fibre.

The most direct evidence for the presence of dendritic impulses in Purkinje cells comes from intradendritic recordings. In in vivo experiments in the alligator, Llínas and Nicholson recorded from presumed dendrites using electrodes filled with the fluorescent dye, procion yellow. Immediately after recording they injected the dye and then fixed the brain so that the dye would not diffuse far from the site of injection. Subsequent microscopical examination confirmed the intradendritic location of the recording electrode. More recently Llínas and Sugimori have worked with in vitro slices of guinea-pig cerebellum and impaled Purkinje cell dendrites under direct vision after injecting the cells with the dye, fast green. In both of these preparations direct evidence for all-or-nothing electroresponsiveness of dendritic

membranes has been observed (Fig. 9.7). In both species the dendritic impulses are large in amplitude (producing a reversal of the membrane potential) and long in duration compared with the impulses evoked at the initial segment. In both species antidromic action potentials set up by stimulation of the Purkinje cell axon do not invade the dendrites. A careful analysis in the alligator showed that dendritic impulses propagated toward the soma of the cell but did not propagate in the opposite direction and therefore did not spread outwards through the dendritic tree. Fig. 9.8 summarizes the probable events that occur in the alligator Purkinje cell with orthodromic and antidromic activation (the orthodromic activation due to parallel fibre firing) and also indicates a role for the inhibitory synapses that are located on the dendrites.

The functional implications of dendritic impulses in neurons such as the Purkinje cell include the possibility that local parts of the dendritic tree can act to integrate localized input in an independent manner. Thus integration in one dendritic branch can occur largely independently of what is happening in others, and the location of synaptic boutons on different parts of the dendritic tree becomes of fundamental importance (see Chap. 10).

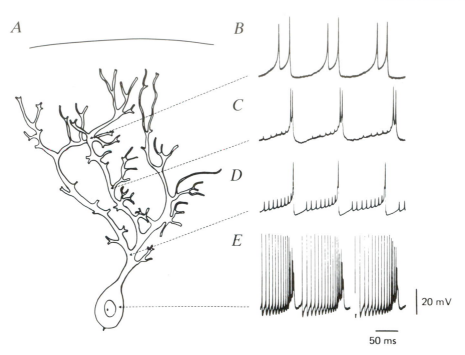

Fig. 9.7. Dendritic action potentials in guinea-pig cerebellar Purkinje cells in vitro. Records were obtained by impaling the cell at the various locations *B–E* and passing a depolarizing current through the microelectrode. When the electrode was in the remote portions of the dendritic tree (record *B*), long-duration calcium action potentials were produced. With intrasomatic recording (record *E*) high-frequency, short-duration sodium action potentials were produced, interrupted periodically by calcium action potentials. Note the passive spread of the sodium potentials into the dendritic tree (records *C*, *D*). (Reproduced with permission from Llínas and Sugimori 1980b.)

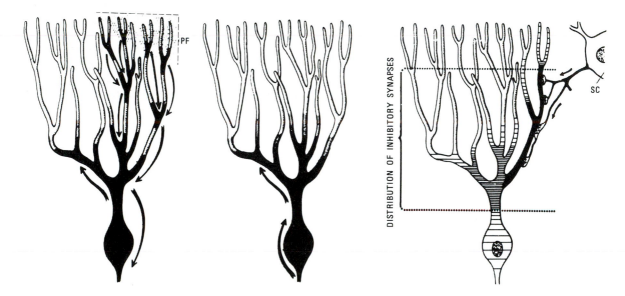

Fig. 9.8. Probable events occurring in a Purkinje cell following orthodromic and antidromic activation. Following orthodromic activation electroresponsive patches of dendrites generate action potentials (calcium spikes) that are conducted electrotonically to the next active patch of membrane and ultimately to the soma. There is little, if any, conduction of these potentials antidromically into the dendritic tree. Following antidromic activation the action potentials (sodium spikes) do not invade the dendritic tree to any great extent. Inhibitory input to the dendrites from stellate cells (*SC*) produces inhibition largely restricted to the sites of synaptic contact. (Reproduced with permission from Llínas and Nicholson 1971.)

The ionic conductances underlying the dendritic and somatic responses of Purkinje cells in the guinea-pig have been analysed by Llínas and Sugimori (1980a,b). They are remarkably complex. In the soma there are two sodium-dependent conductances, one responsible for the short duration action potential and another (non-inactivating) sodium conductance responsible for a plateau-like response. In the dendrites there are an impulse-generating calcium conductance and a plateau-generating calcium conductance brought into action by excitatory input from the climbing fibres. Furthermore, both voltage- and calcium-dependent potassium conductances were observed in these cells.

It is obvious that our concepts of the integrative properties of dendrites has changed quite drastically over the past few years. With the increasing use of various brain slice preparations (and spinal cord slices) it is also obvious that these concepts will change even more dramatically in the next few years. Dendritic membrane differs greatly from somatic, initial segment and axonal membrane. It is useful to visualize dendritic membrane as a mosaic of areas containing different concentrations of chemically gated and voltage-gated channels. At one extreme some dendrites will contain no, or very few, voltage-gated channels, whereas at the other extreme the concentration of voltage-gated channels might be very high.

Summary

1.   In the spinal alpha-motoneuron impulses are initiated at the initial segment of the axon (axon hillock region). Control of the membrane potential at this region is of prime importance for the regulation of impulse initiation.

2.   In spinal motoneurons trains of impulses may be set up by injecting ionic current into the cell. With relatively low currents the firing rate of the impulse trains depends on the strength of injected current – primary range of firing. There is a linear summation between the effects of injected current and of EPSPs and IPSPs. With stronger injected currents there is an abrupt shift of firing frequency into another, higher, linear range – the secondary range.

3.   In the primary firing range, which is responsible for about 85% of steady muscle tension, there is an after-hyperpolarization at the end of the action potential. This potential controls the frequency of discharge within the primary range. There is little or no after-hyperpolarization when the motoneuron is firing in its secondary range.

4.   Neurons belonging to ascending sensory pathways only show a primary range of firing, but this extends to several hundred impulses a second. These neurons are specialized for transmitting high rates of impulse firing.

5.   In many neurons action potentials may be generated in dendrites. Such dendrites have voltage-gated channels in their surface membranes. The ionic mechanism of dendritic action potentials is not necessarily the same as that in the axon of the same neuron. In neurons with dendritic action potentials there are additional opportunities for the individual nerve cell to act as a complex integrating unit.

10 The Neuron as an Integrative Device

Neuron Doctrine and the Law of Dynamic Polarization

Ramon y Cajal, the great Spanish neuroanatomist, enunciated the neuron doctrine at the end of the last century. This states that the nerve cell is the structural (cellular) and functional unit of the nervous system. From his doctrine he inferred the law of dynamic polarization, namely that all neurons are dynamically polarized such that excitation can only be transmitted from the axon of one neuron to the dendrites or soma of another, and, within a neuron, this excitation travels from the dendritic pole to the axonal pole. The doctrine and the law provided the basis for theories of the nervous system and was supported by the classic work of the British physiologist Sir Charles Sherrington. With the advent of electrophysiological techniques, especially their use by Eccles and his collaborators in the study of mammalian motoneurons, it seemed that these ideas were fully validated. Indeed, up to about 1960 the only major additions needed to the neuron doctrine and law of dynamic polarization were that inhibition occurred as a positive process (Sherrington's central inhibitory state) being carried out by a special set of inhibitory interneurons (a concept due essentially to Eccles) and that the nerve impulse originated, in central neurons, at the initial segment of the axon (again largely due to the evidence from Eccles's laboratory). The motoneuron became the standard neuron for ideas about how nervous systems operated. During the past 25 years or so, however, it has become increasingly apparent that these concepts need considerable modification, but it is convenient to begin a discussion of the neuron as an integrative device from a simplified point of view.

The Generalized Neuron Concept

A generalized neuron (see Bullock 1959; Bodian 1962) may be considered in which the neuronal membrane is made up of three distinct components: (1) a receptive component for input to the neuron either from other neurons or for sensory signals, with (2) an impulse-initiating and impulse-propagating component which sends the impulse to (3) a transmitter-releasing component (see Fig. 1.1). The diagrammatic representation of Fig. 1.1 indicates a common anatomical feature of all neurons – the receptive and transmitter-releasing components often have greatly increased surface areas. In the receptive component the membrane contains non-voltage sensitive ion channels that respond to either neurotransmitters or to sensory signals. Thus these ion channels might be chemically gated, thermally gated, mechanically gated etc., and the membrane in this component acts as a passive cable and transmits the voltage changes caused by ionic current flow due to the opening (or closing) of these channels. In the second component, that which initiates and propagates an all-or-nothing action potential, voltage-gated channels occur. In the third component, that which releases neurotransmitter, another set of voltage-gated channels are located. These are voltage-gated calcium channels responsible for the coupling of voltage changes to transmitter release. It will be noted that no mention is made of the cell body, or soma, which contains the nucleus of the cell and the sub-cellular apparatus necessary for protein synthesis etc. This is an important point. The membrane functions of the neuron and the trophic functions are separated in this model, and it is immaterial where in the cell the soma is located. It is a consequence of this functional conceptualization that there are no difficulties such as appear with anatomical conceptualizations: e.g. when is a structure to be called a dendrite?; is the axon of a sensory neuron (such as a dorsal root ganglion cell) really a dendrite? The essence of the scheme, therefore, is the organization of special membrane components in a neuron.

The Generalized Neuron as a Model for the Mammalian Motoneuron

Mammalian motoneurons are located either in the ventral horn of the spinal cord or in the various cranial nerve motor nuclei. They consist (see Figs. 1.1, 1.2) of a cell body or soma containing the nucleus, the endoplasmic reticulum and Golgi apparatus etc. From the soma a number of processes are given off. In spinal alpha-motoneurons there are about 7–18 dendrites that extend for about 1 mm from the soma, branching as they do so to give rise to up to about five or six orders of daughter branches (Fig. 10.1). Also from the soma, or sometimes from the initial part of a stem dendrite, an axon arises. The axon often gives off a few branches (axon collaterals) near the soma but ultimately leaves the central nervous system either via the ventral roots of the spinal cord or through one of the cranial nerves to run, in a peripheral nerve, to its target skeletal muscle, where it breaks up into branches that innervate the muscle at the neuromuscular junctions.

A first approximation of the generalized neuron concept applied to the motoneuron is shown in Fig. 1.1. The dendrites and soma form the receptive surface for input from other neurons and are studded with synapses. The impulse originates at the axon initial segment (axon hillock and first part of the axon) and propagates to the axon terminals, where transmitter is released. Consideration of the anatomy of the motoneuron, especially of where on its surface there are synaptic contacts, and also of the evidence of soma-dendritic invasion by the impulse discussed in the previous chapter, will lead to the realization that the above description is an oversimplification. If the impulse can invade the soma and the basal dendritic tree there must be voltage-gated

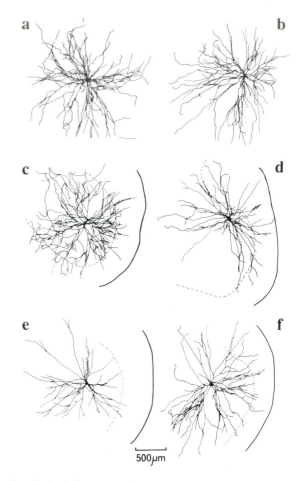

Fig. 10.1a–f. Reconstructions of lumbosacral alpha-motoneurons from the cat following intracellular injection with horseradish peroxidase. **a,b** are reconstructed from serial sagittal sections and **c–f** from serial transverse sections. In **c–f** the surface of the spinal cord is shown as a *thick solid line* and the border of the ventral horn by a *dashed line*. Note the numerous dendrites in the white matter. The initial few hundred micrometres of the axons are indicated by *broken lines*. (Reproduced with permission from Brown and Fyffe 1981a.)

channels in this part of the membrane in addition to the chemically gated ones. Furthermore, the location of synaptic terminals on the axon hillock and initial part of the axon (Figs. 10.2, 10.3) indicate that chemically gated channels should be found here as well as the voltage-gated ones. Thus, a more satisfactory concept is to consider the neuronal membrane to be made up of a mosaic of channels with gradients of concentration such that the dendrites (that do not support an action potential) contain a high concentration of chemically gated channels but few voltage-gated ones, whereas at the initial segment there is a high concentration of voltage-gated channels (since this component of the membrane has the

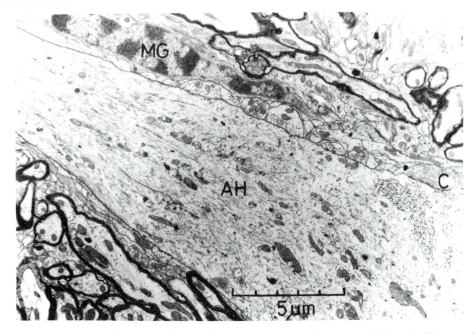

Fig. 10.2. Electron micrograph of the axon hillock region of a motoneuron in the cat spinal cord. The axon hillock (*AH*) receives contacts from several synaptic boutons (one labelled *C*). *MG*, dark glial cell. (Reproduced with permission from Conradi 1969.)

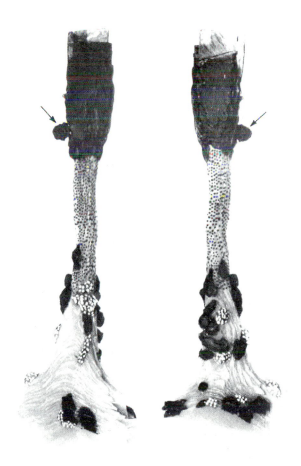

lowest threshold for the initiation of an impulse) but there are still a considerable number of chemically gated channels.

In some respects the generalized neuron is not a satisfactory model for the motoneuron. Or, perhaps more usefully, it should be stated that the motoneuron does not fit the generalized model too closely, since the motoneuron is highly specialized for its function of controlling muscle contraction. If we consider how the above motoneuronal model might need modification in order to provide a general model for other neurons, we find that many neurons have an additional receptive surface on their axon terminals where neuronal control of transmitter release takes place. In these instances the axonal terminals contain chemically gated channels that respond to transmitter released from synapses on the terminals, and voltage-gated calcium channels responsible for excitation–secretion coupling.

If, for the time being, we consider the generalized neuron to be a reasonable concept, then we

Fig. 10.3. Two views of a wax model of the axon hillock (*not painted*) and the initial segment (*stippled*) of a motoneuron. The cell body is at the bottom. The location of synaptic boutons is shown: the F boutons containing flattened vesicles and thought to be inhibitory are in *black*, and the S boutons containing spherical vesicles and thought to be excitatory are *stippled*. (Reproduced with permission from Conradi 1969.)

can conclude that all synaptic boutons ending on a neuron arise from axons. Since boutons may make contact with dendrites, soma, initial segment or axon terminal (the fine terminal part of the axon as well as the synaptic boutons it carries), all synapses may be classed as axo-dendritic, axo-somatic or axo-axonic (it is a matter of preference whether one calls a synapse on the initial segment axo-somatic or axo-axonic). We shall see later that the presynaptic component is not necessarily axonic in origin and that the law of dynamic polarization is no longer valid for all neuronal circuits.

Importance of Synaptic Location

The location of synapses on a neuron is of great importance. This importance is not limited to neurons with only a single site of impulse initiation but is also vital in neurons with more than one site of impulse initiation (those with dendritic action potentials, for example) and, as we shall see, also for those neurons that have presynaptic dendrites. Again it is convenient to consider the mammalian motoneuron first because it is, in many respects, simpler than other neurons and also because there is more experimental data for this type of neuron than for most others.

Excitatory Synaptic Location on Motoneurons

Mammalian motoneurons receive direct excitatory synaptic connexions (monosynaptic connexions) from sensory fibres (Group Ia fibres) that innervate the annulospiral endings of the muscle spindle stretch receptors. Transmission between these two neurons is considered in more detail in Chapter 11. Here it is sufficient to note that a single Ia afferent fibre makes only between one and about ten synaptic contacts with its target motoneuron, with most making less than six contacts, and with the vast majority of contacts being made on the motoneuronal dendrites and with very few on the soma. A single action potential in a single Ia afferent fibre leads to a small excitatory postsynaptic potential (EPSP), with an amplitude ranging from about 100 μV to a millivolt or so. The size of this monosynaptic Ia EPSP is never sufficient to elicit an action potential in the motoneuron. In order for a Ia input to fire a motoneuron there has to be either simultaneous activity in a number of Ia fibres, probably

at least about 20, so that their individual EPSPs can sum over the dendritic membrane in space (spatial summation) to reach firing level at the initial segment, or there has to be summation of EPSPs over time (temporal summation) due to individual Ia fibres carrying a train of impulses.

Detailed electrophysiological analysis of single-fibre Ia EPSPs in mammalian motoneurons, together with direct observations of the contacts made between Ia axons and motoneurons by injecting both the axon and the motoneuron with horseradish peroxidase, have shown that the synaptic contacts are made at various distances out on the dendrites (up to about halfway along the dendritic tree) and with a few on the cell soma. In most examples studied so far there has been a tendency for all the synapses from a single Ia axon to be located fairly close together, often on a single dendrite or its branches (see Fig. 11.6).

Because the motoneuronal impulse is elicited at the initial segment and since the dendritic and soma membrane has resistance and capacitance and therefore acts like an electric cable (see Chap. 2), those EPSPs set up nearest to the initial segment should be both larger in amplitude and also shorter in duration (with a faster rise time and shorter decay time) than those set up more distally). The underlying assumptions necessary for this to happen are that activity at each synapse injects the same amount of current into the motoneuron and that the motoneuronal dendritic membrane has the same resistance and capacitance throughout its extent. Since individual Ia afferent fibres make different numbers of contacts with different motoneurons it should also be necessary that there is no systematic correlation between the numbers of boutons and their location on the motoneuron (for example, there should not be more contacts if they are made distally on the dendrites).

Examination of single-fibre Ia EPSPs in motoneurons (see Fig. 11.10) shows that they vary both in amplitude and also in duration. Furthermore, those with a fast rise time also have a fast decay time, as shown by plotting the half-width (duration at half maximal amplitude) against their rise times (see Fig. 11.8). These results are as predicted from cable theory and show that synapses located distally on the dendrites produce EPSPs that have slower rise and decay times and therefore longer durations than those located nearer, or on, the soma. (This analysis also assumes that the intracellular recording micro-electrode is located in the soma, or possibly in a basal dendrite. This is a reasonable assumption, since the soma provides the largest target for the microelectrode. Also, such a location for the microelectrode means that what the microelectrode "sees" in terms of synaptic activity is very similar to what the initial segment "sees".) Since the excitatory input to the motoneuron is integrated at the initial segment, an EPSP elicited by synaptic activity close to the initial segment will cause a briefer effect than one elicited far out on a dendrite. EPSPs with a distal origin will have a far more long-lasting effect at the initial segment and could be responsible for fine tuning of the membrane potential at the impulse-initiating zone.

As described in Chapter 11, a single Ia fibre can produce EPSPs with quite different shapes in different motoneurons, which suggests that a single Ia afferent fibre distributes its input to different motoneurons in different ways and that it does not always have synaptic boutons limited to the same part of the motoneuronal receptive surface. Single-fibre EPSPs elicited from two different Ia afferent fibres may not add linearly when evoked simultaneously, even though their shapes are quite different. Different EPSP shapes indicate a different localization for the respective synapses. Such observations suggest that some of the individual synaptic sites from each afferent fibre are located close together and that there is shunting of ionic current between the synapses so that the synaptic potential is less than expected. More unexpected has been the observation that single-fibre EPSPs with slow rise and decay times, indicative of a distal synaptic location, often have maximal amplitudes greater than expected. This observation leads to questioning of the assumptions that (1) activity of any Ia synapse, wherever its location, always injects the same current into the motoneuron; (2) a single Ia afferent does not have more synapses on a motoneuron if they are located distally; and (3) the dendritic membrane is the same throughout its extent. Direct observation has provided no support for any anatomical differences in distally located synapses (such as different bouton size or more synapses from single Ia fibres if distally located), and it may be that the compensating mechanism resides in the dendritic membrane. It is of interest that a similar observation of larger than expected EPSP amplitudes for distally elicited EPSPs has been observed in pyramidal cells of the hippocampus. Whatever the mechanism that produces this effect may be, operationally it means that synapses located even very far out on a dendrite can have a significant action at the level of the initial segment.

Inhibitory Synapses

The location of inhibitory synapses on neurons is, if anything, even more critical than the location of excitatory synapses. In those neurons in which impulses arise at the initial segment of the axon it is obvious that a preferential location of inhibitory synapses at this site would be very powerful indeed in preventing the setting up of impulses. It is a common anatomical observation that inhibitory synapses are concentrated on the axon hillock and initial part of the axon in very many different types of neurons (Figs. 10.3, 10.4). Inhibitory synaptic action at or near the locus of impulse initiation can prevent impulses in two ways:

1. The inhibitory postsynaptic potential (IPSP) holds the potential at the impulse initiation site below threshold for an action potential.
2. More importantly, by increasing the conductance of the membrane it short-circuits the EPSP and also reduces the space constant of the membrane, thus cutting down the spread of EPSPs along the membrane.

Inhibitory synapses are not exclusively located at and near the axon hillock but occur, as far as is known, on all parts of a neuron, even on distal dendrites. Wherever they occur they will affect the membrane in the same two ways, as described above. Thus they can, locally, decrease or nullify the effects of excitatory inputs within their area of influence and prevent excitatory actions influencing the impulse-initiation zone. Where there are highly organized excitatory inputs to particular dendrites of a neuron, a strategically placed set of inhibitory synapses (for example more proximally on the dendrites) can selectively inhibit the effects of these excitatory inputs. In neurons that have dendrites capable of supporting all-or-nothing action potentials such selective location of inhibitory synapses can prevent the setting up of such dendritic impulses or, if located on the base of a dendrite, can prevent the impulse invading the initial segment region where the neuron's "output impulse" is initiated.

Consequences of Synaptic Location Specificity

In addition to the functional effects of synaptic location outlined above there are other consequences of selective location of synapses. In order that these sorts of functional effects can occur

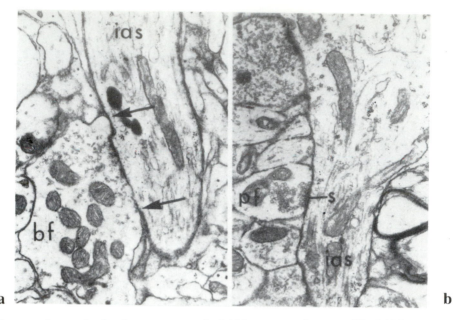

Fig. 10.4a,b. Electron micrographs showing synapses on the initial segments of axons. **a** The initial segment of a cerebellar Purkinje cell (*ias*). It receives a symmetrical (Gray type II) synapse from a basket fibre (*bf*). **b** The initial segment (*ias*) of a basket cell receives an asymmetrical (Gray type I) synapse from a parallel fibre (*s*). (Reproduced with permission from Mugnaini 1970.)

there must be great precision in the way neurons are connected to one another; particular neurons must be connected to other particular neurons and in a highly precise fashion in terms of the numbers and locations of the synapses. Many instances of such precision can be found: for example the Mauthner cell in teleost fishes, cerebellar Purkinje cells and, perhaps one of the most striking of all, the organization of synaptic inputs to the large pyramidal cells of the cerebral cortex, especially those of the hippocampus (Fig. 10.5). Other consequences follow from these observations in the adult nervous system. Thus, during development the appropriate synapses must be formed on the appropriate postsynaptic membrane between the appropriate neurons. Very little is known about how such precise "wiring" comes about.

Dendritic Spines

A further specialization of the receptive surface of some neurons (on dendritic and somatic membranes but much more common on dendrites) is the development of spines. These are evaginations of the surface membrane forming a sack-like protrusion, often with a narrow neck and enlarged head (Fig. 10.6). Such dendritic spines tend to form during the early life of the organism, often at the times of most rapid learning, and become reduced in number in old age and also after experimental loss of input to the neurons on which they occur. The spines are postsynaptic to boutons; often there are excitatory synapses on the spine head and inhibitory synapses on the neck. The role(s) of dendritic spines is (are) not clear, although there have been many hypotheses that they have a part to play in memory and learning mechanisms. The neck of the spine provides a very high resistance path between the spine head and the dendritic shaft, and current injection (excitatory action) at the head should produce a large potential change (EPSP) in the head itself but a reduction in the amount of synaptic current injected into the dendritic shaft. The membrane of the spine head is also relatively well isolated from the rest of the dendrite by this high resistance neck so that synaptic actions on the spine are protected from events occurring elsewhere in the neuron. The location of inhibitory synapses on the neck of the spine provides evidence that the excitatory input from the spine head may be selectively cut off. It is highly likely that the dendritic spines provide another, largely mysterious, way in which integrative functions can be carried out by single neurons.

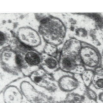

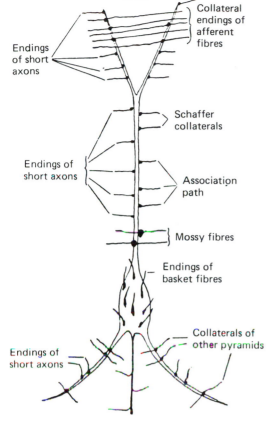

Fig. 10.5. Differential distribution of axon terminals on a pyramidal cell of the hippocampus. (Reproduced from Lorenté de Nó 1934.)

Dendrodendritic Interactions

All of the discussion in this chapter so far has been in terms of Ramon y Cajal's law of dynamic polarization. But it has become apparent that this "law" no longer holds for all neuronal interactions. In many parts of the vertebrate nervous system dendrites may form synapses with other dendrites with one, or both, dendrites being presynaptic to the other (Fig. 10.7). Here we have the possibility for local interactions. Thus, the dendritic tree is not solely a receptive surface for input but may, in addition, be an output membrane akin to axon terminal membrane. Study of these dendrodendritic interactions has also shown that impulse activity is not necessary for transmitter release since many dendrites release transmitter without having the ability to generate action potentials.

One of the best known examples of dendrodendritic interactions occurs in the olfactory bulb

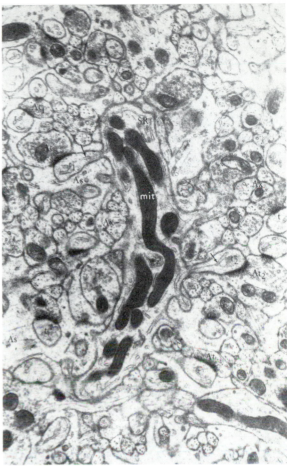

Fig. 10.6. Dendritic spines on a Purkinje cell. Extending down the middle of this electron micrograph is a spiny branchlet of a Purkinje cell, containing mitochondria (*mit*) and cisternae of the smooth endoplasmic reticulum (*SR*). Two spines (t_1 and t_2) emerge from the dendrite and form asymmetrical synapses with the axon terminals (*At*) of parallel fibres (*Ax*). *As*, processes of Golgi epithelial cells. (Reproduced with permission from Peters et al. 1976.)

(Fig. 10.8). In the olfactory bulb primary sensory afferent fibres from the olfactory mucosa make monosynaptic excitatory connexions with the mitral cells at a complex synaptic structure called a glomerulus. The glomerulus (Fig. 10.8) consists of the specialized dendrites of the mitral cell (dendritic tufts at the distal extremities of the mitral cell apical dendrite), the axon terminals of the olfactory nerves and the dendrites of a small cell in the olfactory bulb, the periglomerular cell. The olfactory nerve makes excitatory synapses with the periglomerular cell as well as with the mitral cell. There are dendrodendritic synapses between the dendrites of the mitral and periglomerular cell. The mitral cell has a further set

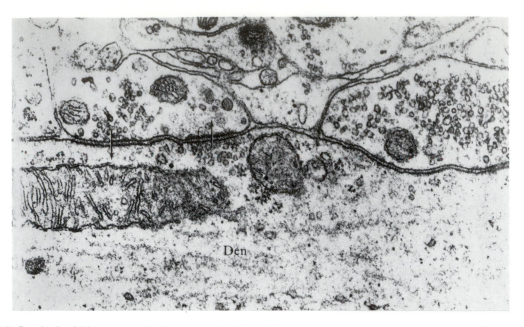

Fig. 10.7. Dendrodendritic synapses. In the lower half of this electron micrograph is the secondary dendrite (*Den*) of a mitral cell of the olfactory bulb. It forms a synapse with a gemmule (*gem*) protruding from a granule cell dendrite. At the synaptic junction there are two synaptic complexes with different polarities, as indicated by the *arrows* and as deduced from the accumulation of synaptic vesicles on the presynaptic side of each complex. There is also a postsynaptic thickening (*f*) at one synapse. (Reproduced with permission from Peters et al. 1976.)

of dendrites, the basal dendrites, which do not take part in the glomeruli but which form dendro-dendritic synapses with the dendritic spines of another cell, the granule cell, which has no axon and is incapable of generating impulses. The

mitral cell has an axon that arises from an axon hillock and projects away from the olfactory bulb to the cerebral cortex. The mitral cell axon gives off collaterals that terminate on cells of the anterior olfactory nucleus and these cells project

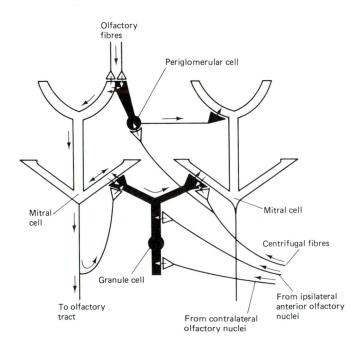

Fig. 10.8. The organization of the mammalian olfactory bulb. Olfactory axons from sensory receptor cells in the olfactory mucosa terminate in a layer of approximately spherical structures called glomeruli, where they make excitatory synaptic contacts with the dendrites of mitral and periglomerular cells. There are reciprocal dendrodendritic synapses between the periglomerular and mitral cells in the glomeruli. There are also reciprocal dendrodendritic synapses between the mitral cell and another cell, the granule cell. For further description see the text. The *arrows* indicate the direction of neural information flow. (Modified from Shepherd 1972.)

to dendritic spines of the granule cell dendrite close to the dendrodendritic synapses with the mitral cell.

The operation of this small group of neurons appears to be as follows. Input along the olfactory nerves produces an EPSP in the mitral cell dendritic tufts which has two actions:

1. It spreads passively to the initial segment of the mitral cell axon and generates an impulse.
2. It activates the dendrodendritic synapse with the periglomerular cell and causes an EPSP in that cell.

Both the mitral cell impulse and the EPSP in the periglomerular cell also have dual functions. The mitral cell impulse (1) propagates to the cortex and excites its target neurons, and (2) excites the granule cell, either directly or via the anterior olfactory nucleus, causing it to inhibit the mitral cell, in a negative feed-back fashion, via its dendrodendritic synapses. The EPSP in the periglomerular cell (1) excites the cell and causes it to initiate an impulse at its axon initial segment, and (2) activates the reciprocal dendrodendritic inhibitory synapse with the mitral cell dendritic tuft. The impulse in the periglomerular cell propagates to the target cells of the periglomerular cells and, in addition, may propagate back to the dendrites and reinforce the inhibitory action on the mitral cell. Thus, there are a series of negative feed-back pathways controlling the firing of the mitral cells. The dendrodendritic reciprocal synapses (both sets of dendrites are pre- and postsynaptic to one another) provide the most compact synaptic circuitry that exists, and the flow of information, from dendrite to dendrite, is against the law of dynamic polarization.

Summary

1. It is convenient to consider a neuron's membrane as consisting of three components: a receptive component, an impulse-initiating and impulse-propagating component and a transmitter-releasing component. Each of these components contains characteristic ion channels. In real neurons these components are not restricted to particular anatomical parts of the cell but intermingle with each other.

2. The location of a synapse on a neuron is of great importance. The closer a synapse is to the impulse-initiating zone the greater is its effect on neuronal firing. Strategically placed inhibitory synapses can nullify particular inputs or prevent neuronal firing. The synaptic connexions to many neurons are very precisely organized.

3. The flow of activity through many neurons is not unidirectional. Dendrodendritic interactions allow for bidirectional influences. Some small neurons do not have axons and do not have the ability to initiate all-or-nothing impulses.

11 Transmission Between Identified Pairs of Neurons

In the previous two chapters the initiation of impulses and the importance of synaptic location were discussed. The present chapter will be concerned with transmission between identified pairs of neurons and will put the previous discussion in the context of normal function. The examples to be considered have been chosen from the mammalian nervous system. This may seem strange to those readers who consider that working with identified neurons is a specialty confined to research on the invertebrate nervous system, where individual neurons may be recognized in living preparations and examined in different members of the same species or, in the case of neurons in ganglia, in different ganglia in the same animal. In vertebrates, identification of neurons is usually in terms of the type of neuron, e.g. motoneurons, and the identification is carried out by a variety of means such as a careful examination of the inputs to the cell, stimulation of the axon terminals of the cell at known sites of projection and the recognition of an antidromic action potential recorded at the cell body, and intracellular staining of the neuron with subsequent histological verification of the cell type and location. With techniques such as this it is perfectly possible to make a rigorous identification of the type of neuron, and indeed this approach is now a most important element in many experiments, both in vivo and also in preparations where slices of nervous tissue are studied in vitro.

Transmission Between Ia Afferent Fibres from Muscle Spindles and Spinal Motoneurons

A well-known spinal reflex (see Chap. 13 for a discussion of reflexes) is the knee-jerk. The knee-jerk is one of a set of reflexes much used by the neurologist to assess motor function. To elicit these reflexes a sharp tap is given to a tendon of a muscle, with the patient and the muscle relaxed, whereupon the muscle reacts with a very brief contraction – the muscle or tendon jerk. Muscle jerks are of use to the physician but not to the patient: absence of the reflexes indicates damage to either peripheral nerves or to the spinal cord, whereas exaggerated reflexes indicate damage to motor systems of the brain. However, the reflexes are produced by activity in a neural circuit that under physiological conditions produces reflex action of use to the organism in posture and locomotion. Such reflex action is the stretch reflex or myotatic reflex.

Stretch reflexes were studied in great detail by Sherrington in the early part of this century in cats and dogs in which the front part of the brain had been removed by decerebration. In these preparations stretch reflexes are greatly exaggerated (in antigravity muscles), and stretch of a

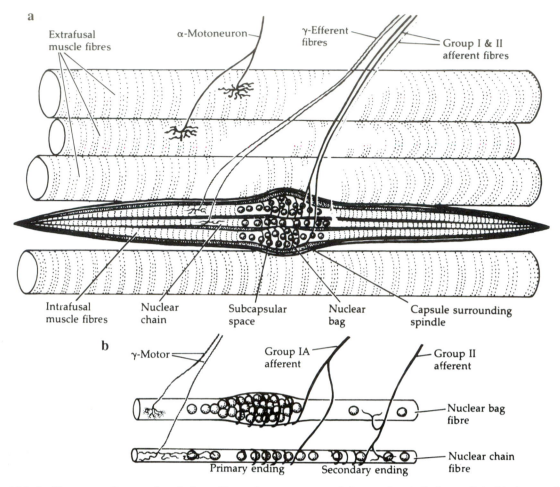

Fig. 11.1a,b. The mammalian muscle spindle. **a** Shows the arrangement of the muscle spindle in parallel with the extrafusal muscle fibres. The spindle is innervated by Group Ia and Group II afferent nerve fibres and by the axons of gamma-motoneurons (efferent fibres). **b** Shows a simplified diagram of the different intrafusal (spindle) fibres and their innervation. (Reproduced with permission from Kuffler et al. 1984, after Matthews 1964 (**b**).)

muscle elicits a reflex contraction of the same muscle and its synergists. This is the stretch reflex (at the same time there is an active inhibition of motoneurons that innervate the antagonist muscles about the same joint). Since the early experiments of Sherrington detailed knowledge of the structural and functional aspects of the stretch reflex has been built up and it is one of the most intensely studied components of nervous action.

The reflex circuit underlying the stretch reflex is indicated in Fig. 8.5. Stretch of the muscle activates mechanoreceptors in the receptor organs known as muscle spindles, which are contained within the body of the muscle. Muscle spindles are extremely complex organs (Fig. 11.1) containing two types of mechanoreceptors – the primary or annulospiral endings and the secondary or flower-spray endings – as well as modified striated muscle fibres that are under the control of small (gamma) motoneurons in the spinal cord. The two types of sensory receptors are innervated by separate afferent nerve fibres – the primary or Group Ia afferent fibres and the secondary or Group II afferent fibres respectively. Group Ia afferent fibres are the largest in peripheral nerve, having diameters of 12–20 μm and therefore have the fastest conduction velocities of all fibres – up to 120 m/s in the cat. Group II fibres are smaller (4–12 μm) and conduct slower (24–72 m/s). Both the primary and secondary endings are sensitive to the degree of stretch of the muscle, and the primary endings, in addition, are sensitive to the rate of stretch (Fig. 11.2). It is convenient to consider the stretch reflex as being due to activity in the primary afferent fibres,

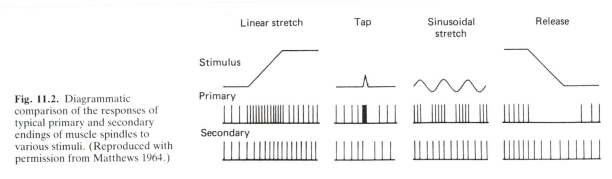

Fig. 11.2. Diagrammatic comparison of the responses of typical primary and secondary endings of muscle spindles to various stimuli. (Reproduced with permission from Matthews 1964.)

although, as we shall see (Chap. 13), a contribution from the secondary afferents is also made. Furthermore, both the whole of the muscle jerk and also the initial parts of the stretch reflex are due to firing of the large (alpha) motoneurons that innervate the muscle fibres (extrafusal fibres) brought about by direct connexions between the primary afferent fibres and the motoneurons. In other words, the stretch reflex is an example of a monosynaptic reflex, and no interneurons are intercalated between the primary afferent fibres and the motoneurons. Some more information about the muscle spindle as a sensory receptor and the control of its sensitivity by the central nervous system are given in Chapter 12, and details of the role of the stretch reflex and also the control of motoneuron output are given in Chapter 13. Here the transmission between the Ia afferent

fibres and the motoneurons with which they make synaptic contact will be discussed. In order to understand this it is necessary to know something of the anatomy of the system as well as the physiology.

Anatomy of the Ia – Alphamotoneuron System

Motoneurons

Spinal motoneurons are located in the ventral horn of the spinal cord, each set of motoneurons that innervates a particular muscle being aggregated in longitudinally running columns of cells, the motor nuclei (Fig. 11.3). Their cell bodies are amongst the largest in the central nervous system, being 30–70 µm in diameter with a sur-

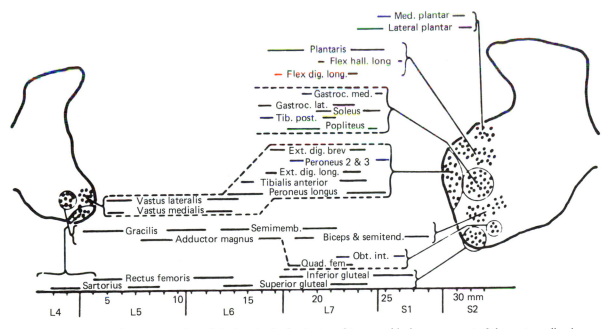

Fig. 11.3. Diagrammatic representation of the longitudinal extents and topographical arrangement of the motor cell columns in the lumbosacral spinal cord of the cat. The segmental levels are indicated at the *bottom* of the figure and the extents of cell columns for each muscle are shown *above*. (Reproduced with permission from Romanes 1951.)

face area of some $10^{-5}-10^{-3}$ cm^2. In addition to a large cell body, motoneurons also have very extensive dendritic trees (see Fig. 10.1). The true extent of the dendritic trees has only recently been realized with the advent of the technique of intracellular staining with the enzyme horse-radish peroxidase (HRP). In this technique a microelectrode filled with a solution containing the enzyme in inserted into the neuron. The microelectrode may be used for standard electrophysiological recording and then, by either passing current through the microelectrode or by applying pressure to it, the HRP is injected into the neuron. Subsequent histochemical reactions generate a reaction product that allows the full dendritic extent of the neuron to be visualized. Furthermore, the reaction product is electrondense, and stained neuronal profiles may therefore be examined with the electron microscope. In the lumbosacral spinal cord of the cat each alpha-motoneuron has between 7 and 18 dendrites originating from the cell body (mean about 11) and these divide and subdivide a number of times producing the extensive dendritic tree. The total dendritic lengths of these neurons is of the order of 100 000 μm (i.e. 100 mm!) and their total dendritic area about 500 000 μm^2.

Ia Afferent Fibres

The anatomy of Ia afferent fibres from muscle spindle primary receptors has been determined by injecting HRP into the axons just after they have entered the spinal cord through the dorsal roots. After entering the cord the axons usually bifurcate into a caudally and a rostrally running branch, and each branch gives off a number of collateral branches at intervals of 100 to about 2500 μm, with a mean spacing of about 1 mm. Each collateral runs ventrally through the grey matter of the spinal cord and produces three main areas of terminal arborization (in the vicinity of the entry of the Ia afferent into the cord) (Fig. 11.4). The deepest of these arborizations is in the region of the motor nuclei and it is here that contacts with motoneurons are made. It is worth noting at this point that intra-axonal HRP injection experiments, in which the various types of primary afferent fibre (from skin and muscle), each innervating different types of sense organs, have been studied, have demonstrated unequivocally that each type gives rise to a specific branching pattern of collateral axons and areas of termination in the spinal cord.

Ia Afferent Contacts upon Motoneurons

By combining intra-axonal staining of Ia afferent fibres with either counterstaining of motoneuronal cell bodies or with intracellular staining of motoneurons, Brown and Fyffe (1981a) were able to reveal the numbers and distribution of Ia synapses on motoneurons. Only a minority of Ia synaptic boutons located within the motor nuclei are in contact with motoneuronal cell bodies (Fig. 11.5). Brown and Fyffe calculated that about 10% of Ia synapses were on the motoneuronal somata. When both the Ia afferents and motoneurons were stained with HRP it was possible to determine the organization of boutons located on the motoneuronal dendrites (Fig. 11.6). Again, there were relatively few contacts between an individual Ia afferent fibre and a single motoneuron – about three to four on the average – and most contacts were located within about 600 μm of the cell's soma, i.e. on the proximal geometrical half of the dendritic tree, and tended to be clustered together.

When all the anatomical observations are considered together with electrophysiological results about the percentage of motoneurons in which responses (excitatory postsynaptic potentials; EPSPs) can be recorded upon stimulating single Ia afferent fibres, the following conclusions can be drawn for the medium to large muscles of the cat's hind limb:

1. Most Ia afferent fibres give less than six boutons to a single motoneuron; on the average about three to four.

2. Each Ia afferent fibre has between 1000 and 2000 boutons in contact with motoneurons.

3. Each motoneuron receives between about 200 and 450 boutons from Ia afferent fibres that innervate spindles in both the muscle that the motoneuron innervates and synergistic muscles.

With this anatomical baseline in mind it is now possible to consider the physiological aspects of transmission in the system.

Actions of Ia Afferent Fibres on Motoneurons

Activity in afferent fibres from the primary endings in muscle spindles leads to the production of a depolarizing potential (the monosynaptic EPSP) in the motoneurons that innervate the same muscle as contains the muscle spindles and

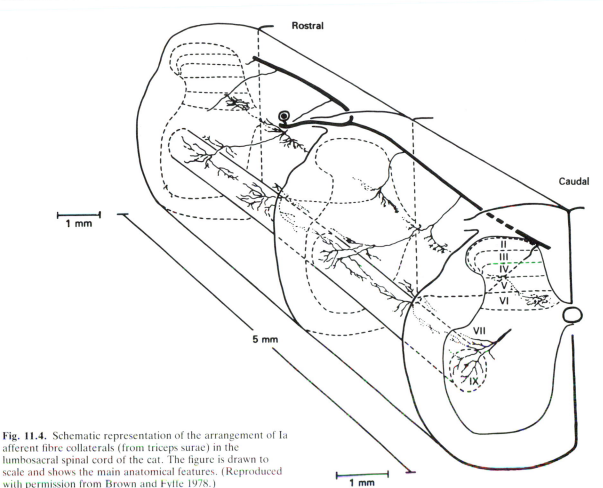

Rostral

Caudal

1 mm

5 mm

II
III
IV
V
VI
VII
IX

1 mm

Fig. 11.4. Schematic representation of the arrangement of Ia afferent fibre collaterals (from triceps surae) in the lumbosacral spinal cord of the cat. The figure is drawn to scale and shows the main anatomical features. (Reproduced with permission from Brown and Fyffe 1978.)

also in motoneurons that innervate synergistic muscles. These Ia EPSPs are made up of a hierarchy of components:

1. *Composite EPSP*, produced by impulses arriving more or less synchronously in two or more afferent fibres. It may be produced by electrical stimulation of muscle nerves or by sudden stretch of the muscle.

2. *Single-fibre EPSP*, produced by activity in a single Ia afferent fibre.

3. *Single terminal EPSP*, produced by transmitter release from a single Ia terminal (i.e. at a single synapse).

4. *Quantal EPSP*, produced by liberation of a single quantum (package) of transmitter by analogy with quantal release at the neuromuscular junction.

It should be realized that this hierarchy is, in part, theoretical. Only the first two categories have been demonstrated unequivocally.

The composite EPSP was the first to be studied (especially by Eccles and his colleagues). The original observations indicated that the composite EPSP, evoked by electrical stimulation of muscle nerves near threshold so that only the Ia fibres were activated, rose to a maximum within about 1 ms of onset and then decayed with a time course longer than that of the single exponential time course expected from measurements of the membrane time constant (Fig. 11.7; see also Fig. 8.6). It was suggested that this was due to some sort of delayed transmitter action, but it is now known that the delayed decay is due to synaptic actions on (electrically) distant dendrites. Early observations also indicated that individual composite EPSPs could summate linearly with one another, suggesting that the active synaptic sites were far enough apart from each other to reduce any interaction to a minimum (no short-circuiting of synaptic current), but more recent studies have shown that some composite EPSPs may add non-linearly, suggesting that synaptic sites are

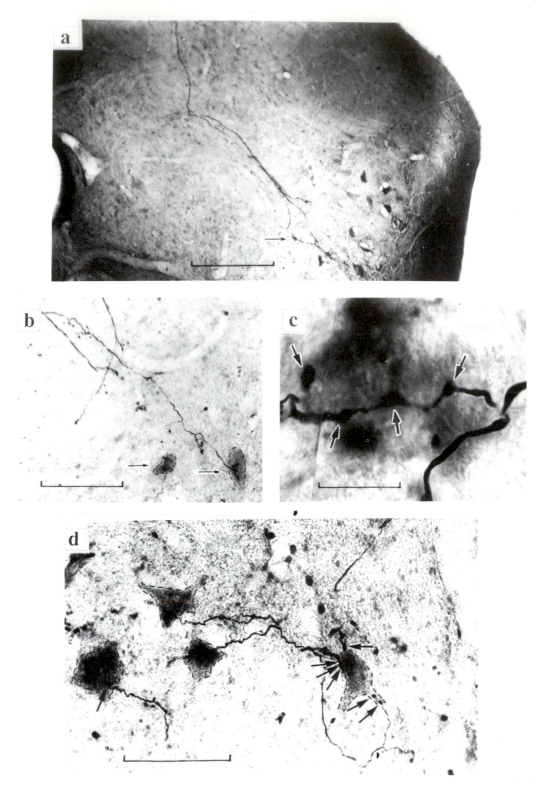

Fig. 11.5a–d. Photomicrographs from 100 μm transverse sections of HRP-stained Ia afferent fibre collaterals terminating on counterstained motoneurons. **a** Low-power view showing a collateral running to the motor nuclei. **b–d** Synaptic boutons on motoneuronal somata and proximal dendrites. The *arrows* in **c** and **d** indicate sites of contact. (Reproduced with permission from Brown and Fyffe 1981a.)

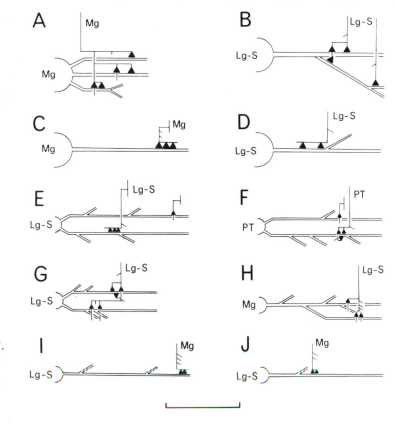

Fig. 11.6. Diagram of the locations of Ia synapses on the dendrites of motoneurons. The motoneurons and Ia fibres are identified: *Mg*, medial gastrocnemius; *Lg-S*, lateral gastrocnemius-soleus; *PT*, posterior tibial. The scale bar represents 50 μm in diagrams *A* and *B* and 500 μm in diagrams *C–J*. (Reproduced with permission from Brown and Fyffe 1981a.)

located close enough together (in electronic terms) to allow interaction of conductances, and therefore voltage, changes.

Studies of single-fibre EPSPs have been of special importance in showing that Ia synapses are distributed on motoneuronal surfaces from proximal to distal sites. Single-fibre EPSPs can be set up by carefully dissecting away most of the fibres in a peripheral nerve, or dorsal root, until only one functioning Ia fibre remains. This can then be excited either by stretching the muscle it innervates or by electrical stimulation of the nerve. Alternatively, the activity of a single Ia fibre, recorded from a slip of nerve or dorsal root, can be used to trigger an averaging device that sums the EPSPs evoked by it in a time-locked fashion (spike-triggered averaging). Single-fibre Ia EPSPs range from those with fast rise times and fast decays (indicative of proximal synaptic location) to those with slow rise times and long

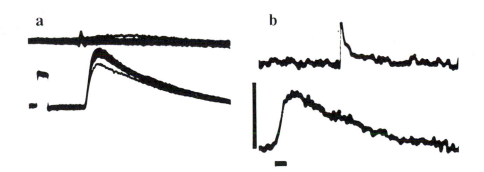

Fig. 11.7a,b. Composite and single-fibre EPSPs in a motoneuron. **a** Shows a composite EPSP in a plantaris motoneuron evoked by electrical stimulation of the plantaris nerve. Calibration pulse 5 mV and 1 ms. **b** Shows two single-fibre Ia EPSPs recorded from the same plantaris motoneuron. Note the wide difference in time course between the two examples. Calibration 1 mV, 1 ms. (Reproduced with permission from Burke 1967.)

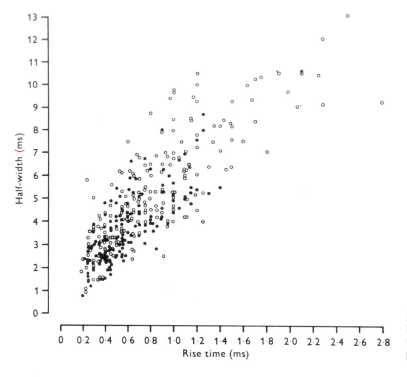

Fig. 11.8. Relationships between the half-widths of single-fibre Ia EPSPs and their rise times. (Reproduced with permission from Jack et al. 1971.)

decay times (indicative of distal locations), as shown for single-fibre EPSPs (Fig. 11.7). The data in Fig. 11.8 are plotted as half-width (duration at half maximal amplitude) against rise time, which demonstrates the positive correlation between these two variables and the wide range of values. Both of these findings suggest that the Ia synapses are found at various spatial locations on the motoneurons.

A single Ia fibre can produce EPSPs with quite different shapes in different motoneurons (Fig. 11.9). This suggests that a single Ia afferent fibre distributes its input to different motoneurons in different ways and that it does not always have synaptic boutons limited to the same part of the motoneuronal surface.

Single-fibre EPSPs are not as simple as they might appear at first sight. If all single Ia fibres terminated on motoneurons with a single synaptic bouton then the situation would be straight-

forward. But, as described above, single Ia fibres terminate usually with a number of boutons on each motoneuron. For convenience it is often assumed that there is a single locus of action for Ia fibres on motoneurons. But electrophysiological data show the complexity of single-fibre EPSPs. Such potentials may not add linearly even when their shapes are quite different, suggesting that some synaptic sites from single fibres are situated close together, even though the majority may not be. Also, it is a common observation that some single-fibre EPSPs with slow rise and decay times, indicating distal locations, have much larger amplitudes than expected on the basis of the measured membrane properties of the motoneurons (for a discussion of this see Chap. 10).

Careful examination of single-fibre EPSPs has shown that each is composed of smaller unitary EPSPs (Fig. 11.10). Between 1 and 15 unitary EPSPs make up a single-fibre EPSP, with the

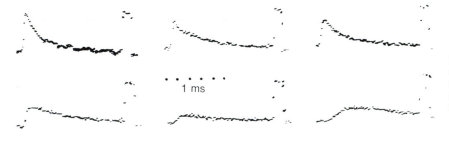

Fig. 11.9. EPSPs produced by a single Ia afferent fibre in six different motoneurons. (Reproduced with permission from Mendell and Henneman 1971.)

Transmission Between Hair Follicle Afferent Fibres and Spinocervical Tract Neurons

The second example of transmission between identified pairs of neurons (hair follicle afferent fibres and neurons of the spinocervical tract) is also taken from the mammalian spinal cord and serves to stress that not all neurons behave like motoneurons in requiring activity in many afferent fibres before they can be caused to fire impulses. Indeed, the motoneuron is probably at or near one end of a spectrum of responses and the spinocervical tract neuron at the other end.

Anatomy of Hair Follicle Afferent Terminations and Spinocervical Tract Neurons

Primary afferent nerve fibres that innervate sense organs in the skin may be divided into several categories according to the sensitivity of the sense organ. Thus some innervate mechanoreceptors, others innervate thermoreceptors and others innervate nocireceptors that respond to damaging stimuli. Within the class of mechanoreceptors there are several divisions according to the detailed response properties and anatomy of the sense organs, e.g. into those afferent fibres innervating the hair follicles and responding to hair movement, those innervating various well-recognized structures such as Pacinian corpuscles (responding to vibration), Ruffini endings (responding to stretch), and so on. A consideration of sensory mechanisms in general is given in Chapter 12. Here we are concerned with primary afferent fibres that innervate the hairs and respond during hair movement. Within this set of afferent fibres there are some that have quite thick myelinated axons (Group II) and some that have thinner myelinated axons (Group III). The Group II hair follicle afferent fibres make monosynaptic excitatory connexions with spinocervical tract neurons, and this system has been investigated in some detail.

Anatomy of Hair Follicle Afferent Terminations in the Spinal Cord

By means of the intra-axonal injection of the enzyme HRP and subsequent histochemistry the light and electron microscopy of these termina-

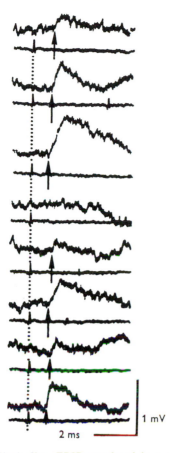

Fig. 11.10. Single-fibre EPSPs produced in a motoneuron. In each pair of records the *upper trace* is the EPSP and the *lower trace* a recording of the single Ia afferent impulse recorded from a dorsal root filament. Note the different amplitudes of the evoked single-fibre EPSPs and the two failures (*4th* and *7th records* from the *top*). The average amplitude of the EPSP was 0.18 mV. (Reproduced with permission from Kuno and Miyahara 1969.)

usual range being between 1 and 5. There are a number of possible interpretations of this observation. Each component might reflect the release of a single quantum of transmitter as at the neuromuscular junction, or it could reflect the release from single boutons, with failure to release occurring randomly. An alternative explanation could be failure of the nerve impulse in the afferent fibre at branch points. Unitary Ia EPSPs in motoneurons are of the order of 100 μV in amplitude, and it is now believed that they represent the release of a single package of transmitter from a single bouton. Furthermore, the variation in the number of unitary potentials evoked by a single impulse in a single Ia fibre is thought to indicate failure of release from individual boutons rather than failure of impulse propagation at branches in the axon near its terminal.

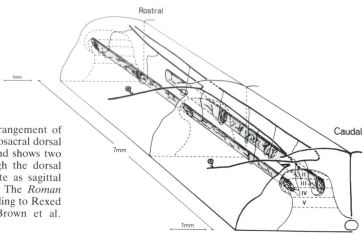

Fig. 11.11. Schematic representation of the arrangement of hair follicle afferent fibre collaterals in the lumbosacral dorsal horn of the cat. The figure is drawn to scale and shows two afferent fibres entering the spinal cord through the dorsal roots and giving off collaterals which terminate as sagittal sheets of arborizations centred on lamina III. The *Roman numerals* indicate the spinal cord laminae according to Rexed (1952). (Reproduced with permission from Brown et al. 1977.)

tions in the cord have been established. Not only are the sense organs of the skin highly selective in their response properties but the central terminals of the different classes of primary cutaneous afferent fibres are also highly specific. Indeed, so specific is the general organization of the central branching pattern and area of termination for each type of afferent fibre that an experienced observer can easily identify which sense organ was innervated by looking at the central terminations of an individual cutaneous (or muscle) nerve fibre. Hair follicle afferent axons enter the cord and give off collateral branches as they run up (and down) the length of the cord. These collaterals run ventrally through the dorsal horn, make a U-turn and ascend to more superficial levels, where they break up into their terminal arborization (Fig. 11.11). The terminal arborizations of adjacent collaterals from the same parent axon form a more or less continuous column of terminations running up and down the dorsal horn for distances sufficient to include two or three spinal cord segments (Fig. 11.11). Within the area of termination an individual hair follicle axon gives off thousands of synaptic boutons.

Anatomy of the Spinocervical Tract

The spinocervical tract (SCT) is part of a somaesthetic pathway present in all mammalian species that have been examined. It is especially well developed in carnivores such as the cat. The SCT neurons are located in the dorsal horn of the spinal cord and have their dendrites ideally placed to receive direct connexions from the hair follicle afferent fibres (Fig. 11.12). SCT neurons send their axons up the spinal cord, via the most superficial and dorsal part of the dorsolateral white matter on the same side as the cell bodies, to the lateral cervical nucleus in the upper few cervical segments. From the lateral cervical nucleus the pathway crosses to the other side and ascends with the medial lemniscus (from the dorsal column nuclei) to the thalamus and thence to the somaesthetic cortex.

Physiology of Hair Follicle Afferent Fibres and Spinocervical Tract Neurons

Hair Follicle Afferent Fibres

In general, the responses of hair follicle afferent fibres code the rate of hair movement quite precisely – the faster the rate of movement the higher the frequency of discharge in the fibre (Fig. 11.13). (There are some exceptions, e.g. some hair follicle receptors are relatively insensitive and other special types innervating the vibrissae respond throughout a maintained displacement of the hair.) Each individual hair follicle afferent fibre innervates a number of hair follicles (between 2 and about 20 hairs for the larger axons to the skin of the hind limb of the cat) contained within an oval or round area of skin. This area of skin (receptive surface) from which the afferent fibre may be excited by natural stimulation, i.e. movement of hairs, is called the receptive field of the neuron.

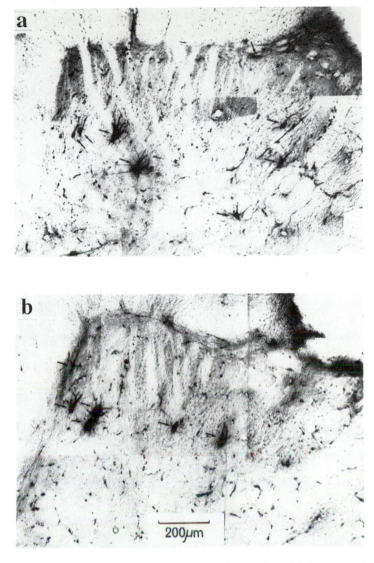

Fig. 11.12a,b. The locations of SCT neurons in the cat's dorsal horn. The neurons were labelled by retrograde transport of HRP and are indicated by *arrows* in these photomicrographs of 100 µm transverse sections of spinal cord. (Reproduced with permission from Brown et al. 1980.)

Spinocervical Tract Neurons

The vast majority (about 90%) of SCT neurons respond to hair movement within their excitatory receptive fields. The receptive fields are, in general, larger than those of hair follicle afferent fibres, but approach them in size on the distal parts of the limbs. For about 30% of SCT neurons the only excitatory input from the skin is via the hair follicle afferent fibres. The remaining 60% or so that respond to hair movement also are excited by noxious stimuli to the skin. The responses to hair movement of SCT cells also code the rate of hair movement. In fact, these responses are often at least as sensitive as those of the afferent fibres and may be more sensitive. As shown in Fig. 11.13 the stimulus–response relations of SCT cells to hair movement

can have a greater slope, indicating this increased sensitivity, which may be due to either convergence of input onto single SCT neurons from a number of afferent fibres or (more likely) to the properties of the synaptic linkages between the afferent fibres and the tract cells.

Hair Follicle Afferent Fibre Synapses on SCT Neurons

By means of intra-axonal HRP injections into hair follicle afferent fibres and intracellular injection of the enzyme into SCT cells in the same preparation it has been possible to study the distribution of hair follicle afferent synapses on the SCT cells. Also, the experiments allowed an

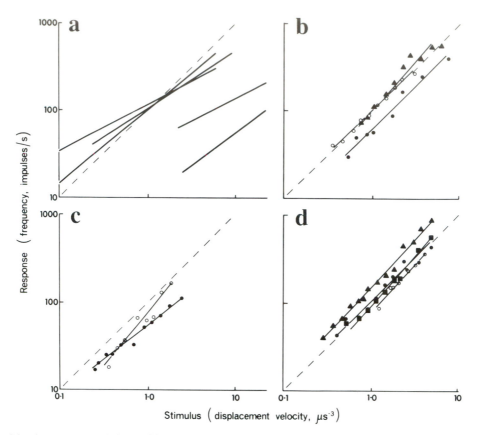

Fig. 11.13. Stimulus response relations of hair follicle afferent fibres (graph *A*) and SCT neurons (graphs *B–D*) to constant velocity hair movement. (Reproduced with permission from Brown and Franz 1969.)

examination of the relationship between this anatomical data and the receptive fields of the afferent fibre and the central neuron, since the HRP-containing microelectrode was also used for standard electrophysiological recording.

When the receptive field of the hair follicle afferent fibre was outside the excitatory receptive field of the SCT neuron no signs of synaptic contacts between the two were seen, even if the separation of fields was minimal (Fig. 11.14). This is an interesting observation since it suggests, for this pair of cells at least, that there are no "silent synapses" between them when the receptive fields are separate. When the hair follicle afferent's receptive field was contained within the excitatory field of the SCT cell then there were monosynaptic connexions between them. More interesting than this, however, was the relationship between the numbers and distribution of these synapses on the SCT neuron and the relative positions of the receptive fields. When the hair follicle afferent fibre had a receptive field at or near the centre of the SCT cell's field then there were between 40 and 60 synapses

located on the proximal part of the cell's dendritic tree. When the afferent fibre's field was at or near the perimeter of the cell's field then there were few contacts (2–10) and these were located distally on the dendritic tree (Fig. 11.15). There is thus a very precise organization of the monosynaptic excitatory connexions between single hair follicle afferent fibres and SCT neurons. It would be expected that excitation of a hair follicle afferent fibre at or near the centre of a SCT cell's excitatory receptive field would have a much more effective action than excitation of an afferent fibre at or near the periphery. However, the situation is more complicated than this description indicates, and only when the actions of single hair follicle afferent fibres on single SCT neurons were studied did this become apparent.

Actions of Single Hair Follicle Afferent Fibres on SCT Cells

Figure 11.16 shows the experimental arrangements used to study the actions of single hair

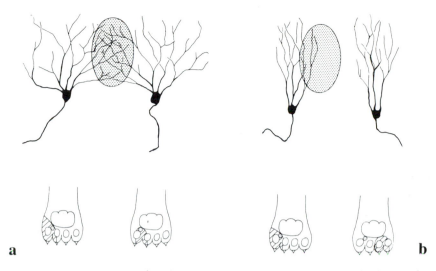

Fig. 11.14a,b. Diagrammatic representation of the relationships between the dendritic trees of adjacent SCT neurons and the terminal arborizations of hair follicle afferent fibres. In **a** the dendritic trees interdigitate and the tract cells' receptive fields overlap; the hair follicle afferent contacts both dendritic trees. In **b** there is no dendritic interdigitation and no receptive field overlap for the tract cells; the hair follicle afferent fibre contacts only the cell on the left. (Reproduced from Brown 1981.)

afferent fibres on SCT cells. A microelectrode was placed inside the cell body of a hair afferent fibre in the dorsal root ganglion. This electrode was used to pass current pulses through the cell and cause it to fire impulses, either single impulses, or pairs or trains of impulses. Simultaneously a second electrode was used to record the responses of a single SCT neuron, either its im-

pulse discharge (by recording from its axon as it ascended the spinal cord) or its synaptic potential responses (by recording from the cell body intracellularly).

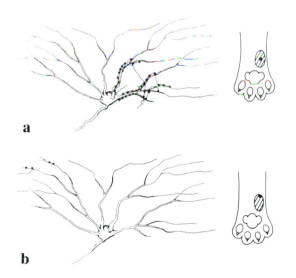

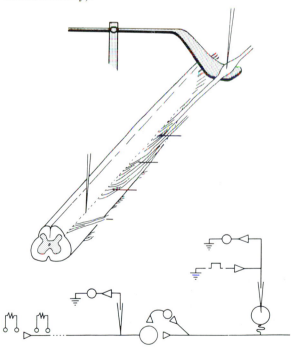

Fig. 11.15a,b. Diagrammatic representation of the relationships between hair follicle afferent fibres and SCT neurons. When the hair follicle afferent has a receptive field at or near the centre of the neuron's receptive field there are many contacts located proximally to the dendritic tree (**a**); when the hair follicle afferent's field is peripherally placed in the neuron's field there are few, distally located contacts (**b**).

Fig. 11.16. Experimental arrangement used to study the effects of impulses in single hair follicle afferent fibres on single SCT cells. The microelectrode used for recording the tract cell reposes could be placed either against the cell's axon (as shown) or inside the cell body. (Reproduced with permission from Brown et al. 1987a.)

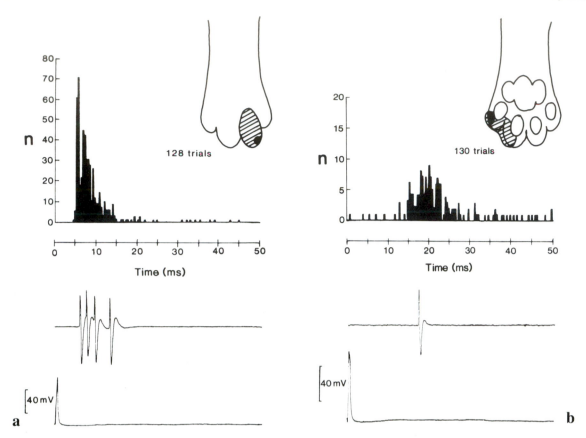

Fig. 11.17a,b. Responses of single SCT neurons to single hair follicle afferent impulses. In both **a** and **b** the *upper part* shows a post-stimulus time histogram of the responses with the receptive fields indicated on the *figurines*, the tract cell's field shown *cross-hatched* and the afferent fibre's field as a *filled area*. The *lower part* of each figure shows a typical single response and, at the *bottom*, the intracellularly elicited and recorded action potential in the afferent fibre. (Reproduced with permission from Brown et al. 1987a.)

The results of such experiments were surprising. A single impulse in a single hair follicle afferent fibre (Group II conduction velocity) produced at least one impulse from the SCT neuron in more than half the pairs of cells investigated, if the SCT neuron's excitatory receptive field contained the field of the hair afferent fibre. In all such pairs the probability of firing of the SCT neuron was increased (Fig. 11.17). In some pairs a single hair afferent impulse always led to at least one impulse in the SCT neuron, and the maximum number of impulses evoked could be as high as five or six. The efficacy of the synaptic linkage must be very great indeed.

In spite of this obviously most efficient coupling between the two elements, the latency of the impulse discharge in the SCT cells was only rarely short enough to have been caused by monosynaptic excitation, even though there are mono-

synaptic connexions between the two elements. Intracellular recording from the SCT cell provided the answer to this puzzle. A single impulse in a hair follicle afferent fibre produced a monosynaptic EPSP (when the SCT cell's receptive field included the field of the afferent), but, in addition, this monosynaptic EPSP was followed by later EPSPs which were often of greater amplitude than the monosynaptic component, and it was from this later EPSP complex that the impulses arose (Fig. 11.18). Thus, in addition to the monosynaptic connexion between the two neurons there must be additional interneuronal connexions, as shown in Fig. 11.16. The electrophysiological results also confirmed the previous anatomical observations – when the hair afferent fibre had a receptive field at or near the centre of the SCT cell's field the monosynaptic component was often of greater amplitude and faster rise

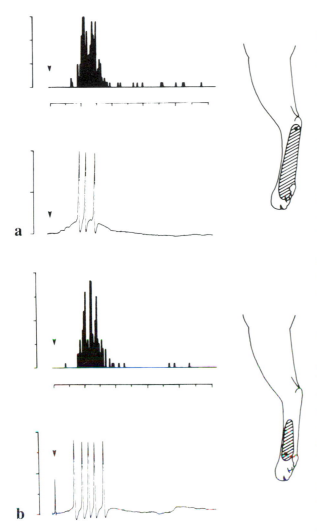

Fig. 11.18a,b. Intracellular recording of the response of a SCT cell to a single hair follicle afferent impulse. In each figure part the *upper record* is a post-stimulus time histogram and the *lower trace* a single response. The receptive fields of the cell (*cross-hatched*) and the fibre (*filled area*) are shown in the *figurine*. Note the EPSP arising at about 3 ms after the onset of the action potential in the fibre (*arrow*) and the cell's impulses coming off the EPSP at about 10 ms. (Reproduced with permission from Brown et al. 1987b.)

and other tract cells in the spinal cord and also between Pacinian corpuscle afferent fibres and neurons in the dorsal column nuclei. Indeed this remarkable ability to transmit input faithfully and also to amplify it appears to be a general property of sensory pathways.

Summary

1. The monosynaptic excitatory connexions between Ia afferent fibres from muscle and the alpha-motoneurons innervating the same muscle and its synergists have been well studied.

2. Each Ia afferent fibre makes rather few (about one to five) contacts with each motor neuron, and these contacts are usually clustered fairly close together. Each Ia afferent fibre carries 1000–2000 boutons that contact motoneurons, and each motoneuron receives some 200–450 boutons from some 50–90 Ia afferent fibres.

3. Each Ia afferent synaptic bouton can eject enough current into a motoneuron to evoke an EPSP of about 100μV (at the soma) and, since the threshold for initiation of an impulse in the motoneuron is about 15 mV above resting level, this implies that about 150 Ia boutons have to release transmitter more or less simultaneously to lead to firing. Thus, in order to cause a motoneuron to fire, about 20–50 Ia afferent fibres need to fire a single impulse more or less synchronously.

4. Connexions between hair follicle afferent fibres and neurons of the SCT have also been examined in some detail.

5. Hair follicle afferent fibres make monosynaptic excitatory connexions with SCT cells, and these connexions are made with a high degree of specificity – fibres from the centre of the cell's receptive field make more contacts (about 40–60) that are located on proximal dendrites, whereas fibres from the periphery of the cell's field make fewer contacts (2–10) on distal dendrites.

6. A single impulse in a singe hair afferent fibre from within a SCT cell's receptive field can cause the SCT cell to fire in more than 50% of trials (in more than 50% of neuron pairs). This remarkable efficacy of synaptic transmission is largely due to the addition of excitatory interneurons between the afferent fibre and the SCT cell, although the monosynaptic EPSP generated between them is considerably larger than single-fibre EPSPs generated by Ia afferent fibres in motoneurons.

time, whereas with a peripherally located hair follicle afferent fibre field the EPSPs included the smallest and slowest potentials.

These experiments demonstrate a very precise organization of the connexions between these afferent fibres and central neurons. Furthermore, the quite remarkably efficient excitatory linkages between them, which contrast strongly with the connexions between Ia muscle afferent fibres and motoneurons, are not exceptional. Similar strong excitations are seen between other afferent fibres

Sense Organ Specificity

Sense organs, or sensory receptors, form the interface between the animal's environment on the one hand and its nervous system on the other. This interface is with both the internal and external environments and it is the function of the sense organs to monitor these environments. The limits of sensitivity of an organism to its environment are set by the sensitivities of the various sense organs, and the nervous system works within these limits. In addition to the role of monitoring the environment, a sense organ must either directly or indirectly convert an energy change (or energy level) into a form which the nervous system can handle. That is, sense organs transduce energy from one form into another and specifically into a form that can influence neurons. As we shall see, the transduction process results in a receptor potential in the sensory receptor cell. This receptor potential may lead to the generation of impulses within the receptor cell or, in other instances, may be transmitted (synaptically) to a nerve cell, where a generator potential is set up, and this generator potential may be responsible for the initiation of impulses.

It is a characteristic of sensory receptors that they are highly specialized in terms of the types of stimuli to which they respond. Thus, some respond to mechanical stimuli, others to thermal or chemical or light stimuli. Within these broad categories there is much further subdivision, so that, for example, thermoreceptors only respond within a fairly narrow temperature range and either to warming or cooling but not both, and

chemoreceptors respond quite specifically to a few structurally related chemicals. Because sensory receptors are innervated by afferent nerve fibres in such a way that only receptors of the same kind are connected to a single neuron (or there is a one-to-one connexion) it follows that the quality of a stimulus (warming, cooling, light of a particular wave-length, a mechanical stimulus of a particular strength etc.) is encoded by the sense organ and transmitted to the central nervous system along a so-called labelled line. The principle of modality specificity that results from labelled lines was first enunciated in 1826 by Johannes Müller as his Doctrine of Specific Nerve Energies – an obvious example of this in operation is the fact that a blow on the eyeball leads to the unfortunate recipient "seeing stars". Because stimulus quality (the "what is it?") is encoded by labelled lines, there remain only two properties of the stimulus that these lines can transmit – the occurrence in time of a stimulus (the "when" of a stimulus) and the intensity of a stimulus (the "how much" of a stimulus).

The sensory receptors that monitor the external environment or that are concerned with the relationships of the animal's body in space are either located within a receptor sheet (e.g. the photoreceptors in the retina, the cutaneous receptors of the skin) or are located in particular body parts whose position the animal needs to be informed about (e.g. individual muscles, joints, the head etc.). As we shall see (Chaps. 14 and 15), the relationships of receptors in space or on the receptor sheet are maintained in the relationships of the neurons within the nervous system to which the receptors send their messages. In other words, the place at which a stimulus acts (the

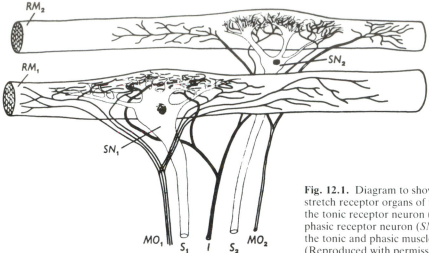

Fig. 12.1. Diagram to show the structure of the abdominal stretch receptor organs of the crayfish. RM_1, muscle bundle of the tonic receptor neuron (SN_1); RM_2, muscle bundle of the phasic receptor neuron (SN_2; MO_1 and MO_2, motor fibres of the tonic and phasic muscle bundles; I, an inhibitory axon. (Reproduced with permission from Burkhardt 1958.)

"where is it?") is encoded in the way in which the sense organs are connected to the central nervous system.

Sensory Transduction Mechanisms

Most sensory receptors are small cells and are relatively, or at present completely, inaccessible to experimental attack. Few receptors have been examined in any degree of detail. Those that have, however, all show the same principles of operation, even though there have been some surprises. Essentially, the specific stimulus acting on the sensory receptor produces a potential change within the sensory cell – the receptor potential – by means of opening or closing ion channels. These ion channels are gated channels but are not voltage-gated or (except in chemoreceptors) chemically gated. Rather, they are mechanically gated, thermally gated etc., according to the specific sensitivity of the sense organ. Knowledge of receptor mechanisms is increasing at a rapid rate; however, at present, most detail is known about the operation of certain mechanoreceptors and photoreceptors, and examples will be considered from these categories.

Crayfish Stretch Receptor

Stretch receptors responding to muscle stretch in crayfish were amongst the first sense organs to be studied. The receptors are specialized neurons with their cell bodies situated close to the muscle fibres that they innervate with their dendrites (Fig. 12.1). From the cell body an axon arises and this projects centrally to a segmental ganglion, where it makes synaptic contacts with other neurons. An advantage of this preparation is that the cell body can be seen in the living preparation, with the aid of a microscope, and can be penetrated with microelectrodes. Stretch of the muscle leads to deformation of the membrane of the receptor cell's dendrites and this leads to a depolarization within the dendrites that propagates passively to the cell body, where it may be recorded (receptor potential, Fig. 12.2)

There are two types of stretch receptor cells in the crayfish, the rapidly adapting and the slowly adapting receptors. The term "adaptation" refers to a property of all receptors – with the passage of time the response of the receptor (or the impulse firing associated with receptor activation) becomes less, even though the stimulus is maintained. Some receptors, however, show rapid adaptation and others slow, or almost no, adaptation.

The precise mechanism that links mechanical deformation with the generation of a receptor potential is not known. It is likely, however, that mechanically gated sodium channels are opened, since the amplitude of the receptor potential is reduced if the sodium in the external solution is replaced with an impermeant ion. These sodium channels are not blocked by tetrodotoxin (TTX), which blocks the voltage-gated sodium channel. It is likely, however, that in this receptor, ions other than sodium are involved. The reversal potential for the receptor potential, determined by voltage clamp experiments, is about +15 mV

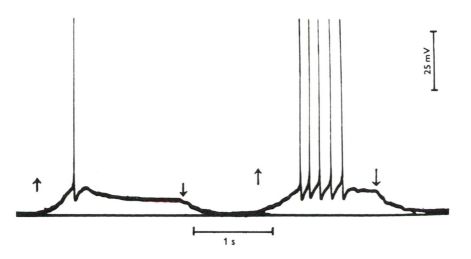

Fig. 12.2. Intracellular records from a crayfish stretch receptor cell. The receptor muscle was stretched between the times marked by the *arrows*, the stretch on the right being greater than that on the left. (Reproduced with permission from Eyzaguirre and Kuffler 1955.)

and this is somewhat lower than the sodium equilibrium potential (Fig. 12.3). With very small stretches the receptor potential can be seen in isolation. Usually, however, the stretch produces a receptor potential that generates action potentials by opening voltage-gated channels in the excitable membrane of the cell body, or rather in the initial segment or axon hillock. In this sense organ the receptor potential produced in the dendrites is propagated electrotonically to the initial segment where it acts as the generator potential. The two potentials are essentially one and the same, and

the initiation of impulses occurs by the same mechanisms as excitatory postsynaptic potentials (EPSPs) initiate impulses in neurons. As will be discussed below, there is a precise relationship between the intensity of the stimulus (degree of muscle stretch in this case) and the amplitude of the resulting receptor potential, and between the amplitude of the receptor potential and the frequency at which nerve impulses are generated in the initial segment.

In the crayfish stretch receptor, therefore, the receptor cell and the sensory neuron are one and the same. In many other sense organs the receptor cell is a separate cell from the first (afferent) neuron that transmits the sensory messages to the rest of the nervous system. In such instances the receptor potential set up by the adequate stimulus spreads passively to a synaptic region of the receptor cell, where contact is made with the sensory neuron. Here, synaptic transmission occurs, leading to the production of a generator potential in the neuron, and this generator potential is responsible for initiating the nerve impulses. Sense organs that have separate receptor cells include the eye (where the rods and cones of the retina are the photoreceptors) and the inner ear (where the cochlear hair cells are the mechanoreceptors sensitive to movement caused by sound waves).

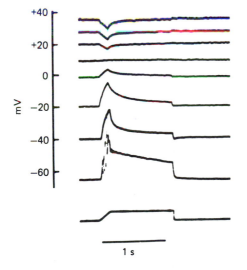

Fig. 12.3. Reversal of the receptor potential of the crayfish stretch receptor. The potential was evoked by stretch and recorded at the different membrane potentials indicated at the *left*. The reversal potential was at about +15 mV. (Reproduced with permission from Brown et al. 1978.)

Vertebrate Photoreceptors

Vertebrate photoreceptors are examples of receptor cells that are separate from the neurons that send the sensory messages into the central nervous system. Much is now known about the photochemical processes involved in the transduction of light energy (photons) into the receptor potential, and also how the receptor potential is transmitted to the next cells (neurons) along the sensory processing chain. Furthermore, the receptor potential in photoreceptors has been shown to be a hyperpolarizing potential in contrast to the depolarizing potential observed in most other sensory receptors. How such a hyperpolarizing potential comes about and how it affects its target cells is a fascinating story.

Figure 12.4 shows, diagrammatically, the general structure of the vertebrate retina. The photoreceptor cells, the rods and cones, form a light-sensitive receptor sheet on the back of the retina, and in front of them are several layers of neurons, the horizontal cells, the bipolar cells, the amacrine cells and the ganglion cells. It is from the last of these, the ganglion cells, that the axons of the optic nerve arise. All of these neurons are in front of the photoreceptors, and light has to pass through the neural layers to reach the rods and cones. However, these layers are translucent, and in the most sensitive part of

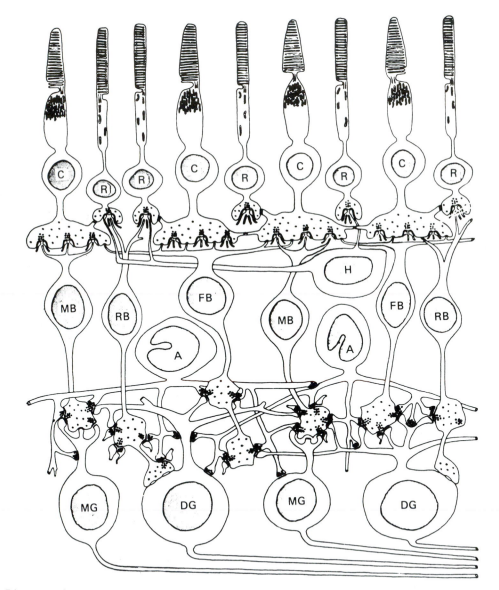

Fig. 12.4. Diagrammatic representation of the organization of the primate retina. *R*, rod; *C*, cone; *MB*, *RB* and *FB*, bipolar cells; *H*, horizontal cell; *A*, amacrine cell; *MG*, *DG*, ganglion cells. (Modified with permission from Dowling and Boycott 1967.)

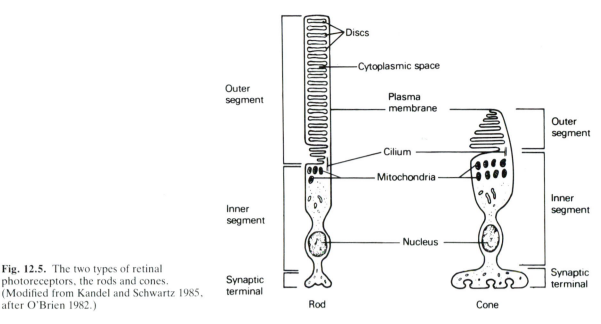

Fig. 12.5. The two types of retinal photoreceptors, the rods and cones. (Modified from Kandel and Schwartz 1985, after O'Brien 1982.)

the retina (the fovea), which contains mainly cones, the layers are thinnest or moved aside.

The rods and cones are both structurally similar and different (Fig. 12.5). They are similar in both having three main parts: an outer segment, an inner segment and a synaptic terminal. The outer segment is the specialized photoreceptive part of the rods and cones and is connected to the inner segment by a narrow bridge of cytoplasm containing a modified cilium. It is the outer segment where the main structural differences between rods and cones occurs. The outer segments contain an elaborate set of membranous specializations (discs) stacked on top of one another, and the photopigments that catch the photons are contained within the membranes of the discs. In rods the outer segment is longer than in cones and also the membranous discs are pinched off from the outer cell membrane, whereas in cones the discs remain connected with the surface membrane (Fig. 12.5). The inner segment contains the nucleus of the cell and many mitochondria and ribosomes. The synaptic region makes presynaptic contact with bipolar cells and (in rods) with horizontal cells and is itself post-synaptic to horizontal cells.

Photochemical Process

The photopigments in rods and cones each contain two parts, a protein called opsin (cone opsin in cones) and a form of vitamin A, 11-*cis*-retinal. All rods contain the same pigment –

rhodopsin, whereas there are three types of cone pigment, each with a different cone opsin (the different cone opsins preferentially absorb light best in different parts of the visible spectrum and therefore it is the cones that are responsible for colour vision). However, it is the 11-*cis*-retinal that is the component that reacts with the photons (retinal is a chromophore). When the *cis* form of retinal reacts with light it is converted to the all-*trans* form and undergoes a conformational change. This conversion from the 11-*cis*- to the all-*trans*- form of retinal is the only light-dependent stage in vision (Fig. 12.6). Ultimately this biochemical reaction leads to the appearance of the hyperpolarizing receptor potential in the photoreceptors, and, in fact, the capture of a single photon of light by a rod is transduced into a receptor potential. The intermediary steps involve an enzyme cascade in which cyclic GMP plays an important role.

Enzyme Cascade

In rods the rhodopsin is contained within the membranous discs of the outer segments. But these discs are separated from the outer cell membrane of the rod, and yet the receptor potential (hyperpolarizing in this instance) is presumably set up by ionic current flow across the cell membrane. The link between the photochemical reaction and the receptor potential is provided by a second-messenger system involving an enzyme cascade. The basic series of events is

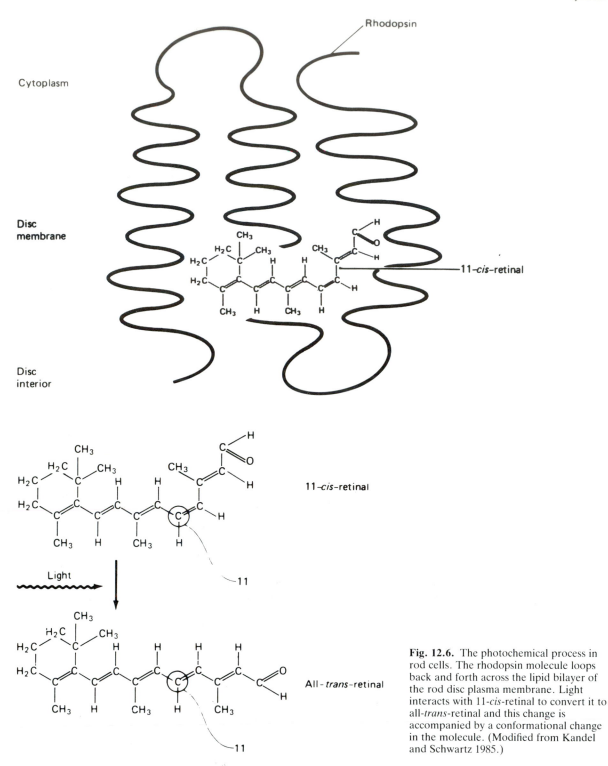

Fig. 12.6. The photochemical process in rod cells. The rhodopsin molecule loops back and forth across the lipid bilayer of the rod disc plasma membrane. Light interacts with 11-*cis*-retinal to convert it to all-*trans*-retinal and this change is accompanied by a conformational change in the molecule. (Modified from Kandel and Schwartz 1985.)

indicated in Fig. 12.6. A single photon can interact with a rhodopsin molecule to excite it (convert its 11-*cis*-retinal to all-*trans*-retinal. The activated rhodopsin molecule in turn activates a

protein (transducin) from a state in which it binds guanosine diphosphate (GDP) to one in which it binds guanosine triphosphate (GTP). The activated transducin in turn activates a photodiesterase

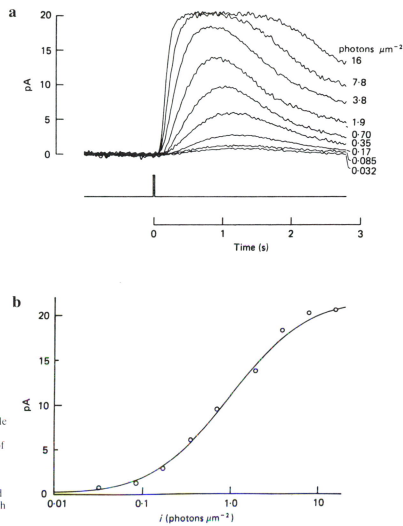

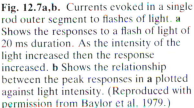

Fig. 12.7a,b. Currents evoked in a single rod outer segment to flashes of light. **a** Shows the responses to a flash of light of 20 ms duration. As the intensity of the light increased then the response increased. **b** Shows the relationship between the peak responses in **a** plotted against light intensity. (Reproduced with permission from Baylor et al. 1979.)

which begins to cleave many molecules of cyclic GMP. All of the protein molecules (rhodopsin, transducin and photodiesterase) are contained within the membranous discs, and have been isolated from them and shown to carry out the required reactions. The cyclic GMP is present in the cytoplasm of the outer segment and provides the link to the cell membrane. The absorption of a single photon leads to the cleaving of very many cyclic GMP molecules.

Receptor Potential

As mentioned above, the receptor potential in photoreceptors is a hyperpolarizing potential. When first recorded this was a very surprising observation, because excitatory processes (and this surely is an excitatory process) were generally held to produce depolarizations in the excited cell. The answer to this paradox is that in the dark a continuous depolarizing current flows through the membrane of the receptor and exposure to light leads to a turning off of this "dark current", leading to a hyperpolarization. In comparison with most other receptors it is as if the vertebrate photoreceptors were excited by dark (absence of stimulus) and inhibited by light (presence of stimulus)!

The "dark current" of rods and cones is due to a passive leakage of sodium ions into the cell. Exposure to light leads to the closure of the sodium channels and therefore a reduction in the sodium current and a hyperpolarization. It has been shown by Baylor and his colleagues (Fig. 12.7) that measurable electric currents, of the

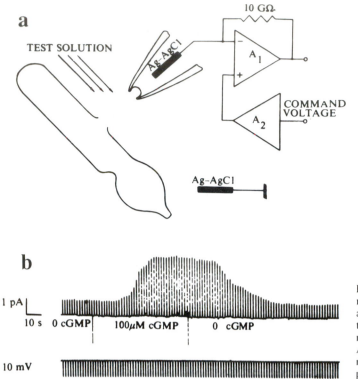

Fig. 12.8a,b. Effect of cyclic GMP on a patch of retinal rod outer segment. **a** Shows the recording arrangement. **b** Shows the current flowing through the patch (Na^+ current mainly) in response to 10 mV command voltage pulses (*lower record*). Addition of cyclic GMP (*cGMP*) produces a marked increase in current flow. (Reproduced with permission from Fesenko et al. 1985.)

order of 1 pA, occur in rod outer segments when a single photon combines with the rhodopsin. The sophisticated techniques used to make these observations include the use of fine suction electrodes to suck up a single rod outer segment into the electrode, and the illumination of the single outer segment by slits of light. The suction electrode fits very tightly around the outer segment and the current flowing into or out of the rod can be recorded.

The final link in the story was provided by experiments carried out by Fesenko and his colleagues. They showed, using the patch clamp technique, that a patch of rod outer segment became permeable to sodium when exposed to cyclic GMP (Fig. 12.8). Thus, exposure to light leads, via the various biochemical processes, to the removal of cyclic GMP from the cytoplasm and to its removal from the outer cell membrane, where, in the dark, it keeps the sodium channels open.

Output from the Rods and Cones

Transmission from the rods and cones to their target neurons, the bipolar and horizontal cells,

is by chemical means. In the dark, transmitter is continually being released. The hyperpolarizing receptor potential reduces the amount of transmitter released. The further processing of visual information will be considered in Chapter 15.

Adaptation of Sensory Signals

As described above for the crayfish stretch receptor, receptors may be classed as slowly or rapidly adapting, and this property may depend on the characteristics of the receptor membrane, rapidly adapting receptors producing a receptor potential that decays rapidly even in the face of a maintained stimulus. This is not the only mechanism of adaptation, however, and both neural and external factors may be involved.

There are two types of crayfish stretch receptor cell, one that adapts rapidly and the other that adapts slowly. The rapidly adapting cell shows rapid adaptation of its firing rate even to injected currents (Fig. 12.9), and therefore part of the adaptation is due to the properties of the neuronal membrane at the site of impulse initiation. In

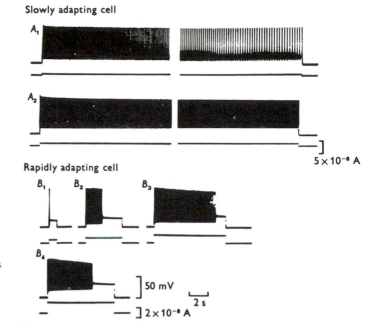

Fig. 12.9. Repetitive impulse discharges evoked in crayfish stretch receptor cells by intracellular current pulses. The slowly adapting cell responds throughout the pulse, whereas the rapidly adapting cell only fires to the initial part of the pulse (Reproduced with permission from Nakajima and Onodera 1969.)

the slowly adapting receptor there is a slow build-up of intracellular sodium, due to impulse activity, and this activates a sodium pump to drive the ions out of the cell. Activity of the pump causes a hyperpolarization and therefore a reduction in impulse frequency.

In vertebrates there are some specialized mechanoreceptors called Pacinian corpuscles. In mammals they occur in the dermis, and in various connective tissue sheets such as in ligaments between bones and in the peritoneum of the abdominal cavity. They are exquisitely sensitive to vibratory stimuli, and the impulse discharge along their afferent fibres can follow vibration in a one-to-one fashion at frequencies of several hundred a second (Fig. 12.10). They are the most rapidly adapting receptors known. This rapid adaptation depends not on the properties of the sense ending or the afferent neuron but on the mechanical properties of a connective tissue capsule that surrounds the nerve ending and gives the structure its corpuscular appearance (Fig. 12.10). Pacinian corpuscles are surrounded by a series of connective tissue sheaths organized in an "onion skin" arrangement. This connective tissue capsule filters out low-frequency mechanical disturbances and only lets through, to the receptor, high-frequency displacements. In the absence of the capsule the sense ending can respond to a maintained displacement with a maintained receptor potential (Fig. 12.10).

Stimulus Encoding

The fact that the great majority of sensory receptors only responds to a particularly narrow range of stimuli (the adequate stimuli), and that individual receptors or a small number of like receptors are connected to the central nervous system by a single nerve fibre (the labelled lines), means that it is the intensity of a stimulus that is encoded by the receptor potential and, ultimately, by the discharge of impulses in the afferent fibres. The amplitude of the receptor potential is a function of the stimulus intensity, and in some receptors this relation is a linear one over most of the sensitive range (Fig. 12.11). In other receptors the relation is non-linear, saturating at the upper end of the range. Generally, the relationship between the impulse discharge frequency in the afferent axon from a receptor and the stimulus intensity is similar to the relation between the stimulus amplitude and the receptor potential amplitude (Fig. 12.11b).

In many sense organs the discharge of impulses in their afferent axons encodes stimulus amplitude as a power function (Stevens 1961), that is, as a function of the form

$$F = k \cdot (S - S_o)^n$$

where F is the frequency of discharge, k is a constant, $(S - S_o)$ the stimulus intensity expressed

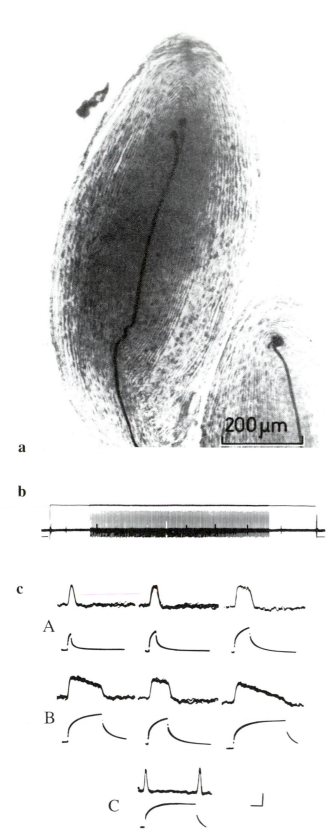

a

b

c

A

B

C

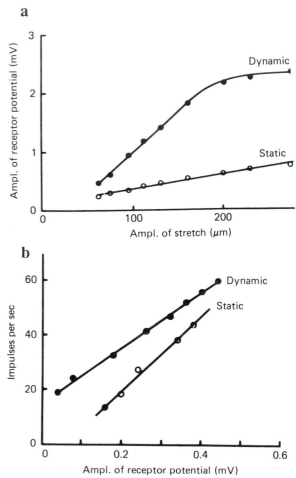

Fig. 12.10a–c. Pacinian corpuscle and their responses. **a** Shows a Pacinian corpuscle from a cat. This is a teased preparation stained with a silver stain to show the afferent fibre entering the corpuscle. **b** Shows the response of a Pacinian corpuscle afferent fibre innervating a monkey's hand. The corpuscle follows a vibration at 150 Hz in a one-to-one manner. **c** The bottom set of traces show (A, B) the receptor potentials recorded from a decapsulated Pacinian corpuscle (*upper records*) to series of displacements of increasing amplitudes and durations. Note the receptor potential lasting as long as the displacements. The lowermost set of traces (C) shows the receptor potential of an intact corpuscle. Note the responses at the on and off of the displacement but no maintained potential. Calibrations 10 ms and 50 µV (for receptor potential) [Reproduced with permission from Barker 1974 (**a**), from Talbot et al. 1968 (**b**) and from Loewenstein and Mendelson 1965(**c**).]

a

b

Fig. 12.11. **a** Shows the relation between the amplitude of the receptor potential in a frog muscle spindle and the amount of stretch of the spindle, for both the dynamic (during stretching) and static (during maintained stretch) components of the response. **b** shows the corresponding relationships between the frequency of firing in the afferent nerve fibre and the receptor potential amplitude. (Reproduced from Ottoson and Shepherd 1971.)

as the stimulus strength above threshold level, and n is a positive number (Fig. 12.12). When n = 1 the relation is linear with a slope of k. It is of some interest that the response of cortical neurons in primates and the relation between stimulus amplitude and the subjective experience of the strength of the stimulus in man can also be described by such a power function (Fig. 12.12). It seems unlikely that such an observation is a coincidence and implies that the mean frequency of discharge in a sensory axon does code the stimulus intensity in a way that is meaningful to the nervous system.

Dynamic and Static Components of the Response

It is obvious that the above general discussion is a gross over-simplification. Consider, for example, two sets of different mechanoreceptors responding to displacements of the skin, some with a rapidly adapting response and others a slowly adapting one. What might the two sets of receptors be encoding? Consider the stimulus to be a controlled "ramp and hold" displacement of a blunt-ended probe that indents the skin. This stimulus has several components. There is the dynamic component, that is, the initial rate of displacement during the ramp part of the stimulation, and the static component, the maintained displacement. Finally, at the end of the period of maintained displacement there is the removal of the stimulus, which may be a reversal of the ramp. Now, if the rapidly adapting receptors are suitably attuned they may only respond during the movement of the skin and could code the rate of skin displacement. Such mechanoreceptors are common and are found, for example, as receptors responding to movement of the hairs of the coat of mammals (see Fig. 11.13). The situation with the slowly adapting receptors is more complex. It is conceivable that some filtering mechanisms might be present to filter out the dynamic component and that the receptors might then only respond to the static (maintained displacement) component of the stimulus. Generally, slowly adapting mechanoreceptors respond to both the dynamic and static components with an initial dynamic response during the change in the stimulus and then with a static component during the maintained stimulus (Fig. 12.13). Both components of the stimulus are encoded in the afferent fibre discharge from such receptors, the dynamic response encoding both velocity and amplitude of displacement and the static com-

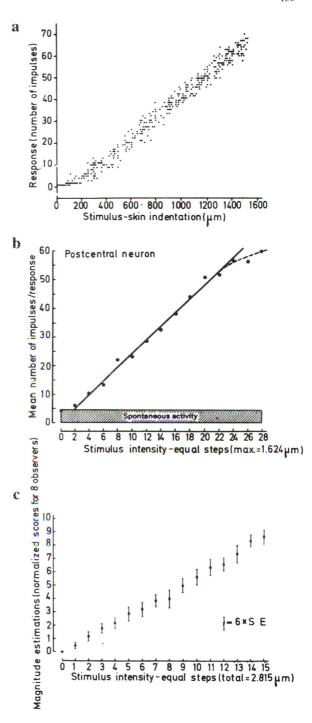

Fig. 12.12a–c. a The linear relation (power function = 1) between stimulus and response for a slowly adapting cutaneous mechanoreceptor of the skin of a monkey's hand. **b** The stimulus–response relation of a slowly adapting neuron in the somatosensory cortex of a monkey. The neuron responded to maintained indentation of the hand skin. **c** Relation between human magnitude estimation and the indentation applied to the hand. (Reproduced with permission from Mountcastle et al. 1966 (**a**) and from Mountcastle and Darian–Smith 1968 (**b**, **c**).)

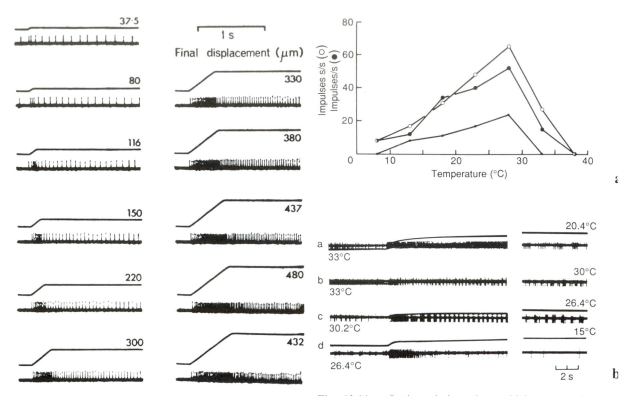

Fig. 12.13. Responses of a slowly adapting (Type II) receptor in the skin of a cat. The records show the impulses, recorded from a single afferent fibre innervating the receptor (*lower traces*), in response to a series of vertical displacements of the skin over the receptor (*upper traces*). The fibre fires rapidly during the dynamic phase of the stimulus and then adapts to a steady discharge during the maintained displacement. The final amplitude of displacement (in micrometres) is indicated for each pair of records. (Reproduced with permission from Chambers et al. 1972.)

Fig. 12.14. a Static and dynamic sensitivity curves for a primate cold receptor. The lowest curve shows the response after adaptation to the temperature. The upper curves show the dynamic response during the first few seconds after the temperature was reduced by 5 °C. **b** Impulses recorded from an afferent fibre innervating a cold receptor in the hairy skin of a monkey. Note the grouped discharges at static temperatures between about 20 °C and 30 °C. (Reproduced with permission from Iggo 1969.)

ponent encoding amplitude alone. For such a receptor it is possible, therefore, that a particular frequency of impulse discharge in its afferent fibre might occur both during the dynamic and the static phases of a response, and it thus seems unlikely that sufficient information is encoded in the discharges of a single afferent fibre for the nervous system to determine whether a dynamic or static stimulus has impinged on the skin. There are a number of ways out of this dilemma: for example, usually several different sensory receptors will be excited by a particular stimulus and some may only code one aspect of the stimulus (such as its velocity); alternatively, further processing in the central sensory systems may allow differentiations to be made (some central neurons may not respond to the initial discharge but require considerable temporal summation and therefore will respond predominantly to the static components).

Encoding by Grouped Impulse Discharges

Thermoreceptors respond to both static and dynamic components of temperature and temperature changes. In addition, their stimulus–response relations to static temperatures take the form of bell-shaped curves (Fig. 12.14). Thus, for both cold and warm receptors there are two points (two different static temperatures) on the stimulus–response relations of their afferent fibre discharges where the same mean frequency occurs. Similar problems of analysis for the central nervous system must occur as for the input from mechanoreceptors described above. Individual stimulus–response curves of single afferent fibres from thermoreceptors differ, and it is likely that the central nervous system analyses the population response. There is another possibility, however, at least for the analysis of the afferent fibre discharges from cold receptors in primates. In primate species, over part of the static sensitivity curve, usually at and near its most sensitive part, the impulse discharge occurs in groups of impulses, with the number of impulses in the group, their frequency within the group and the interval between groups varying with the static temperature (Fig. 12.14). It is not known if the central nervous system makes use of this additional information in the afferent input (although signs of the grouping can be seen in the responses of central neurons at early stages in the processing of thermosensory input), but it is a possibility.

Centrifugal Control of Sense Organs

The central nervous system actively controls the responses of many sense organs. It does so by a number of different mechanisms such as direct innervation of the sensory receptor cells themselves, by affecting neurons associated with the receptor cells or by altering the physical environment of the receptor cells. Thus, there is direct innervation of the hair cells (the receptor cell) of the inner ear, and activation of this pathway causes a large reduction in sensitivity of the receptors by means of a hyperpolarizing inhibitory potential. In the retina of birds there is an innervation, by fibres from the isthmo-optic nucleus, of the amacrine cells, and this innervation controls the sensitivity of the system. Perhaps the best known example of this sort of control by the nervous system over its own input (centrifugal control) is in the mammalian muscle spindle, where the mechanism of control alters the mechanical environment of the spindle mechanoreceptors. The following account of the muscle spindle, its responses and its control by the central nervous system is much simplified and is aimed at presenting the basic principles of centrifugal control.

Mammalian Muscle Spindles and their Centrifugal Control

Mammalian muscle spindles are mechanoreceptors that respond to changes in muscle length, tension and velocity of movement. They are complex structures containing two main types of mechanosensitive receptors and are innervated by two main types of efferent axons from the central nervous system.

Structure of Muscle Spindles

Mammalian muscle spindles (see Fig. 11.1) are located within the fleshy parts of skeletal muscles. Each is surrounded by a connective tissue sheath and is made up of modified muscle fibres that run from end to end of the muscle, that is, the muscle spindle is situated in parallel with the muscle fibres of the muscle in which it lies. The modified muscle fibres of the spindle are called intrafusal fibres to distinguish them from the extrafusal fibres of the main body of the muscle. The intrafusal fibres are contractile but do not contribute to the overall tension produced by the muscle. Rather, their contraction affects the sensitivities of the spindle mechanoreceptors.

There are two main types of intrafusal fibres – the nuclear bag and the nuclear chain fibres, so-called because of their appearance. The bag fibres have nuclei clustered in small groups at their central (equatorial) region, whereas the chain fibres have their nuclei in single file. Around the equatorial region of each type of fibre are wound the terminals of an afferent fibre (the Ia afferent fibre; see Chap. 11) forming the primary or annulospiral ending. Slightly away from the equatorial region of the chain fibre (and less often the bag fibre) are the endings of another afferent fibre (from a somewhat thinner, Group II, axon) forming the secondary or flower-spray ending. Like all striated muscle, and the intrafusal fibres are modified striated muscle, each intrafusal fibre receives an efferent innervation (a fusimotor fibre) from a motoneuron in the central nervous system. These motoneurons that innervate intrafusal fibres are called gamma-motoneurons since their axons conduct within the gamma component of the A wave of the compound action potential. The nuclear bag fibres are innervated by dynamic fusimotor fibres and the nuclear chain fibres by static fusimotor fibres. The fusimotor fibres receive their names from their actions on the intrafusal fibres and on the afferent discharges. There are further subdivisions of the intrafusal bag fibres and of the fusimotor neurons but these will not be described here.

Responses of Muscle Spindle Afferent Fibres

When a muscle is stretched passively, both the Group Ia fibres, from the primary endings, and

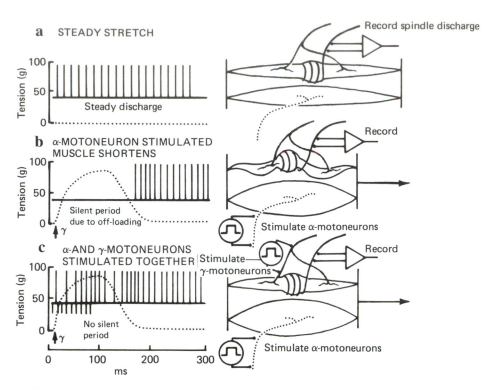

Fig. 12.15a–c. Effect of fusimotor stimulation on the response from the muscle spindle during contraction of the extrafusal muscle fibres. **a** During steady stretch of the muscle the spindle afferent fibres fires regularly. **b** During muscle contraction caused by stimulation of the axons of alpha-motoneurons the spindle afferent fibre ceases to fire because it is off-loaded. **c** If the axons of both the alpha- and gamma- (fusimotor) motoneurons are stimulated together, the spindle afferent fibre maintains its discharges as it is no longer off-loaded by the muscle shortening. (Modified from Kuffler et al. 1984, after Hunt and Kuffler 1951.)

the Group II fibres, from the secondary endings, respond to both the dynamic and static components of the stretch (see Fig. 11.2). The primary endings are much more sensitive to the dynamic component of passive stretch and the secondary endings respond primarily to the static component. That is, the primary endings are sensitive to both the rate of change in length of the muscle and to its length, whereas the secondary endings are sensitive primarily to muscle length only.

At resting length of the muscle (when there is no active tension) there is a resting discharge along the afferent axons from the spindle. Because the spindle is in parallel with the extrafusal fibres of the muscle, active contraction of the muscle from its resting length, or from some length shorter than resting, will lead to an off-loading of the intrafusal fibres, which will shorten, and this will lead to a period of silence in the afferent discharge (Fig. 12.15). During this silence there will be no message being sent to the central nervous system about the state of the muscle. As

will be seen, one of the roles of the centrifugal control is to "fill-in" this silence.

Actions of Gamma-motoneurons

Activation of the fusimotor fibres alters the sensitivity of the muscle spindle receptors. As shown in Fig. 12.16, the static and dynamic fusimotor fibres have different effects on the discharges of the primary endings. Fusimotor stimulation causes contraction of the intrafusal muscle, static fibre activation causing an increase in the signal coding for muscle length and dynamic fibre activation causing a preferential increase in the discharge during active stretch.

As mentioned above, one role for the fusimotor fibres is to "fill in" the silence that would otherwise occur during active contraction produced by activation of the extrafusal fibres (see Fig. 12.15). In fact, it appears that during the majority of voluntary movements both alpha- and gamma-motoneurons are caused to fire

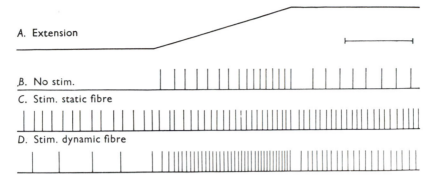

Fig. 12.16. Effects of stimulating static and dynamic fusimotor fibres on the responses recorded from a muscle spindle primary ending to stretching the muscle. In the absence of fusimotor stimulation (record *B*) the primary ending responds with an increasing discharge during stretching and settles down to a steady response after the stretch has reached its final value. Stimulation of a single static fusimotor fibre (record *C*) leads to an increased discharge during the steady phases of stretch with little effect during active extension. Stimulation of a single dynamic fusimotor fibre (record *D*) has relatively little effect on the discharges at constant length but results in a marked increase in the response during active stretching. (Reproduced with permission from Crowe and Matthews 1964.)

simultaneously (leading to co-contraction of extra- and intrafusal muscle fibres), preventing this unfortunate possibility that the muscle spindles might be silenced. Such a mechanism would be especially important if, during a muscle contraction, an unexpected load were encountered. Such a load would lead to the slowing of extrafusal muscle contraction but, with the gamma co-activation, the intrafusal fibres would continue to shorten and would stretch the sensory endings, thereby increasing the afferent discharge from the spindles. This increased afferent discharge would reflexly increase the discharge of the alpha-motoneurons (through various spinal reflex mechanisms; see, for example, Chaps. 11 and 13) and overcome the opposition to movement.

Summary

1.   Sense organs, or sensory receptors, transduce energy from one form (the stimulus) to another that can be handled by the nervous system. The transduction process results in a potential change (receptor potential) within the sensory receptor cell. Receptor potentials may be depolarizing or hyperpolarizing.

2.   Sensory receptors are highly specific for the forms of energy to which they respond – they show modality specificity. Thus, there are mechanoreceptors, thermoreceptors, photoreceptors, and chemoreceptors etc., with further specialization within each group.

3.   Receptor potentials are caused by the opening or closing of ion channels by the adequate stimulus for the sense organ. These ion channels are gated by the adequate stimulus.

4.   Sense organs may be classed as rapidly or slowly adapting according to whether they respond essentially only to rate of change of a stimulus or to a steady maintained stimulus, respectively. The adaptation process may be a property of the receptor cell itself or of the tissues surrounding the receptor cell.

5.   The intensity of a stimulus is encoded in the frequency of discharge of nerve impulses carried by the afferent nerve fibre that innervates the sensory receptor.

6.   Many sensory receptors receive an innervation from the central nervous system that can control the sensitivity of the receptor. This centrifugal control is important in setting the sense organ sensitivity in the light of prevailing stimuli and also allowing sense organs to function in the face of self-imposed alterations in the working conditions of sense organs, e.g. such as might be caused by muscle contraction.

13 Functional Organization in Groups of Neurons

So far, the properties of single neurons and transmission between pairs of neurons have dominated the discussion. Elementary consideration has been given to the stretch reflex in Chapter 11 (with some detail of transmission in the pathway in Chapter 10 and of the workings of the muscle spindle in Chapter 12) and some aspects of neuronal group organization in Chapter 11. It is now time to examine how the interconnexion of excitatory and inhibitory neurons leads to the emergence of particular operating characteristics of nervous systems and how such interconnexions of groups of neurons in a modular fashion form the basis of much nervous system organization.

Properties of Small Neuronal Circuits

In unicellular (or acellular) organisms responses to the environment are generally straightforward, such as taxis towards or away from external stimuli. Even in such organisms, however, more complex behaviour like the gradual reduction in a response to repeated stimuli (habituation and/or fatigue) can often be observed. Multicellular organisms with nervous systems, however, are capable of diverse forms of behaviour which are due, essentially, to nervous system organization and function.

The Two-Neuron Reflex Arc

Consider a system such as that depicted in Fig. 13.1a, consisting of a sensory receptor (R) and an effector cell (E), which could be either a muscle cell or a gland cell, and with the sensory and effector cells connected by two neurons. Assume also that all interactions between these four elements are excitatory, that is, stimulation of the receptor leads to excitation in the first (or afferent) neuron. The afferent neuron has excitatory actions on the second (or efferent) neuron and the efferent neuron, in turn, excites the effector cell causing it either to contract, if a muscle cell, or to secrete, if a gland cell. What properties might such a simple system express?

If the sensory receptor is specific for some adequate stimulus and responds only to one form of energy (say mechanical rather than thermal, chemical, or light energy) then the system will display specificity of response. The system depicted in Fig. 13.1 will also show specificity of effect since the efferent neuron is connected to a single effector. Because of the anatomical arrangement of this simple reflex arc the effector will only be caused to contract or secrete if the particular receptor of the arc is excited. That is, the reflex displays local sign. This phenomenon may be better appreciated if a set of similar sensory receptors on a receptor sheet is considered, as in Fig. 13.1b. Here each member of a set of receptors is connected, via a two-neuron arc, to one of

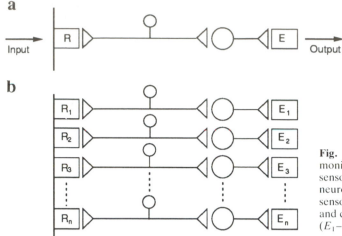

Fig. 13.1a,b. The two-neuron reflex arc. a Sensory input is monitored by the sensory receptor (R), transmitted to the sensory (afferent) neuron and then to the motor (efferent) neuron, which, in turn excites the effector cell (E). b The sensory receptors (R_1–R_n) are located in a sheet of tissue and connected, by sets of neuron pairs, to a set of effectors (E_1–E_n).

a set of effectors. A particular effector will only be excited if a particular sense organ has been stimulated. This simple example stresses just how important are the anatomical connexions within the nervous system. Sense organs are often organized in sheets (the retina, in the skin, etc.) and well-ordered connexions form the basis for the nervous system's ability to localize a stimulus.

Other important properties of this simple two-neuron arc depend on the efficacy of each of the junctions (synapses) between the four elements. If each synapse transmits in a one-to-one fashion, then once an above-threshold stimulus has acted on the receptor the system will operate to cause excitation of the effector cell. Such one-to-one operation is the exception rather than the rule in real nervous systems. One-to-one transmission occurs between motor nerve fibres and skeletal muscle in vertebrates and also in certain reflex arcs that control escape reactions to potentially damaging stimuli, for example the giant fibre systems of annelids and arthropods. At most synapses, especially where chemical transmission takes place, a single impulse in one neuron will evoke a subthreshold excitatory postsynaptic potential (EPSP) in its target neuron. In order to cause the postsynaptic neuron to fire an action potential a series of impulses in the presynaptic neuron is required. This phenomenon is known as temporal summation. Usually activation of a sensory receptor will lead to the initiation of a train of impulses in the afferent neuron and temporal summation occurs at the synapses between the afferent and efferent neuron.

The efficacy of transmission between two neurons at any time also depends on the previous history of the system. Since transmitter release depends on the free calcium level in the nerve

terminals and depolarization produced by the nerve impulse opens voltage-sensitive calcium channels (see Chap. 6), a train of impulses may lead to a build-up of calcium and each succeeding impulse may lead to more transmitter being released and therefore to successively greater postsynaptic actions. This phenomenon is known as post-tetanic potentiation and may be considered as a simple form of learning. Alternatively, successive responses may become smaller (show decrement). This may be due to a variety of causes, including reduction in the availability of transmitter for release if the pool of readily available transmitter is severely restricted, a shutting of the voltage-sensitive calcium channels in the presynaptic terminals, or interference with the ability of the postsynaptic transmitter receptors to combine with transmitter, perhaps due to them being already occupied by transmitter.

Convergence and Divergence Within the Two-Neuron Arc

A reflex arc consisting of just two neurons is an abstraction, useful for discussion, which does not exist in nature. Even in those systems, such as the reflex arc underlying the monosynaptic myotatic reflex in mammals, many neurons are involved. Thus a single efferent neuron is usually excited by more than one afferent neuron, and usually by many. This is shown in the diagram of Fig. 13.2a, where a number of afferent neurons, each innervating a sense organ located at a different place on the receptor sheet, converge onto a single efferent neuron. This convergence is a very common principle of organization in the nervous system. If forms the anatomical basis for

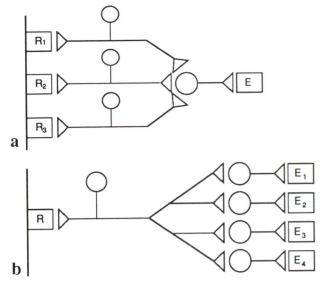

Fig. 13.2. **a** Convergence in a two-neuron reflex arc. **b** Divergence in a two-neuron reflex arc. (Labelling as in Fig. 13.1.)

a number of possible functional properties. For example, since activity in a single presynaptic neuron may be insufficient to cause the postsynaptic neuron to fire, the simultaneous activity of a number of presynaptic excitatory neurons can overcome this problem and raise the postsynaptic neuron's membrane potential above firing threshold. This phenomenon is known as spatial summation (or facilitation). Another possible outcome of convergence is heterosynaptic facilitation, where activity at one set of synapses between a presynaptic and a postsynaptic neuron leads to facilitation between another presynaptic neuron and the same postsynaptic neuron.

Another common anatomical arrangement is shown in Fig. 13.2b, where a single neuron sends axonal terminals to many postsynaptic neurons. This organization is called divergence. Obviously it leads to a single afferent neuron being able directly to influence a large number of other neurons and can be looked upon as a form of amplification of the afferent signals.

A considerable degree of both convergence and divergence is found between neurons in reflex arcs, and in ascending and descending relays in sensory and motor subsystems etc. At first sight such an arrangement may seem to negate an advantage noted above for the simple two-neuron pathways described earlier, that is, the ability to localize the site of a stimulus. The nervous system overcomes this problem in other ways, such as by the use of inhibition (see below

and Chap. 15). Also, the efficacy of the excitatory connexions between different neurons can be weighted, for example, by the numbers of synapses made between a pair of neurons, by the location of the synapses on the postsynaptic neuron, by the amount of transmitter released, by the amount of ionic current injected at the postsynaptic membrane, by the presence of dendritic impulses and so on.

Addition of Interneurons to the Two-Neuron Arc

Both excitatory and inhibitory interneurons may be found added on to the two-neuron arc (Fig. 13.3). Excitatory neurons intercalated between the afferent and efferent neuron, in addition to the monosynaptic excitatory connexions, are commonly found in both spinal reflex pathways and also in sensory pathways. Organization of this type has already been discussed (Chap. 11) for the hair follicle afferent fibre – spinocervical tract neuron circuit and is also found in the Ia afferent fibre – alpha-motoneuron reflex arc (see below). The addition of this excitatory interneuron (Fig. 13.3a) may have several effects:

1. It may lead to amplification of the response, as exemplified in the hair follicle afferent – spinocervical tract neuron system.

2. It adds an additional synaptic delay into the circuit so that the early monosynaptic EPSP is followed by later EPSP components, especially if the intercalated neuron fires repetitively to the afferent input, and in this way it will prolong the firing of the target neuron; in other words, it will increase the temporal facilitation in the system and also make post-tetanic potentiation more likely.

3. With appropriate connexions there may be increased divergence of the input, and, for some systems, connexions onto neurons that do not receive the monosynaptic excitation from the first neuron.

An inhibitory interneuron may be interposed in the same way. Here the action may be to terminate the excitatory effects of the monosynaptic excitation. Commonly the inhibitory interneuron is intercalated between the pre- and postsynaptic neurons such that neurons not excited monosynaptically are inhibited (Fig. 13.3b). Such an arrangement can form the basis of lateral (or surround) inhibition, commonly observed in sensory pathways (see below). As

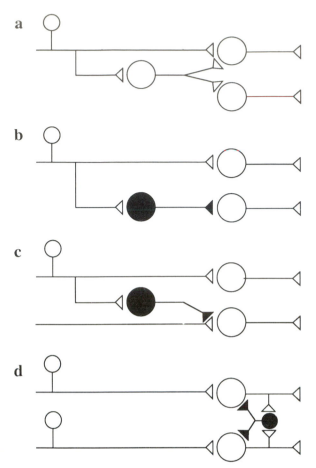

Fig. 13.3. a The addition of an excitatory interneuron to the two-neuron reflex arc. **b** The addition of an inhibitory inter-neuron to the two-neuron arc. The neuron acts postsynaptic-ally on the motoneuron. **c** The addition of an inhibitory interneuron to the arc. The interneuron acts presynaptically on the terminals of the afferent neuron. **d** The addition of an inhibitory interneuron to the arc – feed-back inhibition.

which, in turn, inhibits motoneurons post-synaptically (see Fig. 13.7). A similar arrange-ment of neurons can also give rise to lateral (or surround) inhibition in sensory systems.

It is instructive to consider the differences between feed-forward and feed-back. In feed-forward systems there is usually one set of synapses fewer than in feed-back systems, and so the effects will have a shorter latency (other things being equal). More importantly, feed-forward actions are dependent on the input to the system, whereas feed-back actions are de-pendent on the output from the system.

Further additions of interneurons, both excita-tory and inhibitory, to these simple circuits will increase the possibilities for temporal and spatial facilitation, for convergence and divergence and so on. One special set of connexions produces interesting effects. If a pair of neurons is inter-calated, with the first being an inhibitory neuron and the second either an inhibitory or an excita-tory neuron, the phenomena of disinhibition and disfacilitation may be seen. Disinhibition is the removal of inhibition by inhibiting the inhibitory interneuron and operationally has an excitatory (facilitatory) effect. Disfacilitation, likewise, is the removal of excitation and has an inhibitory effect.

Segmental Motor Apparatus – An Example of the Operation of Small Groups of Neurons

Spinal Monosynaptic Reflex

The monosynaptic excitatory connexions between the Ia afferent fibres from the primary (annulo-spiral) endings of muscle spindles and the alpha-motoneurons are responsible for much of the mechanism underlying tendon jerks (useful clini-cal tests of the function of reflexes etc.) and the stretch reflex. Stretch of a muscle, especially an antigravity muscle, leads to a reflex contraction of that muscle that opposes the stretch. Such stretch reflexes are prominent in animal prepara-tions in which the forebrain has been removed by decerebration. There are two components to the stretch reflex: a phasic component, which is short-lasting (and exemplified by the tendon jerks), and a tonic component, which lasts longer.

The anatomy of the connexions between Ia afferent fibres and motoneurons and the physio-

shown in Fig. 13.3c, the interneuron may act on the terminals of the presynaptic neuron pro-ducing, for example, presynaptic inhibition and thereby reducing the effects of the presynaptic neuron on the postsynaptic one.

These examples of interneurons located on the pathways afferent to a neuron are instances of feed-forward excitation and inhibition, res-pectively. Feed-back from the postsynaptic cell may also take place if the interneuron is inter-calated between the postsynaptic cell and either other postsynaptic cells or the presynaptic cell (Fig. 13.3d). The classic example of feed-back inhibition is in the Ia afferent – motoneuron reflex arc. The axon of the motoneuron gives off branches shortly after its origin and these excite an inhibitory interneuron (the Renshaw cell)

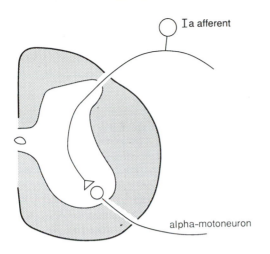

Fig. 13.4. The two-neuron arc in the spinal cord – the basis for the monosynaptic (myotatic) reflex.

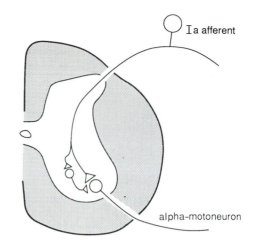

Fig. 13.5. The addition of an excitatory interneuron to the two-neuron arc.

logy of transmission between them have been discussed in some detail in Chapters 10, 11 and 12. Here it is sufficient to summarize this by reference to Fig. 13.4 and to remember that the Ia afferent fibre from each muscle spindle in a particular muscle will make excitatory connexions with nearly every (about 90%) alpha-motoneuron that innervates the same muscle. Each Ia fibre forms a small number of synapses (about two to five) with every motoneuron it contacts: thus the system shows divergence. Also, each motoneuron receives excitatory connexions from nearly every Ia fibre from the same muscle: the system shows convergence. In addition to these connexions between the Ia afferent fibres from a muscle and the alpha-motoneurons of the same (the homonymous) muscle, Ia afferent fibres make monosynaptic excitatory connexions with other motoneurons (heteronymous motoneurons) that innervate muscles having a similar action around a joint (the synergist muscles). Thus there is greater convergence and divergence. It is possible to calculate the probable number of Ia synaptic boutons received by a single motoneuron. Thus, for the triceps surae muscle group of the cat there are about 153 muscle spindles (35 in lateral gastrocnemius, 62 in medial gastrocnemius and 56 in soleus), and each spindle may be assumed to have a single Ia afferent fibre. With projection ratios from Ia afferent to motoneurons of about 90% for the homonymous motoneurons and about 60% for the heteronymous motoneurons and with each Ia fibre giving between two and four contacts to each motoneuron, then each triceps motoneuron will receive between 200 and 450 contacts from triceps Ia afferent fibres. There

are about 750 triceps alpha-motoneurons, and with the above projection ratios this means that between 450 and 500 will receive monosynaptic excitation from a single triceps Ia afferent fibre. Thus the divergence ratio, from a single Ia afferent to motoneurons, is of the order of 1:500, and the convergence ratio from Ia afferent fibres onto a single motoneuron is of the order of 100:1 for this particular muscle group.

Excitatory Interneurons Intercalated in the Monosynaptic Reflex Pathway

It has become obvious in recent years that Ia afferent fibre connexions to motoneurons are not limited to the monosynaptic ones described above. In addition, there are excitatory interneurons interposed between the Ia afferent fibre and the motoneuron (Fig. 13.5). A particular group of such interneurons is located several segments rostral (towards the head) of the appropriate hind limb motoneurons in the cat. Activation via this route will excite the motoneurons at a later time than via the monosynaptic connexions and will provide for the possibility of temporal facilitation. This is an example of feed-forward facilitation.

Feed-forward Inhibition in the Monosynaptic Reflex Pathway

Transmission between the Ia afferent fibres and their target motoneurons is under a feed-forward inhibitory control using presynaptic inhibition.

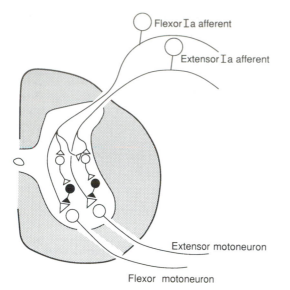

Fig. 13.6. The addition of presynaptic inhibition to the monosynaptic reflex arc. The terminals of Ia afferent fibres from both flexor and extensor muscles receive presynaptic inhibition. Flexor Ia afferent fibres are more effective at producing this action.

As shown in Fig. 8.12, the monosynaptically evoked Ia EPSP in a motoneuron can be reduced by previous activity in other afferent fibres. This reduction in the size of the EPSP is due to presynaptic inhibition of the Ia afferent fibres. It has been proposed, by Eccles and his colleagues, that the interneurons involved consist of a chain of at least two neurons, an excitatory interneuron and the inhibitory neuron responsible for forming the axo-axonic contacts upon the Ia terminals (Fig. 13.6). Analysis of the presynaptic inhibition of Ia afferent fibres reveals that it can be elicited by activity in both group Ia afferent fibres from the primary endings of muscle spindles and also the Ib afferent fibres from the Golgi tendon organs and that both Ia and Ib fibres from flexor and extensor muscles are effective, those from flexor muscles being especially effective.

Feed-back Inhibition in the Monosynaptic Reflex Pathway

Feed-back inhibition in this reflex arc is carried out by a special interneuron, the Renshaw cell, named after its discoverer. Renshaw cells are excited by collateral branches of alpha-motoneurons and, in turn, inhibit motoneurons, including those that provided the excitatory input (Fig. 13.7). The Renshaw cells produce postsynaptic inhibition of their target neurons.

The activity of this recurrent inhibitory pathway is a true feed-back inhibition, since the strength of the inhibition produced is directly dependent on the strength of motoneuronal firing. Recurrent inhibition will tend to keep down the rate of motoneuronal firing and also, since the connexions of the Renshaw cells are such as to provide strong inhibition of neighbouring motoneurons, will lead to a relatively greater output from those motoneurons that are firing the strongest. In other words, recurrent inhibition will highlight the action of the most strongly activated motoneurons at the expense of those less strongly activated. This is a form of lateral inhibition.

It would be a mistake, however, to consider the Renshaw cell simply in the context of recurrent inhibition. Other factors must be taken into account. Thus, excitatory inputs to Renshaw cells come from many diverse sources, such as cutaneous nerves responding to noxious stimuli and to various systems descending from the brain. Furthermore, an important target for Renshaw cell inhibitory action is another inhibitory interneuron, that intercalated between Ia afferent fibres and motoneurons of antagonistic muscles (Fig. 13.8). In this case the action of the Renshaw cell is to inhibit another inhibitory pathway, thus producing disinhibition of the Ia actions on antagonistic motoneurons. Thus when a pool of motoneurons is caused to fire, activity will be evoked in the Renshaw cells leading to recurrent inhibition of that pool of motoneurons (and in motoneurons to synergist muscles), while there will be a concomitant disinhibition of antagonistic muscles. Thus, the Renshaw cells may be con-

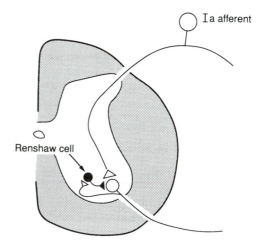

Fig. 13.7. Feed-back inhibition in the spinal cord. Recurrent collateral axons from the motoneuron excite Renshaw cells, which, in turn, produce postsynaptic inhibition of the motoneurons.

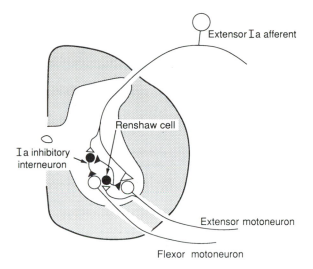

Fig. 13.8. Reciprocal inhibition in the spinal cord. An extensor Ia afferent fibre excites motoneurons innervating the muscle containing the muscle spindles from which the Ia afferent comes (and also motoneurons innervating synergist muscles). The Ia afferent also excites an inhibitory interneuron that inhibits antagonistic motoneurons – this is reciprocal inhibition. The Renshaw cell, activated by feed-back from the extensor motoneuron, also inhibits the inhibitory interneuron, thus disinhibiting the reciprocal inhibition.

sidered as limiting the duration and magnitude of Ia afferent fibre evoked actions, both direct actions on homonymous and heteronymous motoneurons and also their actions via inhibitory interneurons on antagonist motoneurons.

Reciprocal Inhibition of Motoneurons from Ia Afferent Fibres

In many motor acts, for example stepping, contraction of one set of muscles around a joint, such as the extensors, is accompanied by relaxation of their antagonists (flexors in this case). The underlying neuronal organization for this is shown in Fig. 13.8. Ia afferent fibres from the primary endings of muscle spindles make excitatory connexions with a set of interneurons that inhibit, postsynaptically, the antagonist motoneurons. This Ia inhibitory pathway is therefore disynaptic.

As mentioned above, the Ia inhibitory neuron is itself inhibited by Renshaw cells activated by motoneurons excited monosynaptically by the same Ia afferent fibres that excite the Ia inhibitory interneurons. In fact, this Renshaw cell inhibition of the Ia inhibitory interneurons is an important experimental criterion for identification of the Ia inhibitory neuron.

Group II Afferent Fibres from Spindle Secondary Endings and the Monosynaptic Reflex Arc

In addition to the Ia afferent fibres from primary (annulospiral) endings of muscle spindles there is a second category of sensory ending in the muscle spindle innervated by slightly finer afferent fibres conducting in the Group II range of conduction velocities (24–72 m/s in the cat). Spindle secondary endings are mainly sensitive to the length of the spindle (muscle) and have little dynamic component in their discharge. The central connexions of these Group II afferent fibres are not as well worked out as are those for Group Ia afferents, but it has been shown that Group II fibres from spindle secondary endings, like Ia afferent fibres, make monosynaptic excitatory connexions with motoneurons, albeit much more weakly. Furthermore, Group II afferent fibres provide excitatory input to motoneurons via excitatory interneurons. These pathways are indicated in Fig. 13.9. The likely role of Group II afferent fibres from spindle secondary endings was suggested by Matthews as early as 1969, on the basis of the observations that (1) maximal activation of Ia fibres (produced by vibrating the muscle) often evoked a reflex contraction in the muscle that was less than the response to stretch, and (2) during a muscle response to vibration that should have activated all Ia fibres maximally an additional contraction to a superimposed stretch could be elicited. Thus the inputs from Group II afferent fibres from muscle spindle secondary endings are arranged in parallel to those from the Group Ia fibres from the primary

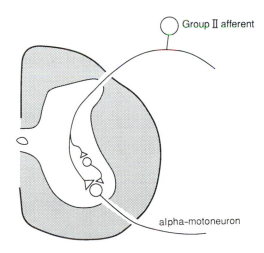

Fig. 13.9. Pathways to motoneurons from Group II afferent fibres innervating the secondary endings of muscle spindles.

endings and have similar actions on their target
motoneurons, both directly and indirectly. The
Group II fibres provide an important excitatory
drive to the tonic component of the stretch reflex.

Reflex Actions of Group Ib Afferent Fibres from Golgi Tendon Organs

The Golgi tendon organs are mechanoreceptors
in the tendinous insertions of muscles that are
innervated by large afferent fibres conducting
impulses in the Group I range (70–120 m/s in the
cat). Activation of these afferent fibres leads to a
disynaptic postsynaptic inhibition of the homonymous and heteronymous muscles and an excitation of their antagonists (Fig. 13.10). On face
value this seems to be the reverse of the actions
of Ia fibres, and indeed their action was termed
the inverse myotatic reflex initially, but this is a
misnomer, since the Golgi tendon organ measures
muscle tension and not length (unlike the spindle).

It was originally thought that the reflex inhibition of muscle produced by tendon organ activation was a protective reflex to prevent excessive
tension being built up in the muscle (Sherrington's "clasp-knife reflex"). However, recent work
has shown that tendon organs are low-threshold
mechanoreceptors which probably inform the
central nervous system of the tension in the
muscle and have a regulatory, rather than
emergency, role to play in motor mechanisms.
The inhibitory interneurons excited by Ib afferent
fibres also receive excitation from cutaneous and
joint receptors, and it is reasonable to suppose

that if a movement meets an obstacle then
excitation of these receptors would occur and
facilitate the Ib inhibition produced by increased
muscle tension as a result of the impediment to
movement.

Flexion Reflex and Crossed Extension Reflex

Many other reflexes (and their underlying neuronal organization) have been described, but it
does not seem relevant to discuss them in the
present context. One set of reflexes, however,
does call for comment. This is the protective
reflex set in play by noxious stimuli. If a harmful,
or potentially harmful, stimulus impinges on a
limb, then that limb is immediately withdrawn.
Usually such withdrawal involves flexion of the
limb, although the initial position of the limb and
the location of the noxious stimulus might lead
to a protective extension. This flexion reflex over-
rides other reflexes – it is imperative that the
limb be removed out of harm's way. Concomitant
with flexion of the limb to which the noxious
stimulus has been applied there is an extension
of the contralateral limb, the crossed extension
reflex. Crossed extension is a necessary postural
adjustment to prevent an animal falling as a result
of sudden flexion of one limb.

The neuronal circuitry underlying these reflex
actions is shown in Fig. 13.11. The afferent limb
of the reflex consists of fibres innervating nocireceptors of skin, subcutaneous tissue and muscle.
These afferent fibres are of smaller diameter than
those considered above. They include the smallest myelinated fibres and the non-myelinated
fibres with a total conduction velocity range of
from less than 1 m/s to about 10 m/s.

Gamma-motoneurons and the Control of Muscle Spindle Sensitivity

As has been discussed in Chapter 12, the muscle
spindle is under centrifugal control from the
central nervous system by the actions of the
gamma-motoneurons on the intrafusal muscle
fibres. Contraction of the intrafusal fibres,
brought about by activity in the gamma-
motoneurons, will obviously affect the functioning
of the muscle spindle sense organs. There are
two main types of gamma-motoneurons, the static
and the dynamic gamma-motoneurons. Their
actions on the response of a primary afferent
fibre from the muscle spindle is shown in Fig.
12.16. Briefly, the static gamma fibre increases

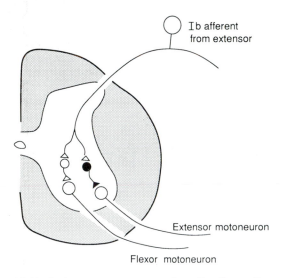

Fig. 13.10. Pathways to motoneurons from Ib afferent fibres innervating the Golgi tendon organs.

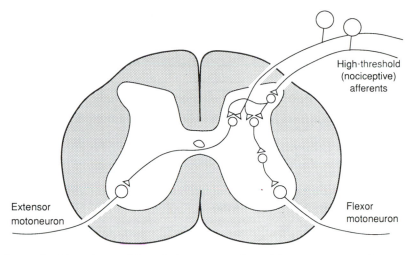

High-threshold
(nociceptive)
afferents

Extensor
motoneuron

Flexor
motoneuron

Fig. 13.11. Pathways responsible for the flexion and crossed extension reflexes.

the static sensitivity and the dynamic fibre increases both the static and dynamic sensitivities of the primary ending. The secondary endings of muscle spindles are influenced almost exclusively by the static gamma-motoneurons.

What are the roles of the gamma-motoneurons? It might be thought that activity in these neurons could be responsible for initiating movement, since their activation would lead to shortening of the spindle with consequent excitation of spindle primary, and secondary, afferent fibres and then the excitation of alpha-motoneurons that would lead to contraction of extrafusal muscle fibres. No clear evidence that this takes place has been found. Rather, as described in Chapter 12, the gamma system seems to have a role in loading the spindles during active muscle contraction when the extrafusal fibre shortening might be expected to "off-load" the spindle to the point where no sensory excitation would exist. Such loading of the spindles allows the system to remain responsive to changes in muscle length even when the muscle is shortening. This role is essentially a function of the static gamma-motoneurons. When voluntary movements are initiated, both the alpha- and the gamma-motoneurons fire together (co-activation of alpha- and gamma-motoneurons). This has been observed by direct recording from single motor nerve fibres in human subjects, and the gamma firing prevents off-loading of the spindles caused by muscle shortening.

Other Influences on the Segmental Motor Apparatus

The above description of the segmental motor apparatus is necessarily sketchy. It may be considered, however, that this apparatus exists at each segmental level in the spinal cord. Obviously the segmental apparatus does not exist in isolation. There is a need, in order to produce limb-to-limb co-ordination of movement, that the segmental apparatus for hind limb control is connected to that for fore limb control. Rather little is known of the mechanisms underlying this. Furthermore, it is obvious that control of the segmental apparatus from the brain must be of overriding importance, and there are many descending pathways that influence motoneurons (both alpha and gamma) directly or indirectly. Finally, there is a need for brain systems concerned with movement and posture not only to receive direct notice of the state of muscle and joint sense organs etc., but also to be informed about the state of the segmental motor apparatus itself. Thus there are many ascending (centripetal) and descending (centrifugal) connexions between the segmental apparatus and the various brain regions concerned with posture and movement. Some principles of the organization of these motor subsystems will be discussed in the next two chapters.

The Modular Design of Nervous Systems

In his important textbook, *Neurological Anatomy in Relation to Clinical Medicine*, Brodal (1981) enunciates three principles:

1.   There is an extremely high degree of order in the anatomical organization of the central nervous system.

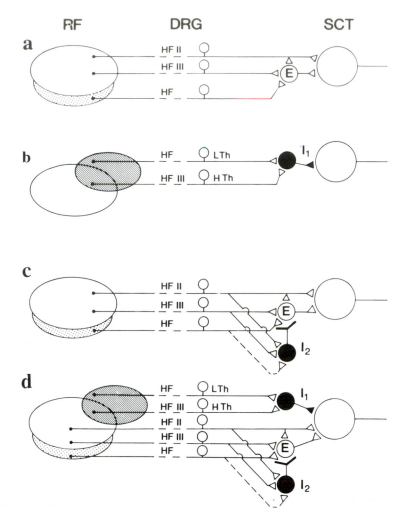

Fig. 13.12a–d. Modular neuronal organization in a sensory system. The diagrams indicate the probable neuronal organization of pathways afferent to spinocervical tract neurons. **a** Excitatory pathways from hair receptors within the excitatory receptive field. **b** Pathways mediating postsynaptic inhibition. **c** The post-excitatory inhibitory pathways from the excitatory receptive field. **d** The sum of **a–c**. *RF*, spinocervical cell receptive field; *DRG*, dorsal root ganglion; *SCT*, spinocervical neuron; *E*, excitatory interneuron; *I*, inhibitory interneurons; *HF*, hair follicle afferent fibre; *LT*, low-threshold mechanoreceptive afferent fibre; *HT*, high-threshold (nociceptive) afferent fibre; *II, III*, Groups II and III afferent fibres. The *cross-hatched area* represents the inhibitory receptive field, the *stippled area* the subliminal fringe from which EPSPs can be evoked; the *open elipse* represents the excitatory receptive field. (Reproduced with permission from Brown et al. 1987b.)

2. The nervous system is composed of a multitude of minor units, each with its specific finer intrinsic organization as well as with its connexions with other units, and there are therefore as many specific functional units as structural ones.

3. Investigation of the structure of the nervous system in all its detail is a prerequisite for progress in studies of its function.

The reader will already have realized just how important the order in neuronal connectivity is,

at both the level of inputs to individual neurons and within neuronal circuits. Also, a number of examples of the "minor units", henceforth called modules, have been described. It is now useful to consider these modules and the modular design of the nervous system in more detail.

Modular Design in the Spinal Cord

The segmental motor apparatus described above is a good example of the modular design of nervous systems. Thus, in Figs. 13.4–13.11, which are abstractions from experimental data, each motoneuron represents a set of motoneurons, each interneuron represents a set of interneurons and each afferent fibre represents a set of afferent fibres. These sets of afferent neurons, interneurons and motoneurons form the modules of the segmental apparatus and are present throughout the length of the spinal cord. Thus, with very few exceptions, what is true for the neuronal organization of afferent fibres from, say, triceps surae muscles and the reflex pathways to motoneurons of the same muscles (and their synergists) and their antagonists is also true for any other muscle of the hind limb or of the fore limb.

There are many other examples of modular design in the spinal cord that do not include pathways to motoneurons. One of these was touched on in Chapter 11 – the module that includes hair follicle afferent fibres, neurons of the spinocervical tract (SCT) and various intercalated neurons between primary afferent fibres and the SCT cells. We have already seen that excitation of a single hair follicle afferent leads to both monosynaptic and polysynaptic EPSPs in SCT neurons. In addition, however, the excitation is followed by a depression of transmission through the system, and the evidence indicates that this is likely to be due to inhibition acting at the excitatory interneurons or on the primary afferent terminals ending on these interneurons. The probable circuitry is shown in Fig. 13.12. Since there are about 3000 SCT neurons on each side of the spinal cord (in the cat) and all but a few (10% or less) appear to have a similar organization of their inputs, then it is necessary to consider the connexions between hair follicle afferent fibres and SCT neurons to be organized in this modular fashion.

Modular Design of the Cerebellum

The cerebellum (Box 13.1) is a most interesting component of the brain of vertebrates, containing an immense number of neurons and having its outer part (the cerebellar cortex) organized in a very regular fashion. Its roles include control of movement and posture, and it appears to do this by affecting the other major motor systems of the brain, that is, it does not affect the segmental motor system directly but rather acts indirectly by adjusting other motor control signals.

BOX 13.1

STRUCTURE OF THE CEREBELLUM

The cerebellum lies below and behind the cerebrum (Fig. 13.Aa). From medial to lateral it consists of three main parts, the vermis, the pars intermedia and the hemispheres (Fig. 13.Ab), and from front to back it is divided into a series of lobes; the primary fissure separates the anterior and posterior lobes and the posteriolateral fissure separates the posterior and flocculonodular lobes.

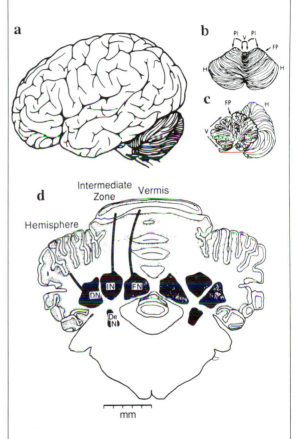

Fig. 13.Aa–d. Parts of the human cerebrum and cerebellum. **a** Cerebrum and cerebellum in position. **b.c** The cerebellum on the same scale, from the dorsal aspect (**b**) and after a sagittal section in the midline (**c**). **d** Drawing of a transverse section through the cerebellum and cerebellar nuclei together with the lines of projection from the vermis, intermediate zone and hemisphere to the respective nuclei. *V*, vermis; *Pl*, intermediate zone; *H*, hemisphere; *FP*, primary fissure; *FN*, fastigial nucleus; *IN*, interpositus nucleus; *DN*, dentate nucleus. (Reproduced with permission from McGeer et al. 1978.)

Continued

Continued

Shallower fissures divide each lobe into a number of lobules. The lobes and lobules are arranged like the branches of a tree when seen in sagittal section (Fig. 13.Ac). On the surface of each branch are a large number of folia producing an enormous expansion of the cerebellar surface (cortex).

The outer part of the cerebellum, the cerebellar cortex, is connected to the deep cerebellar nuclei (the fastial, interpositus and dentate nuclei) by efferent fibres which are the axons of one particular set of cortical neurons – the Purkinje cells (see Fig. 13.13), which are inhibitory neurons. Afferent fibres to the cerebellar cortex are of two types – climbing fibres from the inferior olivary nucleus in the medulla and mossy fibres from a variety of brain stem nuclei and the spinal cord.

The cerebellum consists of an outer region, the cortex, an innermost region, the deep cerebellar nuclei, and a region containing only nerve fibres interposed between these two (and containing fibres afferent to the cortex in addition to connexions between the deep nuclei and cortex in both directions). Afferent fibres from peripheral sense organs, the brain stem and the cerebral cortex project to both the cerebellar cortex and the deep nuclei; the cerebellar cortex projects to the deep nuclei. Thus the deep nuclei may compare the afferent signals reaching them directly with the same signals after processing in the cerebellar cortex.

The cerebellar cortex is remarkable in the regularity of its organization, consisting of an almost crystalline structure of repeated neuronal elements (modules). This regularity suggests that the neuronal operations performed by the cerebellar cortical modules are all similar. Furthermore, an additional remarkable fact about the cerebellar cortex is that all but one of its intrinsic neurons, of which there are four main types, are inhibitory neurons, and the only cell that has an axon leaving the cortex (the Purkinje cell) is also an inhibitory neuron. The output of the cerebellar cortex is inhibitory and whatever operations are performed by the cerebellar cortex are converted into inhibitory action on the target cells of the Purkinje axons.

Cerebellar Cortical Module

The cerebellar cortex is a much folded and fissured structure; the basic subdivision being the folium. The neuronal organization of the cerebellar cortex is shown in Fig. 13.13. The cortex is divided into three distinct layers, the outer molecular layer consisting mainly of the axons of granule cells whose cell bodies are located in the innermost granular layer. The axons of these granule cells ascend to the granular layer, where they bifurcate and (now known as parallel fibres) run in the long axis of the folium at right angles to the dendrites of the Purkinje cells, which have their cell bodies in the middle layer, the Purkinje cell layer. The molecular layer also contains local interneurons, the basket and stellate cells. The basket cells send their axons to the Purkinje cell layer, where they end at and near the initial segments of Purkinje cells at some distance away from the basket cell body in the transverse plane of the folium. As mentioned above, the Purkinje cell layer contains the cell bodies of the Purkinje cells. The axons of Purkinje cells descend through the cortex to the deep nuclei (and also to the vestibular nuclei of the brain stem) and form the only output of the cortex. Deep to the Purkinje cell layer is the granular layer, containing the cell bodies of the granule cells and also a small number of Golgi cells.

The afferent nerve supply to the cerebellar cortex is from two systems of excitatory fibres. These are the mossy fibres and the climbing fibres. Mossy fibres arise from the spinal cord and a variety of brain stem nuclei that in turn receive input from the cerebral cortex and the spinal cord. Mossy fibres enter the cerebellum, give branches to the deep cerebellar nuclei and then proceed to the cerebellar cortex, where they form synapses with the dendrites of the granule cells in special synaptic arrangements called cerebellar glomeruli. From the granule cells the input is conveyed to the Purkinje cells via the parallel fibres. The parallel fibres, as they run along the axis of the folium contact the dendrites of a large number (several thousand) of Purkinje cells all lined up in the foliar axis. Each Purkinje cell receives excitation from a large number of parallel fibres (and therefore from a large number of granule cells); from as many as 200 000. The climbing fibre input is arranged quite differently: all climbing fibres originate from neurons in the inferior olivary nucleus in the medulla; each olivary neuron that projects to the cerebellum excites cells in the deep nuclei and then projects to the cerebellar cortex, where it terminates on

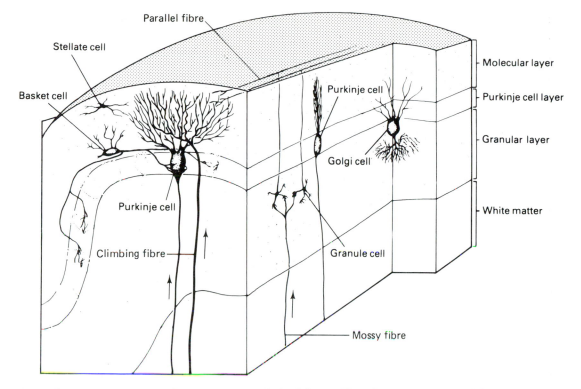

Fig. 13.13. Diagrammatic representation of part of a cerebellar folium to show the neuronal types and their locations and the courses and connexions of the nerve fibres. (Modified from Kandel and Schwartz 1985.)

very few Purkinje cells, about one to ten. Each Purkinje cell receives climbing fibre excitation from only a single climbing fibre, and the climbing fibre terminates on the Purkinje cell in a remarkable way – each climbing fibre makes numerous synaptic contacts with the soma and dendrites of the Purkinje cell (Fig. 13.13). The inferior olive receives its inputs mainly from the spinal cord, the motor cortex and the red nucleus.

Operation of the Cerebellar Cortical Circuitry. It is important to realize that the afferent fibres that excite neurons of the cerebellar cortex do so only after they have already excited neurons in the deep cerebellar nuclei (Fig. 13.14). The neuronal circuits through the deep cerebellar nuclei constitute the primary cerebellar circuits, and the circuits through the cerebellar cortex, activation of which leads to alterations in the firing of Purkinje

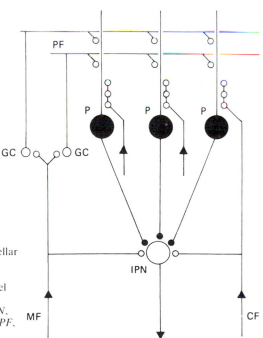

Fig. 13.14. Diagrammatic representation of the inputs to the cerebellar Purkinje cells and to the deep cerebellar nuclei. Excitatory and inhibitory neurons and synapses are represented by *open* and *filled* symbols, respectively. Basket cells (which receive input from parallel fibres) and Golgi cells (which receive input from parallel and mossy fibres) have been omitted. *CF*, climbing fibre; *GC*, granule cell; *IPN*, deep cerebellar nuclear neuron; *MF*, mossy fibre; *P*, Purkinje cell; *PF*, parallel fibre. (Reproduced with permission from Armstrong 1988.)

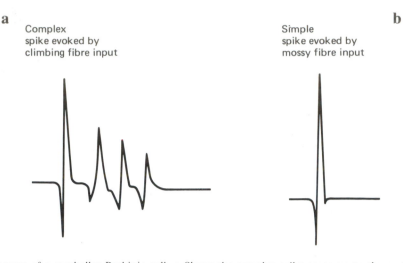

Fig. 13.15a,b. Responses of a cerebellar Purkinje cell. **a** Shows the complex spike response to the excitatory input from a climbing fibre. **b** Shows the simple spike response to the excitatory input from mossy fibres (via the parallel fibres from granule cells). (Modified from Kandel and Schwartz 1985.)

cells with subsequent inhibitory actions on the deep cerebellar nuclei, constitute the secondary cerebellar circuit. The secondary cerebellar circuit through the cerebellar cortex acts to modulate the primary circuit.

Activation of mossy fibre inputs leads, via the granule cells and their parallel fibre excitatory contacts with Purkinje cells, to the excitation of a long row of Purkinje cells. Mossy fibre inputs cause the Purkinje cells to discharge so-called simple spikes – impulses that are essentially similar to those of many other neurons, for example motoneurons (Fig. 13.15). It needs activity in many mossy fibres, and therefore many parallel fibres, to cause a Purkinje cell discharge, since the EPSPs evoked in Purkinje cells by parallel fibres are small. In contrast, a single climbing fibre has very powerful excitatory connexions with each Purkinje cell it contacts, through its many synapses with it, and a single action potential in a climbing fibre will lead to a high-frequency burst of impulses, the so-called complex spike (Fig. 13.15). As has been discussed (Chap. 9), the climbing fibre input to Purkinje cell dendrites is capable of eliciting active responses (dendritic impulses), and these, in turn, are responsible for the "complex spike" response originating at the initial segment region of the cell body and propagated down the axon. During normal movement mossy fibres fire at quite high rates and this leads to Purkinje cells firing simple spikes at about 50–100 Hz. In contrast, cells of the inferior olive, which give rise to the climbing fibres, fire at much lower rates (about 1 per second) and pro-

duce low-frequency firing of complex spikes by the Purkinje cell.

The parallel fibres excite basket and stellate cells in addition to Purkinje cells. The basket and stellate cells are inhibitory neurons that inhibit Purkinje cells to either side of the long row of Purkinje fibres that are excited by the same parallel fibres. This laterally organized inhibition leads to a sharpening up of the row of Purkinje fibres that is excited (Fig. 13.16). The Golgi cells are also excited by parallel fibres but they act back on granule cells (negative feed-back).

The function of this cerebellar cortical module is unknown. The cerebellum itself has important roles to play in the normal control of posture and movement, especially in the initiation of movement, control of muscle tone and coordination of muscle contraction. The cerebellum does not initiate voluntary movement, but lesions of the cerebellum lead to delays in initiating muscle contraction. It seems that the cerebellum, in conjunction with the cerebral cortex, is important for the learning of movements. Once the movement has been learnt it may be that the cerebral cortex instructs the motor apparatus to carry out a particular set of operations and, since the cerebral cortex sends that same message to the cerebellum, the cerebellum checks that the movements are being carried out and makes appropriate adjustments in the face of unexpected muscle loads etc. Indeed it has been shown by Gilbert and Thach (1977) that when monkeys have learned a motor task Purkinje cells fire mainly simple spikes in a repeatable way during the

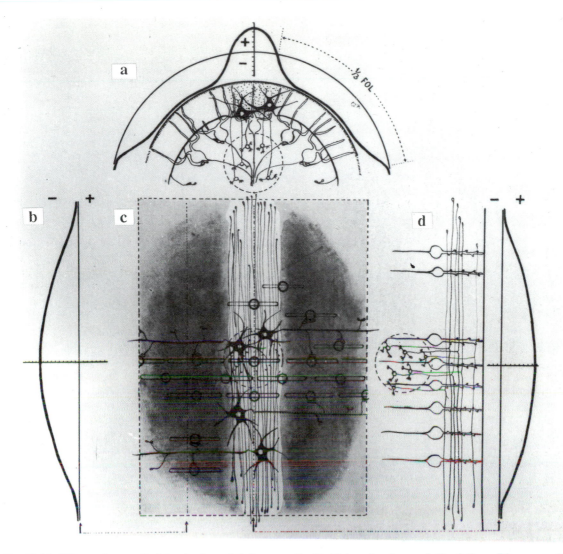

Fig. 13.16. Effects of an excited band of parallel fibres on the Purkinje cells of a cerebellar folium. Diagram **a** shows a transverse section of the folium, diagram **c** shows a plan view and diagrams **b** and **d** show longitudinal sections. A focal input from mossy fibres onto granule cells (outlined by a *dashed circle* in **a, c, d**) set up an excited band of parallel fibres along the folium, flanked on each side by deep inhibition caused by the activity of Basket cells. (Reproduced from Eccles et al. 1967.)

execution of the task, but when an unexpected load is introduced there is an increased firing of complex spikes. If the monkey is allowed to become used to the additional load, then the increased firing of complex spikes is replaced by a new pattern of simple spike discharges with only the occasional complex spike. Furthermore, it has been shown that climbing fibre activity modifies the response of a Purkinje cell to mossy fibre inputs for a long period of time. It is convenient to consider that during learning of a new motor act the neurons of the inferior olive detect a mismatch between the intended motor act and the actual act and then send, via the climbing

fibres, a signal to the cerebellum. As far as the cerebellar cortex is concerned, this signal, which produces complex spikes in Purkinje cells, modifies the responses of some Purkinje cells to mossy fibre inputs.

Modular Organization in the Cerebral Cortex

The cerebral cortex, responsible for the control of voluntary movements, for conscious appreciation of sensory information, for memory and many aspects of learning, for language and for

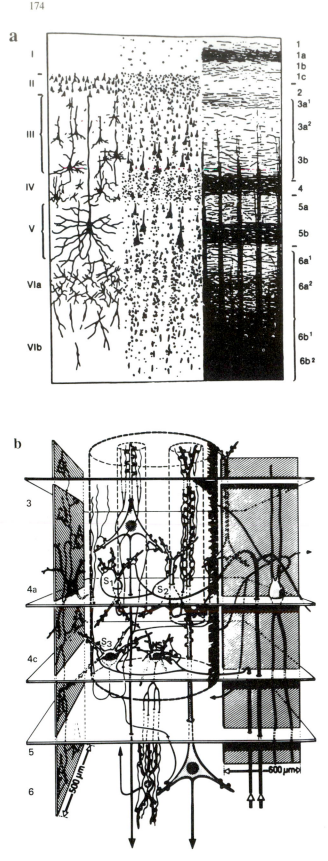

Fig. 13.17a,b. Organization of the cerebral cortex. **a** Basic layered structure of the cortex. To the *left* is a Golgi preparation to show the cell types, in the *middle* a Nissl-stained preparation to show the cell density and shapes of the cell bodies, to the *right* a myelin-stained preparation to show the trajectory of myelinated axons. **b** The neuronal organization in sensory cortical areas according to Szentágothai. The cortical layers are indicated on the *left*. Specific sensory afferents (the *black vertical lines* at the *right*) terminate on spiny stellate cells (S_1, S_2) and star pyramidal cells (S_3) and non-spiny tellate cells (*NS*). Transmission is ultimately to the pyramidal cells which provide the output from the cortical module. [Reproduced with permission from Brodal 1981 (**a**) and from Szentágothai 1975 (**b**).]

other so-called higher functions of the nervous system, is essentially a six-layered structure (Fig. 13.17). Even though different parts of the cortex are concerned with different functions, and in different parts there are modifications in the development of the six layers, the general plan of cortical organization is the same in all areas. Most importantly, it appears that the functional unit of cortical organization is a column of cells running at right angles to the cortical surface (Fig. 13.17). This columnar organization is most easily observed in the main sensory and motor areas of the cortex.

The columnar organization of the cerebral cortex was first recognized by Mountcastle in the somatosensory cortex, and quickly confirmed for the visual cortex by Hubel and Wiesel. The columnar organization was revealed by the use of microelectrodes for recording from single neurons or small numbers of neighbouring neurons and by making long recording tracks through considerable distances in the cortex. Within the somatosensory cortex (Fig. 13.18) each vertical column contains neurons that respond to the same submodality: some columns are activated by moving hairs on the skin, others by gentle pressure on the skin, others by joint movement. Furthermore, each neuron within a column has a similar (not necessarily identical) receptive field on the skin (see the discussion on cortical maps in Chap. 15). Within the visual cortex there are columns whose neurons respond to visual stimuli (bars) of particular orientation (orientation columns), and to input from a particular eye (ocular dominance columns). These two sets of columns are arranged at right angles to each other (see Fig. 15.12). Hubel and Wiesel suggested that the functional unit of the visual cortex (primary visual cortex, striate area, area 17) is a hypercolumn containing a complete set of orientation columns for 360 degrees as well as a set of ocular dominance

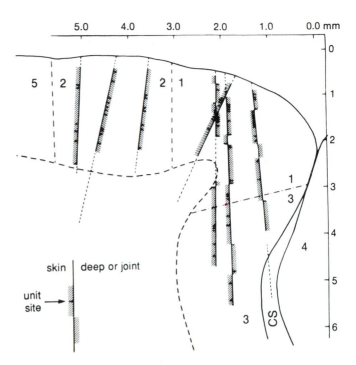

Fig. 13.18. Columnar organization of the somatosensory cortex in the monkey. The figure shows a section through the cortex and the location of recording microelectrode tracks. Penetrations at right angles to the cortical surface record from a column of cells of the same submodality (skin or deep), whereas penetrations that cut across the columns show changes in submodality. The *numbers* refer to cortical areas. *CS*, the cruciate sulcus. (Reproduced with permission from Powell and Mountcastle 1959.)

columns. (It should be noted that this "classical" view of the organization of visual cortex, originally proposed by Hubel and Wiesel, has been made more complex recently with the recognition of cells in the orientation columns that do not respond to orientation! Furthermore, these cells stain specifically for cytochrome oxidase activity and are arranged in "blobs"; see Chap. 15.) At present the mode of operation of cortical columns (or hypercolumns) is unknown, but the fact that this organization appears to be similar for the whole cortex underlines the principle that the nervous system consists of a set of repeating units, each apparently carrying out similar functions.

Summary

1. The specific interconnexion of small groups of neurons leads to the emergence of particular operating characteristics. These characteristics include convergence and divergence of input, temporal and spatial facilitation, post-tetanic potentiation, post-excitatory depression, hetero-synaptic facilitation (and inhibition), feed-forward and feed-back inhibition and excitation, lateral or surround inhibition (and facilitation), disinhibition and disfacilitation.

2. The segmental motor apparatus provides a good example of the characteristics of small groups of neurons having most of the above properties.

3. The nervous system is built up from large numbers of repeating units, or modules, each of which consists of a relatively small number of neurons.

4. Examples of neural modules include the spinal motor apparatus, spinal sensory circuits, the highly ordered circuitry of the cerebellar cortex and the columnar organization in the cerebral cortex.

14 Structural Organization of Specific Sensory and Motor Systems

The neuronal subsystems concerned with sensory mechanisms (somaesthesia, vision, audition, balance, and olfaction and taste) and with motor mechanisms (posture and locomotion) have a number of features in common:

1. They are each organized with chains of neurons connected in an hierarchical (or serial) fashion, transmission between neurons taking place in the so-called relay nuclei.

2. Within each particular subsystem there is a series of distinct parallel pathways.

3. The organization within each subsystem is precise and is arranged in a topographical fashion, that is, within sensory systems the local relationships at the peripheral receptive surface are maintained in the receptive fields of neurons at each level of the system (sensory maps) and within the motor systems there are also motor maps.

4. In bilaterally symmetrical animals most of the specific sensory and motor systems cross the midline, in whole or in part.

Sensory Systems – Hierarchical Organization

As discussed in Chapter 12, the first stage in the sensory analysis of the external, or internal, environment is by the sense organs or sensory receptors. These sense organs are highly specialized and each type responds only over a limited range of the wide spectrum of energy changes that can occur. Thus, some respond to cooling, some to warming, some to mechanical displacement, some to particular chemicals, some to particular wavelengths of light and so on. The sense organs transduce energy changes at their receptive component into a form that the nervous system can handle – electrical potential changes brought about by ionic current flow across their cell membrane. From the sense organs, the first neuronal component of the sensory system (the primary afferent neuron) transmits the neural signals (impulses, usually) to the central nervous system. (The visual system is an exception to this general rule as the first few neurons in the system are located in the retina, which may be considered a part of the central nervous system: the optic nerve, connecting the retina to the brain is formed from the axons of the retinal ganglion cells.) Onward transmission from the primary afferent neuron is via a series of so-called sensory relay nuclei (this term is a misnomer, as will be explained) ultimately to the cerebral cortex. All specific sensory systems "relay" in the thalamus, which is a large collection of individual nuclear masses in the diencephalon (a component of the forebrain). Outlines of the organization of various specific sensory systems in mammals are provided in Boxes 14.1–14.4 (Figs. 14.A–14.D.)

BOX 14.1

THE ANATOMICAL ORGANIZATION OF THE SOMATOSENSORY PATHWAYS

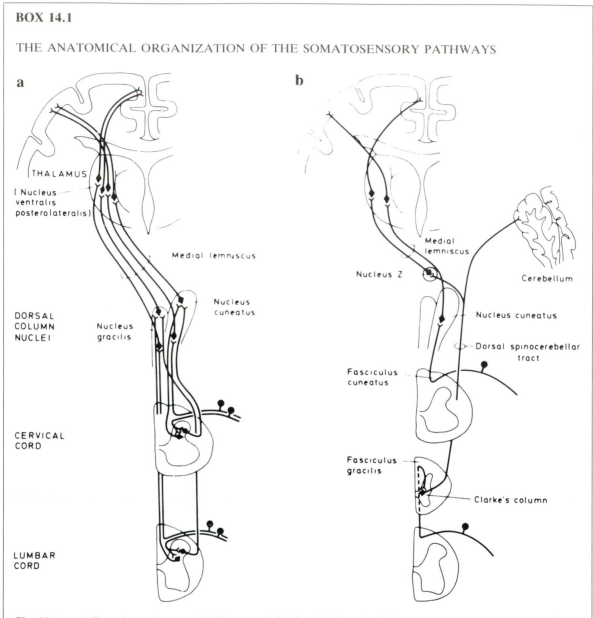

Fig. 14.A. a, b Show the main anatomical features of the dorsal column/medial lemniscal pathway: **a** for fibres carrying impules arising from low-threshold cutaneous mechanoreceptors; **b** for fibres carrying impulses from muscle and joint receptors.

Continued

Primary Afferent Neurons

The cell bodies of primary afferent neurons are located outside the central nervous system, often in collections of cell bodies called ganglia. Such ganglia include the dorsal root ganglia, containing cell bodies of primary afferent neurons innervating sense organs in the skin, muscles, tendons and subcutaneous tissues of the trunk and limbs; the trigeminal or semilunar ganglion, containing cell bodies of afferent fibres innervating similar receptors of the head; the spiral ganglion, containing cell bodies of the auditory nerve; and the

Continued

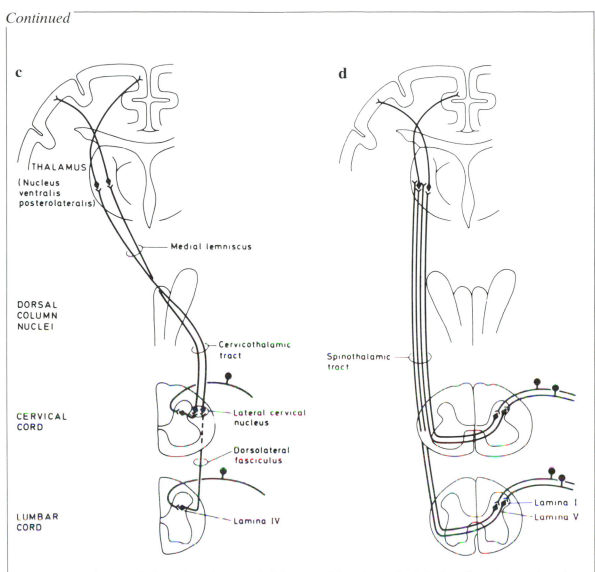

c

THALAMUS
(Nucleus
ventralis
posterolateralis)

Medial lemniscus

DORSAL
COLUMN
NUCLEI

Cervicothalamic
tract

CERVICAL
CORD

Lateral cervical
nucleus

Dorsolateral
fasciculus

LUMBAR
CORD

Lamina IV

d

Spinothalamic
tract

Lamina I

Lamina V

Fig. 14.A. (*continued*) **c,d** Show the main anatomical features of the spinocervicothalamic pathway (**c**) and the spino-thalamic tract (**d**). The termination of spinothalamic fibres in areas other than the nucleus ventralis posterolateralis of the thalamus is not shown. (Reproduced with permission from Brodal 1981.)

nodose, petrosal and geniculate ganglia, contain-ing cell bodies of primary afferent neurons con-cerned with taste. As mentioned above, the optic tract, which connects the retina with the brain, is not composed of the axons of primary afferent fibres but of axons from higher order neurons – the retinal ganglion cells. The primary afferent neurons of the olfactory system are the olfactory receptor cells and they lie within the olfactory epithelium. The axons of the olfactory cells form the olfactory nerve and run to the olfactory bulb of the brain.

Each primary afferent neuron, at its peripheral end, either innervates one or more sensory receptor cells or, itself, has specialized nerve terminals that act as sensory receptors. The primary afferent neuron together with its sensory receptors is known as a sensory unit (cf. the

BOX 14.2

THE ANATOMICAL ORGANIZATION OF
THE VISUAL PATHWAYS

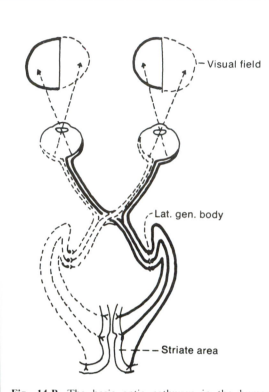

Fig. 14.B. The basic optic pathways in the human, demonstrating the partial decussation (crossing over) of the optic nerve fibres in the chiasma. (Reproduced with permission from Brodal 1981.)

of those that respond to moving hairs on the coat of mammals, where a single afferent neuron may innervate a large number of receptor cells at the bases of many tens of hair follicles, and some (about 10%) of the afferent fibres of the eighth (auditory) cranial nerve, each innervating many outer hair cells in the organ of Corti of the cochlea.

At its central end, each primary afferent axon divides into a number of terminal branches within the central nervous system and makes synaptic contact with many neurons at the first stage of central neural processing. This processing usually takes place within well-defined nuclei, such as the dorsal column nuclei and the main sensory nucleus of the trigeminal nerve (somatosensory system), the dorsal and ventral cochlear nuclei (auditory system) and the nucleus solitarius (gustatory system). In some sensory systems the first set of synapses may be located in less well-defined areas of the central nervous system, such as in the grey matter of the spinal cord (parts of the somatosensory system, for example).

Relay Nuclei

Each of the specific sensory systems, between its primary afferent neurons and the cerebral cortical areas to which the pathway projects, is interrupted a number of times by the "relay nuclei". The systems are therefore organized in an hierarchical fashion from so-called lower to higher levels of the central nervous system. In many systems the first of these nuclei is located in the brain stem, e.g. the dorsal column and trigeminal nuclei, the solitary nucleus, the cochlear nuclei. All sensory systems have relays in the thalamus, which is the penultimate processing station before the cerebral cortex.

As will be discussed in Chapter 15, the relay nuclei do not simply relay sensory messages, but process these messages – by means of the neuronal mechanisms described earlier, such as divergence, convergence, feed-back, feed-forward, summation, facilitation, inhibition etc. Within each nucleus, and in those areas where well-defined nuclei are not obvious, there are two main classes of neurons: those that have axons projecting to the next processing station – the projection neurons – and those with axons that remain within the nucleus – the local interneurons. Projection neurons may also have axon collaterals that are given off near the cell body and terminate on other neurons within the nucleus. As far as is known, within specific

motor unit, which is a single motoneuron together with all the muscle fibres it innervates). At one extreme, therefore, a sensory unit may consist of a single primary afferent fibre and a single sensory receptor. An example of such a sensory unit is the slowly adapting Type II mechanoreceptor unit; each single afferent neuron innervates a single mechanoreceptor (Ruffini ending) in the skin. Also, a single receptor cell may receive innervation from more than one primary afferent fibre. For example, inner hair cells of the cochlea each receive about 10–20 fibres (peripheral processes) from the spiral ganglion, and each fibre innervates only a single hair cell. At the other extreme, a sensory unit may consist of the single primary afferent fibre and a large number, hundreds, of receptor cells that are innervated by it. Examples of such sensory units include some

BOX 14.3

THE ANATOMICAL ORGANIZATION OF THE AUDITORY PATHWAYS

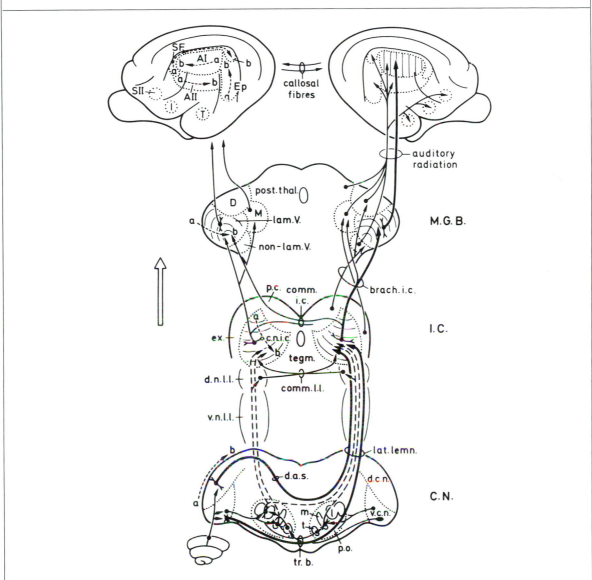

Fig. 14.C. The ascending auditory pathway in the cat. *Thick lines* indicate the major projection to the contralateral primary auditory cortex. Abbreviations for major components: *AI, AII*, primary and secondary auditory cortical areas; *Ep*, posterior ectosylvanian area; *brach. i.c.*, brachium of the inferior colliculus; *C.N.*, cochlear nuclear complex; *I.C.*, inferior colliculus; *lat.lemn.*, lateral lemniscus; *M.G.B.*, medial geniculate body of the thalamus; *SF*, suprasylvanian fringe. Other abbreviations; *comm.i.c.*, commissure of the inferior colliculus; *comm.l.l.*, commissure of the lateral lemniscus; *c.n.i.c.*, central nucleus of the inferior colliculus; *D.*, dorsal division of the medial geniculate body; *d.a.s.*, dorsal acoustic stria; *d.c.n.*, dorsal cochlear nucleus; *d.n.l.l.*, dorsal nucleus of the lateral lemniscus; *ex.*, external nucleus of the inferior colliculus; *I.*, insular area of cortex; *l.*, lateral superior olive; *lam.V.*, laminated portion of ventral division of the medial geniculate body. *M.*, medial division of the medial geniculate body; *m.*, medial superior olive; *non-lam.V.*, non-laminated portion of ventral division of the medial geniculate body; *p.c.*, pericentral nucleus of the inferior colliculus; *p.o.*, periolivary nuclei; *post.thal.*, posterior thalamic group. *SII*, second somatosensory area; *T*, temporal area of cortex. *t*, nucleus of the trapezoid body; *tegm.*, midbrain tegmentum. *tr.b.*, trapezoid body; *v.c.n.*, ventral cochlear nucleus; *v.n.l.l.*, ventral nucleus of the lateral lemniscus. The tonotopical organization is indicated by *broken arrows* from apical (*a*) to basal (*b*) areas of cochlear representation. (Reproduced with permission from Brodal 1981.)

BOX 14.4

THE ANATOMICAL ORGANIZATION OF THE GUSTATORY AND OLFACTORY PATHWAYS

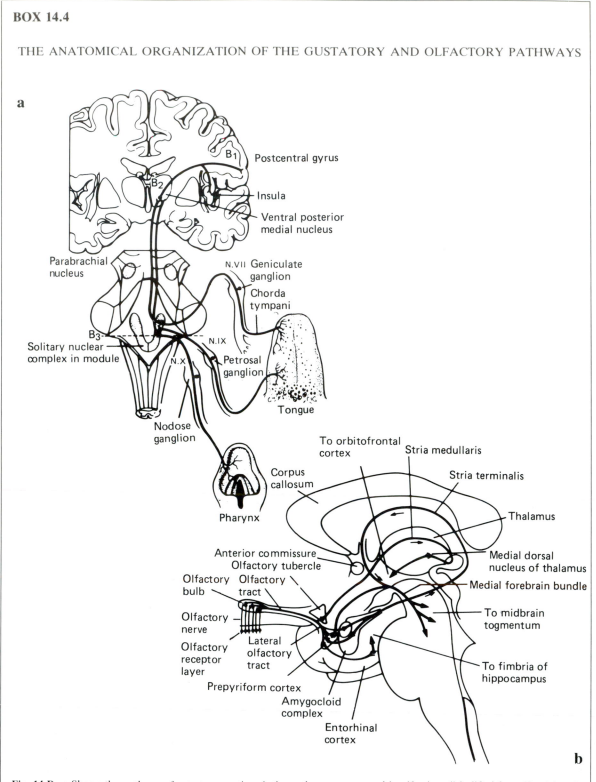

Fig. 14.D. a Shows the pathways for taste sensation; **b** the pathways concerned in olfaction. (Modified from Kandel and Schwartz 1985.)

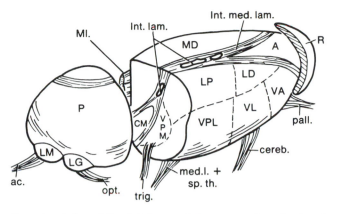

Fig. 14.1. Diagram of a three-dimensional view of the right human thalamus seen from the dorsolateral aspect. The posterior part is separated from the rest to display some features of the internal structure. The main afferent inputs to some of the nuclei are indicated. Abbreviations for thalamic nuclei: *A*, anterior; *CM*, centromedian; *Int. lam.*, intralaminar; *LD*, *LP*, lateralis dorsalis and posterior; *LG*, lateral geniculate body; *MD*, dorsomedial; *Ml*, midline; *P*, pulvinar; *R*, reticular; *VA*, ventralis anterior; *VL*, ventralis lateralis; *VPL*, *VPM*, ventralis posterior lateralis and medialis. Other abbreviations: *ac.*, acoustic input through brachium of inferior colliculus; *cereb.*, cerebellar input; *med. l.*, medial lemniscus; *opt.*, optic tract; *pall.*, pallidal inputs; *sp. th.*, spinothalamic tract; *trig.*, trigeminal input. (Reproduced with permission from Brodal 1981.)

sensory systems the projection neurons are all excitatory in their actions on their target neurons. The local interneurons are of diverse anatomical types and may enter into a variety of synaptic relationships with their target cells. In general, it is convenient to consider them as being either excitatory or inhibitory interneurons, but this is undoubtedly an over-simplification.

The Thalamus

The gross anatomical subdivisions of the human thalamus are indicated in Fig. 14.1. As mentioned above, all specific sensory systems project to the thalamus and from it to the cerebral cortex. This applies not only to the visual, auditory, somatosensory, olfactory, and gustatory system but also to the afferent motor pathways. Each of these specific systems has a specific thalamic nucleus allocated to it and each nucleus projects to a specific area of the cerebral cortex (Table 14.1; Fig. 14.2). (An additional set of specific thalamic nuclei, the anterior nuclei, is concerned in the regulation of emotion in humans and with emotional-type behaviour in animals. The anterior nuclei receive input from the hypothalamus and project to the cingulate gyrus of the cerebral cortex; see Chap. 16.).

In addition to the specific nuclei, the thalamus contains two other important sets of nuclei: the association nuclei and the non-specific nuclei.

Thalamic association nuclei each receive input from several sources and project to the so-called association areas of the cerebral cortex (Table 14.1). Their functions are little known but include some aspects of emotional control and probably the integration of several sensory modalities. The non-specific thalamic nuclei have widespread (distributed) projections to the rest of the thalamus and to wide areas of the cerebral cortex (Table 14.1); they are thought to be concerned with the level of arousal (see Chap. 16.).

Cerebral Cortex

Each of the specific thalamic sensory nuclei projects to a particular part of the cerebral cortex (neocortex) – the primary sensory and motor areas (Fig. 14.2). Each primary sensory area of the cerebral cortex receives a direct input from one of the specific sensory thalamic nuclei; therefore, there are primary visual, auditory, somatosensory, gustatory and olfactory areas where the first stage of cortical processing occurs. (The olfactory system is exceptional in that in addition to its projection to the neocortex via the thalamus it also projects to another part of the cortex, the paleocortex of the piriform lobe.) The afferent motor pathways also project, via specific thalamic nuclei, to the primary motor area of the cortex. The primary cortical areas, in turn, project to other areas of the cerebral cortex, where

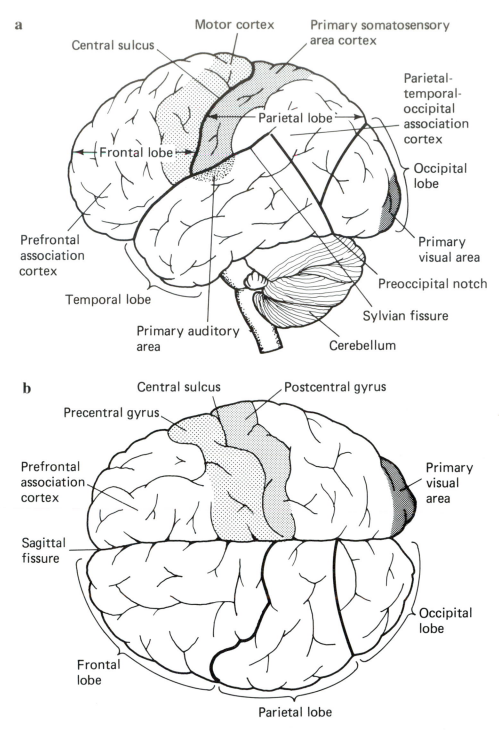

Fig. 14.2a,b. The major divisions of the human cerebral cortex. **a** Lateral view; **b** dorsal view. (Modified from Kandel and Schwartz 1985.)

further processing of sensory messages takes place (Fig. 14.3).

As mentioned in Chapter 13, the cortex is a six-layered structure whose functional unit of organization is a column of cells running at right angles to the cortical surface. Within different cortical areas the six layers are developed to different extents, and it is on the basis of these

Table 14.1. Connexions and functions of thalamic nuclei

Nuclei	Principal afferent inputs	Major projection sites	Function
Specific relay nuclei:			
Anterior nuclear group	Mamillary body of hypothalamus	Cingulate gyrus	"Limbic"
Ventral anterior	Globus pallidus	Premotor cortex	Motor
Ventral lateral	Dentate nucleus of cerebellum through brachium conjunctivum (superior cerebellar peduncle)	Motor and premotor cortices	Motor
Ventral posterior:			
Lateral portion	Dorsal column-medial lemniscal pathway and spinothalamic pathways	Somatic sensory cortex of parietal lobe	Somaesthesis (body)
Medial portion	Sensory nuclei of trigeminal nerve	Somatic sensory cortex of parietal lobe	Somaesthesis (face)
Medial geniculate	Inferior colliculus through brachium of inferior colliculus	Auditory cortex of temporal lobe	Hearing
Lateral geniculate	Retinal ganglion cells through optic nerve and optic tract	Visual cortex of occipital lobe	Vision
Association nuclei:			
Lateral dorsal	Cingulate gyrus	Cingulate gyrus	Emotional expression
Lateral posterior	Parietal lobe	Parietal lobe	Integration of sensory information
Pulvinar	Superior colliculus, temporal, parietal, and occipital lobes, and primary visual cortex	Temporal, parietal, and occipital lobes	Integration of sensory information
Medial dorsal	Amygdaloid nuclear complex, olfactory, and hypothalamus	Prefrontal cortex	"Limbic"
Non-specific nuclei:			
Midline nuclei	Reticular formation and hypothalamus	Basal forebrain	"Limbic"
Intralaminar nuclei: Centromedian and centrolateral	Reticular formation, spinothalamic tract, globus pallidus, and cortical areas	Basal ganglia (striatum)	—
Reticular nucleus	Cerebral cortex and thalamic nuclei	Thalamic nuclei	Modulation of thalamic activity

Modified from Kandel and Schwartz (1985).

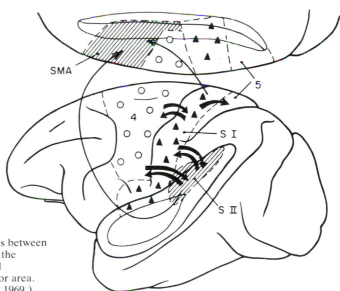

Fig. 14.3. The main ipsilateral association connexions between the major motor and somatosensory cortical areas in the monkey. Note that the connexions are reciprocal and somatotopically arranged. *SMA*, supplementary motor area. (Reproduced with permission from Jones and Powell 1969.)

differences that the cortex has been divided into numerous cytoarchitectonic areas. The major thalamic afferent inputs from the specific sensory systems terminate largely in the third and fourth cortical layer on both the output cells of the cortex (the pyramidal cells) and also on intrinsic cortical neurons (non-pyramidal cells which may be divided into several types; see Fig. 13.17). It is generally accepted that the cortical column is an input–output processing device. In addition to the thalamic inputs it receives inputs from other cortical columns (from various parts of the cerebral cortex of the same side and, usually, from cortex of the opposite side. These afferent inputs terminate in various cortical layers. The axons of pyramidal neurons provide the outputs from cortical columns. In addition to the projections to other cortical columns there are major outputs to non-cortical structures, especially the thalamus (reciprocal connexions with the parts providing input), the basal ganglia, reticular formation, the brain stem sensory and motor nuclei, and the spinal cord.

Specific Sensory Systems – Parallel Pathways

The hierarchical organization described above was stressed, until recently, as the basis of sensory (and motor) processing by the nervous system, with each "higher" level of the system providing more sophisticated feature extraction from the raw sensory input data. It has become apparent, however, that all specific systems although organized in an hierarchical fashion are also organized in a parallel way. What this means in reality is that for every system there is not just one set of ascending neurons, from sense organs to cortex, but a whole array of ascending pathways running in parallel with each other, in some cases through the same sets of relay nuclei and in others through different nuclei, but ultimately reaching the cortex. This sort of organization allows for some interesting and useful properties of sensory systems. Thus the messages from different sense organs in the same receptor sheet (for example retina or skin) may be handled by different, parallel, sensory pathways or the same messages from a set of sense organs may be handled differently by different parallel pathways. In order to illustrate this sort of organization, examples from the visual and somatosensory systems will be discussed.

Parallel Pathways in the Visual System

Photoreceptor mechanisms in the rods and cones of the vertebrate retina have been discussed in Chapter 12, where the general structure of the retina was described (see Fig. 12.4). In addition to the receptor cells, the retina contains four major types of neurons: the bipolar, horizontal, amacrine and ganglion cells. Considerable neural processing occurs in the retina, with the main flow of sensory traffic being from rods and cones via bipolar cells to ganglion cells. The horizontal and amacrine cells mediate lateral interactions between receptor and bipolar cells and between bipolar and ganglion cells, respectively.

Because the rods and cones are selectively sensitive to different wavelengths of light and because the messages from them are kept separated along the visual pathway, there are two major parallel paths: (1) the rod path, with high sensitivity to light but low acuity, which subserves achromatic vision; and (2) the cone path, with relatively low sensitivity and high acuity, which subserves colour vision in those animals with it such as primates, the ground squirrel and some fish.

In addition to the achromatic (rod) and chromatic (cone) pathways or channels in the visual system there is another major classification of pathways. The retinal ganglion cells, whether influenced by rods or cones, fall into one of two functional types: they are either excited by light falling on the centre of their receptive field (for the concept of receptive field see Chap. 15), or they are inhibited by a similar stimulus (Fig. 14.4). The neurons of the thalamic relay nucleus in the visual pathway, the lateral geniculate nucleus, also have a similar functional organization; therefore, in the visual pathways from retina to cortex there are either on-centre neurons or off-centre neurons. (As will be discussed in Chapter 15, the receptive fields of the retinal ganglion and lateral geniculate neurons are organized in a centre–surround antagonistic fashion so that the on-centre cells have an off-surround and the off-centre cells have an on-surround.)

Finally, there are three types of ganglion cells providing a further three parallel outputs from the retina. These are known as X, Y and W ganglion cells. In the cat, X cells are of medium size with small dendritic trees. They are influenced by a small number of photoreceptors and are important in high acuity vision (in primates with a well-developed colour vision which also has high acuity there are no X cells as such).

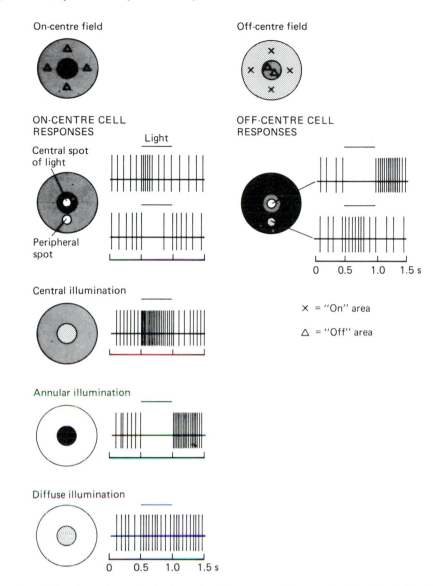

Fig. 14.4. Receptive fields of ganglion cells in the retina. On-centre cells are excited by light falling in the centre of the receptive field and inhibited by light falling in the surrounding area, and off-centre cells show the reverse effects. (Modified from Kuffler et al. 1984.)

Y cells, which are large with large dendritic trees and axons with high conduction velocities, are influenced by a large number of rods over a considerable area of the retina. They respond only to large objects in the visual field and appear to be important for analysis of the gross features of the stimulus and for movement. The third class of ganglion cells, the W cells, which have small cell bodies and large dendritic trees, do not project through the path to cortex via the lateral geniculate nucleus but project to the superior colliculus and are concerned with the control of head and eye movements (some Y cells also

project through this latter pathway). An idea of the anatomical organization in hierarchical and parallel fashion of the visual pathways to the primary visual area of the cerebral cortex and beyond is given in Fig. 14.5.

Parallel Pathways in the Somatosensory System

There are three major specific somatosensory pathways in most mammals, the dorsal column/ medial lemniscal system, the spinothalamic tract

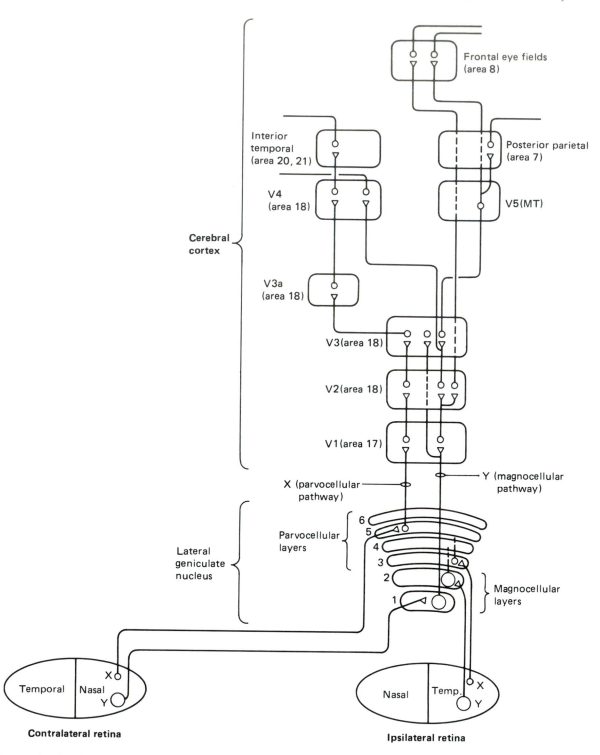

Fig. 14.5. The visual projections from X and Y cells in the retina to the various visual areas of the cerebral cortex in the monkey. (Modified from Kandel and Schwartz 1985, after Van Essen 1979.)

ascending the anterolateral (or ventrolateral) part of the spinal cord, and the spinocervico-thalamic system ascending in the dorsolateral spinal cord.

The Dorsal Column/Medial Lemniscal System

A diagrammatic representation of this system is shown in Box 14.1 (Fig. 14.A). Most of the axons running through the dorsal columns to the dorsal column nuclei in the brain stem are primary afferent fibres innervating sensory receptors in skin, subcutaneous tissue and joints (some nerve fibres from muscle receptors in the fore limb also ascend the dorsal columns). But, as shown in Fig. 14.6, not all of the possible types of primary afferent fibres from these structures take this path. Only nerve fibres innervating sensitive mechanoreceptors do so. In this pathway the dorsal column nuclei carry out the first stage of central processing. (The dorsal columns contain some 10%–15% of axons that arise from neurons in the spinal dorsal horn, forming the postsynaptic dorsal column system, and terminate in parts of the nuclei that do not

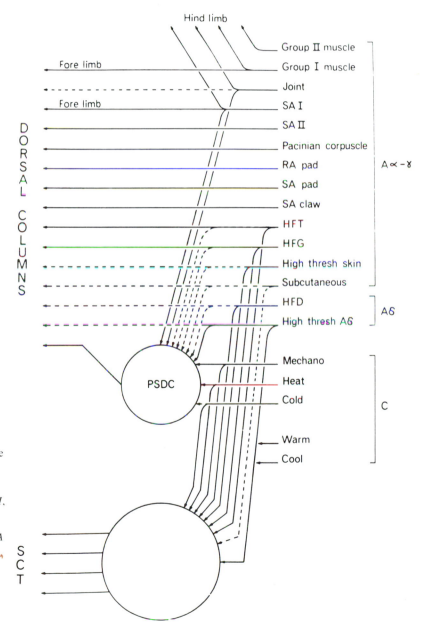

Fig. 14.6. Distribution of afferent fibres to the dorsal columns and spinocervical tract in the cat. The afferent fibre conduction velocities are indicated on the *right*, as are the sensory receptors they innervate. *PSDC*, postsynaptic dorsal column system; *SCT*, spinocervical tract; *SA I*, slowly adapting type I mechanoreceptor; *SA II*, slowly adapting type II mechanoreceptor; *SA pad*, slowly adapting type I mechanoreceptor from glabrous skin; *SA claw*, slowly adapting type II claw receptor; *RA*, rapidly adapting mechanoreceptor from glabrous skin; *HF*, hair follicle receptor. (Reproduced from Brown 1973.)

receive the primary afferent fibres. This system contains neurons responding to additional inputs, such as those from nocireceptors. It is not known whether this input has a role to play in the processing that occurs in the parts of the nuclei receiving primary afferent projections or whether it is kept separate and projected to other parts of the brain).

From the dorsal column nuclei the pathway projects via the medial lemniscus to the contralateral thalmus (the ventral posterior lateral nucleus) and hence to the primary somatosensory cortical receiving area (SI), and also directly to the secondary somatosensory cortex (SII). Within the dorsal column nuclei, the somatosensory thalamic nuclei and the cortex there appear to be separate sets of neurons that handle input from particular groups of mechanoreceptors. Thus there are separate parts of the dorsal column nuclei and the thalamus that are concerned with Pacinian corpuscle input, and separate parts of the first somatosensory cortex dealing with rapidly adapting cutaneous, slowly adapting cutaneous and joint and muscle inputs.

The Spinothalamic Tract

As shown in Box 14.1 (Fig. 14.A), direct connexions between the spinal cord and the thalamus are made by the spinothalamic tract. (This can be subdivided into the neospinothalamic tract and also some parts of the paleospinothalamic tract, most neurons of which do not project as far as the thalamus.) The first set of synapses occurs between primary afferent fibres and neurons of the spinal cord. The axons of these cells cross over to the opposite side of the cord and ascend in the ventro- (or antero-) lateral part of the cord, through the brain stem, where they join and contribute to the medial lemniscus, to the thalamus (ventral posterior lateral nucleus and the posterior nuclear group) and then to the first and second (primary and secondary) somatosensory cortical areas SI and SII. In addition to handling input from some sensitive mechanoreceptors, the direct spinothalamic tracts process input from thermoreceptors and nocireceptors. In other words, the spinothalamic pathway is the pain and temperature path (and also deals with some aspects of touch).

The Spinocervicothalamic Pathway

This pathway (see Box 14.1; Fig. 14.A), which is well-developed in carnivores but also present in primates and rodents as well as a variety of other species including sheep and whales, arises from the dorsal horn of the spinal cord, where the primary afferent fibres make their initial central contacts. The axons of spinocervical neurons ascend the spinal cord (on the same side as their cell bodies) to the lateral cervical nucleus in the upper two segments of the cord. From the lateral cervical nucleus the projection is to the opposite side, where the axons join the medial lemniscus and terminate in the thalamus (ventral posterior lateral nucleus and the posterior nuclear group). From the thalamus the pathway projects to the SI and SII areas of the cerebral cortex.

The spinocervicothalamic system appears to process only the input from two major classes of sensory receptors: in the cat these are those responding to movement of the hairs of the animal's coat (hair follicle receptors) and nocireceptors. Within the system neurons fall into three classes according to their excitatory responses: (1) responding to hair movement alone, (2) responding to hair movement and noxious stimuli and (3) responding to noxious stimuli. The system is obviously highly specialized for extracting certain features from the wide spectrum of possible sensory stimuli acting on the body surface.

Distribution of Input to the Parallel Somatosensory Pathways

Consideration of the above descriptions of the organization of the three specific somatosensory paths allows some conclusions to be drawn about how particular somatosensory inputs are distributed amongst them. Thus, messages from thermoreceptors are sent exclusively to the direct spinothalamic paths. Excitation of nocireceptors, however, will lead to excitation of some neurons in the direct spinothalamic and the spinocervicothalamic pathways and will also excite some postsynaptic dorsal column neurons (see above). Activation of hair follicle receptors will lead to neural activity being distributed to the dorsal column/medial lemniscal system, the spinocervicothalamic system and the spinothalamic system, that is, to all three of the specific somatosensory pathways. At present we have insufficient knowledge to allow us to suggest any particular function or set of functions for the different somatosensory paths, except that sensations of heat and cold and of pain are subserved (in part at least) by the spinothalamic system, and the most sophisticated tactile explorations are dependent on the dorsal column pathway. However, it is obvious that parallel pathways are highly developed in the somatosensory system, and the assumption must be that the different pathways are carrying out different functions.

Descending (Centrifugal) Loops in the Ascending Sensory Systems

The ascending sensory messages are subject to controls from more cranial levels at each of the relay nuclei. These controls are exerted from a variety of locations in the brain, and some of the neural pathways involved parallel the ascending ones but in the descending direction (Boxes 14.1–14.4; Figs. 14.A–14.D). Thus, from each primary sensory receiving area of the cerebral cortex there are descending projections to the specific thalamic sensory nucleus from which the primary cortex obtains its specific sensory input. Within the somatosensory systems there are descending projections from the somatosensory cortical areas to the dorsal column nuclei and also to the spinal cord. Both of these sets of projections provide the anatomical basis for cortical control of sensory input at the first stage of central sensory processing in the dorsal column/medial lemniscal system and in the spinocervical and spinothalamic paths. Activity in the corticospinal tract leads to primary afferent depolarization of the terminals of primary afferent fibres and therefore produces presynaptic inhibition at the first synaptic relays.

Some centrifugal systems actually act at the level of the sensory receptor. The role of fusimotor (gamma) motoneurons in the control of muscle spindle sensitivity has been discussed in Chapter 12, but other examples abound: thus, there is an inhibitory centrifugal innervation of the hair cells in the inner ear in most vertebrates; in birds there is an inhibitory control from the brain (isthmo-optic nucleus) to the retinal amacrine cells, and since the amacrine cells are themselves inhibitory on retinal ganglion cells this centrifugal inhibitory pathway actually has a facilitatory effect by disinhibition of the amacrine cell action.

The action of some centrifugal control systems will be discussed in more detail in the next chapter. But it is important here to stress that the underlying anatomical organization of reciprocal connexions between cortex and thalamus and of various descending neuronal loops between various points in the ascending sensory pathways is an important principle of neuroanatomy. A further extension of this principle is to be found in the cerebral cortex, where a majority of the cortical areas dealing with sensory and motor mechanisms are reciprocally connected.

Motor Systems – Hierarchical and Parallel Pathways

Like the specific sensory systems, the motor systems are organized in both a hierarchical and parallel fashion. It is generally considered that there are four levels of organization in the motor systems (Fig. 14.7). The lowest (or first) level is the spinal motor apparatus that has been discussed in some detail in Chapter 13. This consists of the primary afferent fibres from muscles, tendons, joints, subcutaneous tissue and skin, the motoneurons (which provide the direct control of skeletal muscle and of the sensitivity of the muscle spindle receptors) and the segmental (and intersegmental) neuronal circuitry between them. In "lower" vertebrates, the spinal motor apparatus can, by itself, carry out certain spinal reflex actions and generate locomotor programmes, but in more "advanced" species such as primates, and especially in man, the spinal cord is capable of only very crude responses, often of a hyperactive nature.

The next (second) level in the hierarchy of the motor control systems is the brain stem. Here there are a number of nuclei that both process motor messages descending from higher levels and also handle sensory input from the spinal cord, from cranial nerves and also from the special sensory systems (visual, auditory and vestibular). With the sole exception of the corticospinal tract, originating in the cerebral cortex, all descending motor pathways to the spinal motor apparatus take origin from this brain stem level.

The third level of motor control is the primary motor cortex (cytoarchitectonic area 4), which projects both directly to the spinal cord via some components of the corticospinal tract and also to the brain stem nuclei via the various corticobulbar tracts. The cortex is also the site of the fourth level in the motor hierarchy – the premotor cortical areas in cytoarchitectonic area 6. The premotor areas act on the primary motor cortex and also directly on the brain stem and spinal

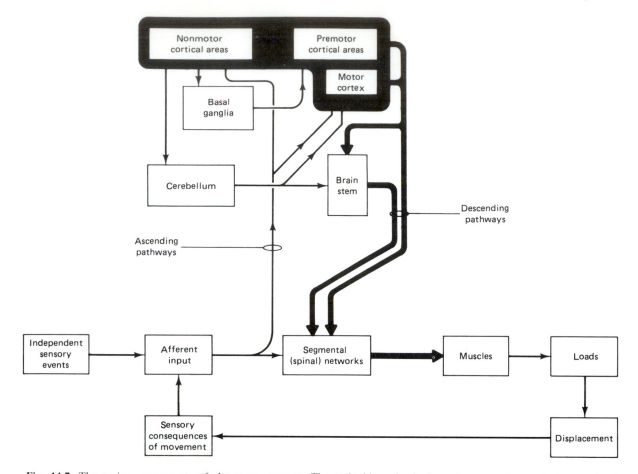

Fig. 14.7. The major components of the motor system. The main hierarchy is from the premotor cortical areas (and supplementary motor areas) to the motor cortex and then, via the brain stem, to the spinal motor apparatus. Note the basal ganglia and cerebellum set off from the main hierarchy but with strong influences at the cortical and brain stem levels. In this diagram non-cortical inputs to the cerebellum have been omitted, as has the thalamus on the afferent pathway to the cortex. The *arrows* denote influences. (Modified from Kandel and Schwartz, 1985.)

levels of the motor hierarchy. In addition, the premotor areas have wide cortical connexions with areas in front and behind them (prefrontal and parietal cortex) and are concerned with programming movements, deciding on motor actions and also identifying targets in space.

It may be seen, therefore, that the motor systems are not only arranged in an hierarchical fashion, from premotor to motor cortex via the brain stem to the spinal motor apparatus, but are also organized in a highly parallel fashion too. Not only that, each level of the motor hierarchy receives input from a variety of sensory receptors and the higher levels may control the sensory messages reaching them. This close relationship between sensory and motor systems should be easily appreciated. Every motor act will lead to sensory input, either directly (for example by

directly affecting muscle, tendon, joint or cutaneous receptors) or indirectly (for example by moving the head and producing changes in the visual field). Furthermore, it is important for the motor systems to be able to compare the sensory input expected from a particular motor act with the sensory input actually evoked, so that compensatory mechanisms may be called into play if necessary.

Systems Controlling the Motor Hierarchy

Set off from the main hierarchical organization of motor systems (premotor cortex, motor cortex, brain stem nuclei and spinal motor apparatus) are two important structures, the cerebellum and

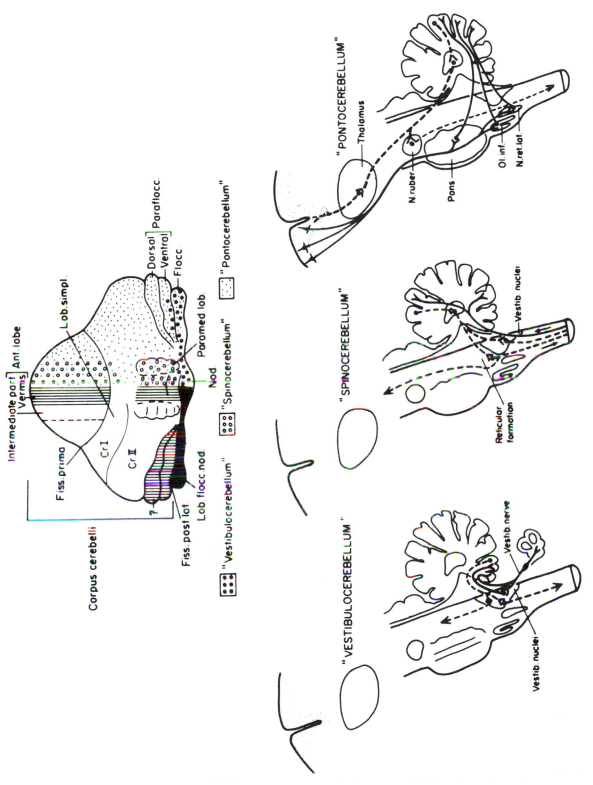

Fig. 14.8. The three major divisions of the cerebellum according to the main afferent and efferent connexions. (Reproduced with permission from Brodal 1981.)

basal gangli, which control the hierarchy (Fig. 14.7). Some aspects of the organization and function of the cerebellum have been discussed in Chapter 13. Here, the more general anatomical interrelationships between the cerebellum and the motor hierarchy will be considered.

The cerebellum may be divided functionally into three zones (which run from rostral to caudal across the cerebellum): the spinocerebellum, the vestibulocerebellum and the cerebrocerebellum or pontocerebellum (Fig. 14.8). The spinocerebellum receives sensory input from the periphery and influences the motor systems at various levels. The vestibulocerebellum receives sensory input from the labyrinth of the inner ear (semicircular canals and otolith organs) and also input from visual pathways and projects to the vestibular nuclei, where it influences the control of eye movements, the coordination of head and eye movements and also the postural control by axial muscles of the body. The cerebrocerebellum, unlike the other functional divisions of the cerebellar cortex, does not receive input directly from sense organs but derives its afferent supply from wide areas of the cerebral cortex, especially the motor and premotor areas and the

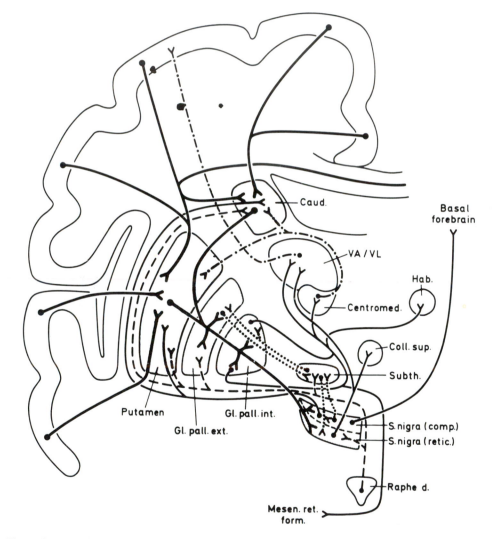

Fig. 14.9. The main connexions of the basal ganglia. Note the major input from the cerebral cortex and the interconnexions between the separate nuclear masses of the basal ganglia (*thick lines*) and the output through the thalamus. *VA/VL*, nucleus ventralis anterior and lateralis; *Centromed.*, centromedian nuclei. Other abbreviations: *Caud.*, caudate nucleus; *Call. sup.*, superior colliculus; *Gl. pall. ext.*, *Gl. pall. int.*, globus pallidus; *Hab.*, habenula; *Mesen. ret. form.*, mesencephalic reticular formation; *Raphe d.*, dorsal raphe; *S. nigra (comp.)*, *S. nigra (retic.)*, substantia nigra. (Reproduced with permission from Brodal 1981.)

sensory and posterior parietal areas. It projects to the motor and premotor areas of the cerebral cortex. Thus the cerebellum, by its connexions, is well-placed to influence motor mechanisms. Its function is best considered as that of a comparator – compensating for errors by comparing the actual performance of a movement with the intended performance (see Chap. 13) – and it receives afferent input from the cortex about intended movement, afferent information from the periphery about the motor performance and, in turn, it provides efferent output that influences the hierarchical motor system at all levels. Finally, as mentioned in Chapter 13, the cerebellum is also involved in the learning of motor skills (see also Chap. 18).

The basal ganglia (the caudate nucleus, the putamen and the globus pallidus) are large nuclear masses in the cerebral hemispheres and together with the subthalamic nucleus and the substantia nigra they are importantly involved in motor control. As shown in Fig. 14.9, they do not receive afferent input directly from the spinal cord or the brain stem motor nuclei, nor do they themselves directly influence these structures. They derive most of their input from wide areas of the cerebral cortex and, in turn, project back to the premotor and prefrontal cortices via the thalamus. Like the rest of the specific motor and sensory systems the basal ganglia are highly organized in a topographic fashion.

The roles of the basal ganglia in motor performance are not well-understood but when affected by pathological processes characteristic motor signs and symptoms are produced. Usually, disorders of the basal ganglia (and associated nuclei) give rise to a variety of involuntary movements (including tremor, writhing movements and sudden flick-like movements), disorders of muscle tone (such as spasticity) and poverty of movements. Parkinson's disease is one of the best known disorders in which there is basal ganglia pathology – a loss of dopamine-containing neurons in the substantia nigra (although other parts of the nervous system and other neurotransmitters are affected in the disease too). Patients with Parkinson's disease show a tremor

at rest, a muscle rigidity and a difficulty in starting movements, and slowness of movement. Another disease due to the loss of specific sets of neurons in the striatum (caudate nucleus and putamen) is Huntington's chorea. The affected neurons contain acetylcholine and gamma-aminobutyric acid (different neurons). Huntington's chorea is an inherited disease that does not manifest itself until about the fourth or fifth decade of life. Sufferers show a progressive series of signs, both motor and psychiatric, starting with clumsiness, forgetfulness and irritability and finishing with chorea (rapid flick-like movements) of a severe form, dementia and ultimately death. In Huntington's chorea there is a loss of cholinergic neurons in the cerebral cortex, and this loss is likely to be mainly responsible for the psychiatric changes in the disease.

Summary

1.   The specific sensory and motor systems are organized in an hierarchical fashion as chains of neurons.

2.   In addition to the hierarchical organization, there are numerous parallel pathways in both sensory and motor systems.

3.   In the sensory systems, in addition to the ascending pathways from sensory receptors to the cerebral cortex, there are parallel descending pathways that can control the flow of sensory messages through the system.

4.   In motor systems, in addition to the descending pathways from one level to the next, each level in the hierarchy receives sensory inputs. These sensory inputs are essential for the successful working of the motor system, since motor acts generate sensory input, and the nervous system must be able to compare predicted sensory messages with those actually occurring.

5.   The cerebellum and the basal ganglia both influence the hierarchical motor systems in important ways.

15 Functional Properties of Specific Sensory and Motor Systems

The specific sensory and motor systems are concerned with the analysis of events in the external (and internal) environment, with the synthesis of some form of abstraction of these events (a process that leads to sensation) and then to the translation of this synthesis into appropriate action. In Chapter 14 the anatomical organization of the mammalian specific sensory and motor systems was discussed, with some indications of certain aspects of functional properties. The mechanisms of action of these systems will form the content of the present chapter, and the approach that will be adopted is to take particular functional properties and discuss them with reference to examples taken from different systems.

Functional Properties of Specific Sensory Systems

Modality Specificity

In all specific sensory systems of mammals there are neurons in the cerebral cortex that are excited by quite specific stimuli, such as by light of a particular wavelength and not by other light, by touch and not by cooling, by sound of a particular frequency and not others etc. This modality specificity is an important functional property of these systems and is due to (1) the properties of the sensory receptors, (2) the organization of primary afferent (sensory) units, and (3) the pathways from the peripheral sense organs to the primary cortical receiving areas that maintain the purity of the responses of sensory receptors.

Sense Organ Mechanisms

The first stage of analysis of events in the environment takes place at the peripheral sense organs. Sense organ mechanisms have been discussed in some detail in Chapter 12. In the present context it is important to realize that sensory receptors are highly specific in terms of the stimuli to which they respond. The synthesis of an organism's abstraction of the environment is limited by the properties of the sensory receptors; only those events that affect the sense organs can lead to afferent input to the nervous system. Thus, the human photoreceptors do not respond to ultraviolet light, whereas those of many insects do; there are electroreceptors in certain fish but these are absent in mammals, and so on. Whatever sensory modalities an organism has are determined by the sensory receptors it possesses. Not only that, but within particular modalities (vision, hearing, taste, somaesthesis etc.) sense organs may only respond to some particular attribute of a stimulus, such as a change in, but not to, a steady level of a stimulus. That is, some sense organs may be rapidly adapting and only respond at the beginning and/or the end of a maintained stimulus, whereas other sense organs may respond similarly to the onset and offset but may, in addition, respond during a maintained stimulus and code its amplitude.

The sense organs, therefore, provide the first level at which feature extraction occurs. The sense organs are responsible for the modality specificity which is such an important property of specific sensory systems; this specificity is maintained through the systems by the way certain chains of neurons are connected. Furthermore, other aspects of the stimulus are also extracted at this level by means of receptor adaptation properties. Rapidly adapting receptors are specialized to react to changes in the environment and will monitor the onset and offset of a stimulus and may also monitor its rate of change, whereas slowly adapting receptors may monitor the duration of a stimulus and its amplitude.

Primary Afferent Units

As mentioned in Chapter 14, primary afferent (or sensory) units consist of a set of sensory receptors and the single primary afferent fibre that innervates them. Each of the sensory receptors within the set is of the same type and therefore the modality specificity of the primary afferent fibre is pure and is determined by the sense organs.

Within a particular class of like primary afferent units there are a number of possible variables important for sensory analysis. Both the number of sensory receptors innervated by a single afferent fibre and the area of the receptor sheet containing the innervated receptors may vary. The primary afferent unit has a receptive field (for a discussion of the important concept of receptive field see below), which may be considered as the area of the receptive sheet enclosing all the receptors innervated by the single fibre or as the individual points on the receptor sheet containing receptors innervated by a single fibre. The latter definition is the more accurate, but the former is often used and is more convenient both for experimental purposes and for ease of description. Receptive field size may vary by either changes in the numbers of individual receptor cells innervated (if the distribution of receptors in the sheet is even) or by changes in the density of receptor cells in the sheet (if the density varies). In fact, both of these mechanisms operate, even though the constraints (of even distribution of receptors or of uneven receptor density) are not exclusive. These points may be illustrated by examples from cutaneous primary afferent units.

The receptive fields of hair follicle primary afferent units from the skin of the limbs vary in

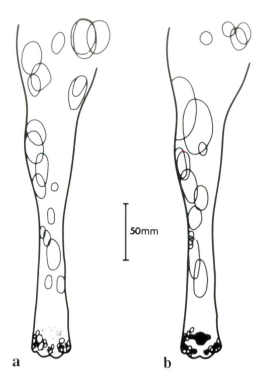

Fig. 15.1a,b. Variation of receptive field size of hair follicle primary afferent units with position on the hind limb of the cat. (Reproduced from Brown 1968.)

size in a systematic way, being very small on the distal parts of the limb (digits) and becoming progressively larger as they are located on more proximal parts (Fig. 15.1). On the digits some hair follicle units have only very few sensitive hair follicles in their receptive fields (less than ten) even though the area containing these follicles contains many others not innervated by the afferent fibre. On the proximal limb, similar afferent fibres usually innervate about the same number of hair follicles as on the distal limb, even though the receptive fields are larger. Within a particular area of the limb, where receptive fields tend to be similar, differences in receptive field size are more likely to be due to differences in the numbers of sense organs innervated. This can be shown for the slowly adapting Type I mechanoreceptive unit, which has between one and seven sense organs for each afferent fibre. (The sense organs are the "touch corpuscles" or *Haarscheiben*, which contain a number of receptor cells, the Merkel cells.)

Usually those areas of a receptor sheet innervated by primary afferent fibres with the smallest receptive fields are those areas of highest innervation density, that is, receiving more primary afferent fibres per unit area. Also, they may have a higher density of sensory receptors. It is these areas, such as the tips of the digits, the lips, the fovea of the retina, that are most sensitive to spatial separation of stimuli and are said to have the highest acuity.

Labelled Lines

In all specific sensory systems there are chains of neurons, connected through the hierarchical pathways, which are excited by activation of a single class of sensory receptor. These "labelled lines" provide the anatomical basis for the perception of particular submodalities of sensation, such as touch, vibration, pressure, warm and cool in the somatosensory system. The presence of these labelled lines, which have been recognized by electrophysiological recording from individual neurons at the various levels of the sensory systems, implies that there is a very strictly specific set of neuronal connexions underlying them – each neuron in the chain, from primary afferent neuron to those in the cerebral cortex, must make synaptic contacts with neurons at the next level with no convergence from neurons excited by activation of other types of sensory receptors.

Not all neurons in specific sensory systems are part of labelled lines. Many neurons in these systems do show considerable degrees of convergence of excitatory inputs from several different types of afferent unit. The benefits of such convergence will be discussed below, as will the problems they pose for our understanding of nervous system function.

Place Specificity

Not only is the modality of a stimulus coded by means of highly specific connexions between the sense organs and the brain, but also the location on the receptor sheet at which the stimulus occurs is similarly coded. At all levels of the specific sensory systems the receptor sheet (retina, basilar membrane, skin etc.) is mapped in terms of the receptive fields of central neurons. Even though there may be considerable distortion in the map, often due to the relative expansion of parts where the receptor density is high, the neighbourhood relations present on the receptor sheet are, in general terms, retained in the central maps. Thus, a stimulus that activates a localized cluster of receptor cells will lead to activity of localized clusters of neurons in the central maps. This

arrangement is known as topographical organization and, like the modality specificity, place specificity is due to the orderly anatomical connexions made between neurons at different levels of the sensory systems (and also between neurons at the same level). Examples of such maps in the somatosensory system (somatotopic maps) are shown in Fig. 15.2. More detailed discussion of both sensory and motor maps will be presented later in this chapter.

The Concept of Receptive Field

So far, the idea of receptive field has been explained for primary afferent units. Such receptive fields consist only of excitatory areas on the receptive surface. This description has tacitly been extended to receptive fields of central neurons. But the receptive fields of central neurons are much more complicated.

The concept of the receptive field of a central neuron derives from observations made during electrophysiological recording from such neurons. Such electrophysiological recordings may be made using either extracellular or intracellular microelectrodes. Extracellular recording reveals only the impulse discharges of a neuron, whereas intracellular recording, in addition, reveals both excitatory and inhibitory postsynaptic potentials. The receptive fields recorded from the same neuron under the two sets of recording conditions may appear quite different, with the extracellular field often appearing as only a part of the field recorded intracellularly (Fig. 15.3). Any definition of receptive field, therefore, must take account of the experimental method used to reveal it. Not only that, but some features of receptive fields, such as responsiveness to a moving stimulus, will only be revealed if the appropriate stimulus is used. It can be seen that the concept of receptive field, while not difficult in the abstract, is difficult to apply in reality to experimental results. To put this another way, the receptive field revealed under one set of experimental conditions may be quite different to the field revealed under some different conditions. A particularly striking example of this occurs in the visual cortex, where cells may respond rather poorly, or not at all, to spots of light shone on the retina but respond briskly and very strongly to lines of particular orientations. For the present purposes the receptive field of a neuron may be defined as that region (area) on the receptor sheet where stimulation can influence the neuron; such influences may be excitatory or inhibitory

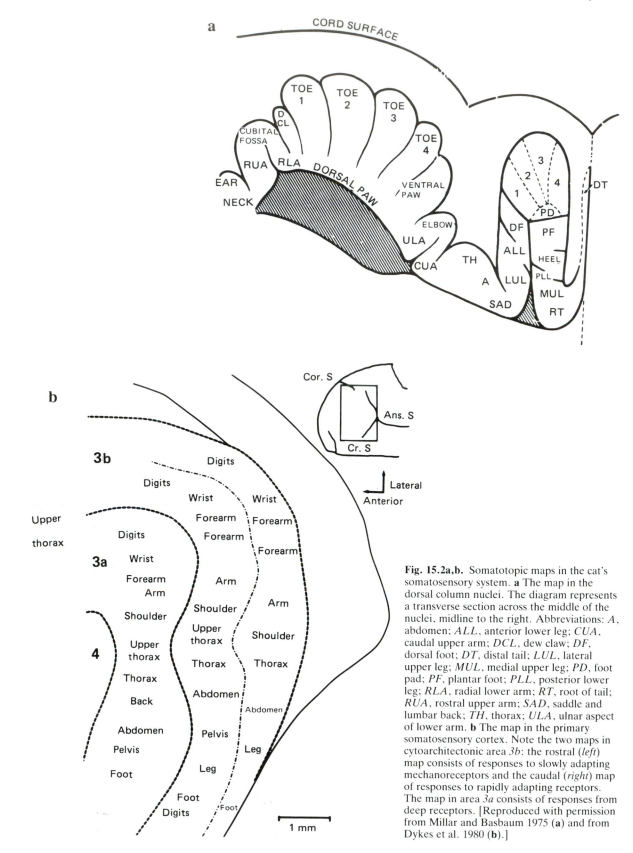

Fig. 15.2a,b. Somatotopic maps in the cat's somatosensory system. **a** The map in the dorsal column nuclei. The diagram represents a transverse section across the middle of the nuclei, midline to the right. Abbreviations: *A*, abdomen; *ALL*, anterior lower leg; *CUA*, caudal upper arm; *DCL*, dew claw; *DF*, dorsal foot; *DT*, distal tail; *LUL*, lateral upper leg; *MUL*, medial upper leg; *PD*, foot pad; *PF*, plantar foot; *PLL*, posterior lower leg; *RLA*, radial lower arm; *RT*, root of tail; *RUA*, rostral upper arm; *SAD*, saddle and lumbar back; *TH*, thorax; *ULA*, ulnar aspect of lower arm. **b** The map in the primary somatosensory cortex. Note the two maps in cytoarchitectonic area *3b*: the rostral (*left*) map consists of responses to slowly adapting mechanoreceptors and the caudal (*right*) map of responses to rapidly adapting receptors. The map in area *3a* consists of responses from deep receptors. [Reproduced with permission from Millar and Basbaum 1975 (**a**) and from Dykes et al. 1980 (**b**).]

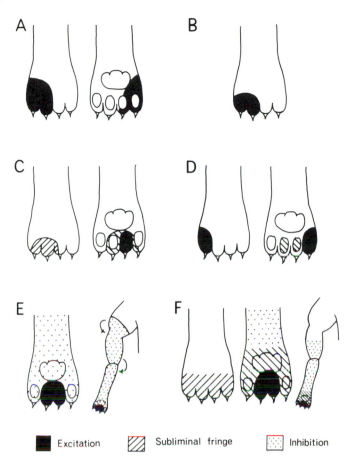

Fig. 15.3. Receptive fields of neurons in the cat's postsynaptic dorsal column system. The subliminal fringe areas (*cross-hatched*) were not apparent during extracellular recording since only excitatory postsynaptic potentials were evoked from these areas and not impulse discharges. (Reproduced with permission from Brown and Fyffe 1981b.)

and may lead to impulse discharges or be subthreshold for such discharges.

Most central sensory neurons have both excitatory and inhibitory components in their receptive fields. Furthermore, since the vast majority of such neurons also has a certain amount of "background" ("resting" or "spontaneous") activity under most experimental conditions, it is possible to recognize some inhibitory components even when extracellular recording is used – inhibition can be seen as a reduction or cessation of this background activity. In other situations it may be necessary to increase the cell's firing (or cause it to fire), either by stimulating the excitatory field or by pharmacological means such as ionophoresis of glutamate (an excitatory amino acid) close to the neuron, in order to reveal inhibition with extracellular methods.

With intracellular recording, areas of the field may be revealed from which excitatory postsynaptic potentials (EPSPs) can be elicited but which, under the conditions of the experiment, do not lead to impulse initiation. These are often at the periphery of the excitatory field and con-

stitute a subliminal fringe. Stimulation at these regions increases the excitability of the cell and, if accompanied by some other stimulation of similar areas, may lead to firing (spatial summation), as may a series of stimuli closely spaced in time at the same position (temporal summation). Moreover, under other conditions, such as in the absence of anaesthesia, or during consciousness with the animal attending to the stimulus, stimulation of such areas may more easily lead to impulse firing.

Receptive Field Organization for Feature Extraction

In this section consideration will be given to how receptive field organization can lead to stimulus feature extraction. Examples will be drawn from the visual and somatosensory systems since we have more knowledge of the neural mechanisms in these systems than in others, although data from the other sensory systems indicate they have similar mechanisms.

Centre–Surround Antagonism in the Visual System

The presence of two major parallel pathways from the retina, via the lateral geniculate nucleus of the thalamus and so to the primary visual cortex, has been described in the previous chapter. These are the on-centre and the off-centre neurons that are excited and inhibited, respectively, by light falling on the centres of their receptive fields. Surrounding these central areas are concentric surrounding areas in which light has the opposite effect, that is, inhibiting on-centre neurons and exciting off-centre ones. The central components of the receptive field of the retinal ganglion cells, which give rise to axons of the optic nerve projecting to the lateral geniculate nucleus, are formed by the direct pathways from photoreceptors via the bipolar cells to the ganglion cells (see Fig. 12.4). The antagonistic surrounds are generated by connexions made by the horizontal cells, which are excited from photoreceptors in the surround field and which inhibit bipolar cells influenced from the centre.

What are the operational effects of this sort of organization? As shown in Fig. 14.4, a small spot of light shone on the centre of the receptive field of an on-centre cell causes a weak excitatory response, whereas a similar small spot shone on part of the surround leads to weak inhibition of the ongoing activity in the neuron. The cell is most strongly excited by illuminating the whole of the central area and most strongly inhibited by illuminating the surround area with an annular stimulus. Diffuse illumination which covers both the centre and surround parts of the field produces very little effect. The opposite actions are observed for off-centre cells. This centre–surround antagonism has the important effect of enhancing contrast (for example in the detection of borders between light and dark). The neuronal organization of inhibitory neurons (horizontal cells in this case) providing inhibitory input from outside a central excitatory region of the receptive field is common in all sensory systems studied and at all levels; a more general term for this phenomenon is surround or lateral inhibition.

In-field Inhibition

In many sensory neurons the excitatory part of the receptive field also contains inhibitory components. That is, stimulation of the excitatory field, in addition to producing excitation often also produces inhibition. Two types of this kind

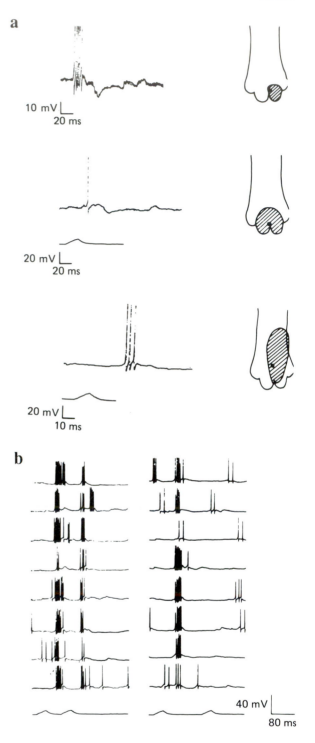

Fig. 15.4a,b. In-field afferent inhibition in the spinocervical tract. **a** Intracellularly recorded response to an air-jet stimulus within the excitatory receptive field (at the *filled circle*). Note the brisk discharge of impulses followed by an IPSP complex. **b** Intracellularly recorded responses to a pair of air-jet stimuli. Note the reduction in response to the second air-jet and the absence of IPSPs. (Reproduced with permission from Brown et al. 1987b.)

of organization have been observed in the spino-cervical tract. In the first (Fig. 15.4a), stimulation of the excitatory field, in addition to producing EPSPs in the spinocervical cells, may produce inhibitory postsynaptic potentials (IPSPs), which usually follow the excitation. The second sort of in-field inhibition in these cells does not appear to produce postsynaptic potentials in the spino-cervical tract neurons themselves but reduces EPSPs in them by acting on the neurons afferent to the spinocervical tract cell (Fig. 15.4b). The operational effects of in-field inhibition are to shorten the duration of the excitatory response, following it with a period of little activity and also to reduce the response to repeated stimuli. Both of these effects will enhance contrast by bringing the onset of the response into relief and also make the first response to a repeated stimulus greater then the succeeding ones and therefore more noticeable.

Further Feature Extraction in the Visual System

The now classic experiments of Hubel and Wiesel in the late 1950s and early 1960s provided important information about how the visual cortex deals with incoming sensory messages and extracts more features from the visual input. The primary visual cortex (area 17 or V1), like all primary sensory cortical areas, is organized in a topographical (retinotopic) fashion and contains a map of the visual field. (Each side of the cortex maps the contralateral visual hemifield in animals with forward-facing eyes due to the crossing of optic fibres from each nasal half of the retina – influenced from the temporal visual field – in the optic chiasm.) Although neurons in the retina and the lateral geniculate are all organized in the centre–surround fashion described above and are influenced very effectively by small spots of light, Hubel and Wiesel found that very few cells in the visual cortex responded to such stimuli. Instead of having circular receptive fields, cells in the visual cortex usually have linear receptive fields (Fig. 15.5) and the most effective sort of stimulus for them is a bar, a line or some sort of edge.

Hubel and Wiesel divided the visual cortical cells into two major classes – simple and complex. Simple cells have receptive fields (Fig. 15.5a) with clearly defined excitatory and inhibitory zones arranged in a linear manner. In order to evoke a response in these cells the adequate stimulus must not only be in the appropriate part of the visual field but must also be a bar or slit of light (or dark) orientated in the correct position. Diffuse illumination is generally ineffective in exciting these cells. Some simple cells have strict requirements for the length of a stimulus, longer stimuli being less effective if the stimulus extends beyond the excitatory component of the receptive field. For many simple cells the most effective stimulus is a moving bar or edge of the correct orientation, and in some cells the direction of movement is critical too. Complex cells also require specific orientation of a dark–light boundary for excitation and also respond weakly, if at all, to diffuse illumination. In addition, they have a much less restricted requirement for position in the visual field, and the receptive fields have no obvious excitatory and inhibitory zones. Thus, complex cells extract the feature of orientation without concern for position. In addition, complex cells may signal increasing length of a stimulus by increasing discharge rate or may have strict requirements for the maximum length of stimulus to which they will respond (Fig. 15.5b). Some complex cells respond best to a moving slit oriented appropriately and moving in a particular direction.

Hubel and Wiesel made further fundamental observations about the functional organization of the monkey's area 17. Shortly after Mountcastle had recognized that the somatosensory cortex was arranged in a columnar manner, with neurons within a column having similar response properties, Hubel and Wiesel made systematic micro-electrode penetrations through the visual cortex of anaesthetized monkeys while presenting visual stimuli (orientated slits and bars of light) to the visual field and to both eyes. They discovered that the primary visual cortex was organized in a columnar fashion into two major sets of columns. One set of columns (Fig. 15.6) contained simple and complex cells in which all the cells had a preference for a particular orientation of the stimulus (orientation columns). The second set of cortical columns (Fig. 15.6) contained neurons that showed preferences for being stimulated through a particular eye (ocular dominance columns). Quite remarkably, these ocular dominance columns may be demonstrated by anatomical means (using a reduced silver histological method), and the complete arrangement of the columns in the exposed part of the primary visual cortex may be reconstructed, as shown in Fig. 15.7. (The columns may also be shown by neuro-anatomical degeneration methods after appropriate lesions in the lateral geniculate body and also by axonal transport methods.)

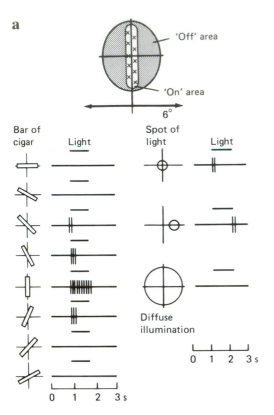

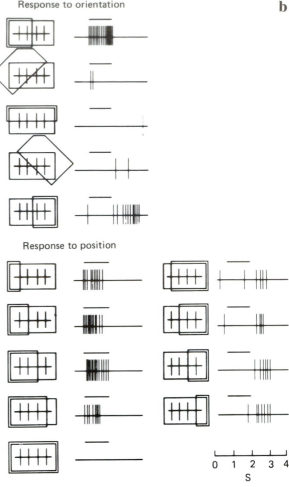

Fig. 15.5a,b. Receptive fields of cells in the primary visual cortex. **a** A simple cell has a linear receptive field responding best to a bar of light oriented in a particular direction. Spots of light and diffuse illumination are ineffective as stimuli. **b** A complex cell responds best to a vertical edge. Orientation is important but position within the field is not. (Modified from Kandel and Schwartz 1985, after Hubel and Wiesel 1962.)

Further meticulous experiments by Hubel and Wiesel revealed that the two sets of columns (orientation and ocular dominance) were arranged at right angles to one another and, in addition, between each set of orientation columns (each about 50 μm wide) there was a systematic shift in preferred orientation of about 10°. Each set of columns, either orientation or ocular dominance, subserved a particular part of the visual field because of the precise retinotopic organization of the primary visual cortex. Hubel and Wiesel called each complete set of columns subserving either all orientations or both eyes (at a particular place in the visual field) a hypercolumn (see Fig. 15.6). Here, therefore, is a scheme whereby inputs produced by stimuli with the same orientation and from the same position in the visual field but via the two eyes can be brought together for processing within a small coherent part of the primary visual cortex.

More recently it has been shown that within the orientation columns in monkeys there are groups of neurons, arranged in blobs, that are not orientation selective (Fig. 15.8). These blobs, first shown by staining for the enzyme cytochrome oxidase, are in the upper and lower layers of the cortex, in exact register with the ocular dominance columns, and contain neurons that show certain selectivities for the wavelength of light. They have a centre–surround organization in which the centre shows colour opponent properties (e.g. red-on/green-off) with a surround that responds to all wavelengths of light.

It would appear, therefore, that within primary visual cortex (V1) processing of incoming visual signals is concerned with orientation (form) and some aspects of wavelength discrimination and also motion of visual stimuli, as well as localization of stimuli in the visual field. The reasons for these conclusions include the presence of neurons

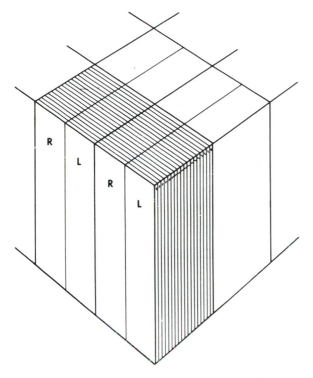

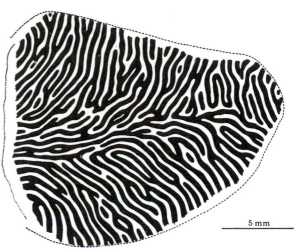

Fig. 15.7. Reconstruction of the ocular dominance columns (in layer IVc of the primate cortex), as seen from the surface of the visual cortex, from a series of reduced silver sections. Every other column has been blacked in to exhibit the nature of the subdivisions into the two sets of columns. (Reproduced with permission from LeVay et al. 1975.)

Fig. 15.6. Model of the primary visual cortex to show the arrangement of the ocular dominance columns (slabs) from the right (*R*) and left (*L*) eyes in relation to the orientation columns (slabs). Note there is a complete set of orientation columns in each pair of ocular dominance columns, making up a hypercolumn. (Reproduced with permission from Hubel and Wiesel 1977.)

selective for: (1) particular wavelengths (in the blobs in layers 2 and 3); (2) orientation (especially concentrated in the inter-blob regions of layers 2 and 3); and (3) motion (in layer 4 throughout V1). Specific connexions with visual cortical areas outside V1 are made from each of these regions (Fig. 15.9).

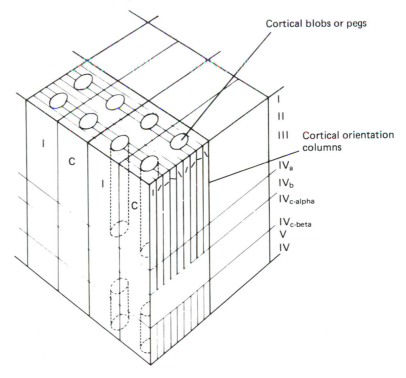

Fig. 15.8. More recent model of the primary visual cortex including the cytochrome oxidase-rich blobs (or pegs) in the upper and lower cortical layers that contain non-orientation selective cells that show colour-opponent properties. (Modified from Kandel and Schwartz 1985, after Livingstone and Hubel 1984.)

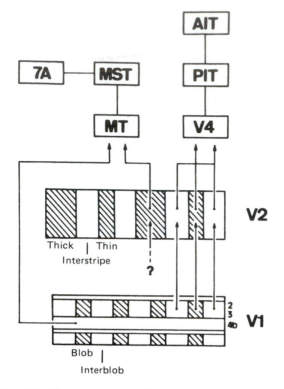

Fig. 15.9. Major components of the motion pathway and the colour and form pathway in the visual cortex. In primary visual cortex (*V1*) the colour and form pathway arises from the blobs and interblob regions in layers 2 and 3. The motion pathway arises from layer 4b. Abbreviations: *V1*, *V2*, *V4*, first, second and fourth visual areas; *MT*, *MST*, middle temporal and medial superior temporal areas; *AIT*, *PIT*, anterior and posterior inferotemporal areas; *7A*, cytoarchitectonic area 7a. (Reproduced with permission from Maunsell and Newsome 1987.)

There are many visual areas in the cortex, 19 having been recognized in monkeys. It appears that these areas are organized for further feature extraction. Indeed, some areas contain neurons that are very rigidly specified in terms of their adequate stimulus, e.g. some respond to a hand or a face. At present, many visual scientists favour ideas that were initially formulated by Zeki (1975), namely, that a major role of V1 is to divide up its outputs into streams projecting to different visual areas of cortex that operate in parallel. But a word of caution should be added here, even in an elementary presentation. Monkeys are very special animals, usually highly dependent on visual signals in their natural arboreal habitat. Indeed, the amount of cerebral cortex given up to visual processing in these animals is enormous – about 20% of exposed

cortex is occupied by V1 alone in macaque monkeys, compared with about 1.5% in humans, and the total amount of neocortex given over to visual processing is about 60% of the total.

Important points to emerge from the electrophysiological analysis of the visual pathways, and also of other sensory pathways, are as follows:

1. Central neurons have particular requirements of a stimulus in order for them to give their best responses – the key pattern of stimulation is known as a trigger feature.

2. As the sensory systems are examined through their hierarchical organization, and especially as the sensory messages are processed through the various cortical areas, the trigger features often become more sophisticated.

3. Although the hierarchical system will allow complex neuronal responses to be built up from preceding simpler ones, this is not the whole story. Parallel processing must also be an important organizational principle, and separate channels of processing for particular stimulus features exist.

Submodality Convergence

Within specific sensory systems not all channels are labelled lines that maintain sensory receptor purity. In many instances there is convergence from different kinds of primary afferent units onto central cells. Examples abound in the somatosensory systems. The possible function of submodality convergence in some cells seems apparent. Thus some cells in the dorsal column nuclei have receptive fields that encompass both hairy and glabrous skin of the distal limbs and are excited by stimulation of both hair follicle receptors and rapidly adapting mechanoreceptors in glabrous skin. Such an arrangement will allow for completion of the somatotopic map in central nuclei and also extract features of stimuli that commonly impinge on both hairy and glabrous skin.

A very common type of submodality convergence found in the spinocervicothalamic and spinothalamic systems is one where neurons respond both to innocuous and noxious stimuli within the excitatory receptive field. Such convergence is more difficult to understand since it is not immediately apparent if the responses to the two importantly different stimuli differ. Either some feature other than the modality of the stimulus is being coded or the nervous system is able to unravel the responses by means not yet recognized. The nervous system can, however, selectively remove one or the other input in such systems (see below).

Centrifugal Control in Sensory Systems

All sensory systems contain descending loops of neuronal connexions that provide for centrifugal control of ascending messages. Unfortunately, although it is generally held that such control must be of fundamental importance, very little experimental evidence is available that throws light on what these descending components actually do. Most is known about centrifugal control of sensory receptors (see Chap. 12). Within the central nervous system itself most detailed evidence comes from work on the descending control of spinal neurons concerned with somaesthesis. Neurons of the spinocervical tract are under the control of a number of descending systems that all seem to have similar actions. Chief among these actions is the ability to inhibit polysnaptic excitatory inputs to spinocervical neurons while leaving monosynaptic inputs unmolested. The operational outcome of such actions therefore depends on the anatomical connectivity in the system. One clear end result is that activity in the descending systems will inhibit input from nocireceptors while leaving input from hair follicle receptors relatively untouched. In the spinothalamic system evidence of the opposite control (inhibition of innocuous inputs, leaving the neuron responding to noxious ones) has also been found. Here we have examples of centrifugal control acting to make a neuron more selective in its responses. It seems likely that mechanisms of this sort underlie attention.

Functional Properties of Specific Motor Systems

Movements may be elicited either in response to some stimulus or by some central commands. Until relatively recently the emphasis was on stimulus-triggered movements, and our knowledge of these is quite well advanced. The recognition that much movement is generated centrally has been more recent, but it is now realized that much stereotyped movement, such as the respiratory movements and locomotion, is generated centrally, even though it can be easily influenced by stimuli acting peripherally.

Stimulus-Triggered Reactions

Spinal reflexes are examples of stimulus-triggered reactions, and the reader is referred to Chapter 13 for an account of such reflexes and the operation of the segmental motor apparatus. Indeed, given the principle of reciprocal innervation, whereby excitation of motoneurons to one set of muscles (say flexors) acting around a joint is accompanied by inhibition of motoneurons supplying the antagonists acting at the same joint (extensors) with concomitant facilitatory and inhibitory action on the appropriate synergistic and antagonistic motoneurons in the same and the contralateral limb, it is not difficult to imagine locomotion being a stimulus-triggered reaction. It is now known that locomotion is centrally programmed. What, therefore, are the roles of stimulus-triggered movements? Obviously, they are important for responses to external stimuli. Furthermore, during centrally programmed, or centrally initiated (voluntary) movements, input from the periphery monitors the performance of that movement and allows adjustments of the motor commands in the face of unexpected deviations from the desired movements.

Centrally Programmed Movements

Many movements are now known to be centrally programmed: for example respiratory movements, movements responsible for bird-song, grooming movements, and eye movements in certain animals. In mammals, locomotion is also possible without sensory feed-back and is based on a central programme, and the neuronal machinery generating this is located in the spinal cord.

Locomotion

Early in this century Graham Brown (1911) observed that immediately after the spinal cord had been transected an animal could show rhythmic walking movements for some time (a minute or so), even when the dorsal roots had previously been cut so that there was no afferent input to the spinal cord. Thus, locomotion is not reflex in origin but generated by neuronal mechanisms within the spinal cord.

Stepping in a spinal preparation is a complex process. Different limb muscles operate with different duty cycles or active periods in a particular sequence (Fig. 15.10). Stepping is not simply a mass contraction of flexors followed by a mass contraction of extensors. It is now believed that in the cord there are sets of premotor inter-

neurons, appropriately connected to one another and to the motoneurons, that are responsible for the complex sequences of motoneuronal firing during stepping. These sets of interneurons are called central pattern generators (CPGs). These CPGs must be linked to one another, for example to allow appropriate coordination of fore limbs and hind limbs. Presumably, neural pathways from the brain to the spinal cord might affect motor performance by influencing either the CPGs or the motoneurons.

In addition to its ability to produce stepping, the spinal cord locomotor apparatus will respond to input from peripheral sense organs to adjust locomotion according to prevailing environmental conditions. Thus, the cord can produce stepping and at the same time produce "paw shake" movements necessary to dislodge a foreign body from the foot (Fig. 15.11). Furthermore, the spinal apparatus can make the necessary adjustments to stepping if the limb is displaced during a stepping movement.

More recently, it has been shown that locomotor movements, or the appropriate locomotor outputs from motoneurons (so-called fictive locomotion) may be elicited by electrical stimulation in various parts of the brain stem. One site is in the subthalamic region and the other in the mesencephalon, just ventral to the inferior colliculus. Stimulation of this latter mesencephalic locomotor region produces stepping. The strength of stimulation determines the force with which the limbs are moved; the speed of the treadmill, on which the preparation is supported, determines the locomotor mode – walking, trotting or galloping. The position of the stimulating electrodes in the brain stem is critical and the mesencephalic locomotor region is now thought to be in the pedunculopontine nucleus, which contains cholinergic neurons.

The cerebellum is also involved in the control of the spinal locomotor apparatus. Input reaching the cerebellum from sense organs in muscles, joints and skin provides information about the movements and any sudden unexpected obstacles. Furthermore, the output of the spinal motor apparatus itself appears to be copied and sent to the cerebellum (via the ventral spinocerebellar tracts) to allow comparison between programmed movement and the actual movement.

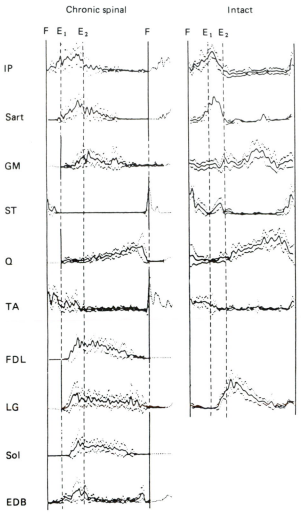

Fig. 15.10. Electromyographic (EMG) signals from a range of cat hind limb muscles during stepping (chronic spinal preparation on the *left*, intact animal on the *right*). Mean EMG signals, averaged over a number of steps, are shown as a *continuous line*. Flexion of the limb begins at *F*, footfall occurs at E_2. Abbreviations: *IP*, ilio psoas; *Sart*, sartorius; *GM*, gastrocnemius medialis; *ST*, semitendinosus; *Q*, quadriceps; *TA*, tibialis anterior; *FDL*, flexor digitorum longus; *LG*, lateral gastrocnemius; *Sol*, soleus; *EDB*, extensor digitorum brevis. (Reproduced with permission from Forssberg et al. 1980.)

Voluntary Movement

Voluntary (purposeful) movement is a function of the motor cortex. It was recognized in the

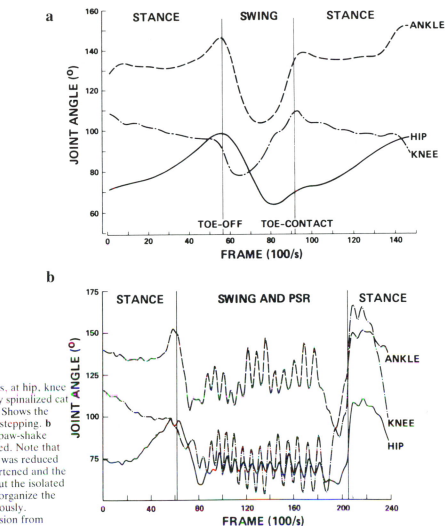

Fig. 15.11a,b. Joint angles, at hip, knee and ankle, of a chronically spinalized cat stepping on a treadmill. **a** Shows the angles during unimpeded stepping. **b** Shows the angles when a paw-shake response (*PSR*) was elicited. Note that the frequency of stepping was reduced with the stance phase shortened and the swing phase prolonged, but the isolated spinal cord is still able to organize the two behaviours simultaneously. (Reproduced with permission from Carter and Smith 1986.)

latter part of the nineteenth century that motor functions were localized to particular parts of the cortex. Clinical observations on the spread of muscle contractions during epileptic attacks and experimental observations on the effects of electrical stimulation of the exposed cortex in dogs and primates provided the initial evidence for this localization. Modern approaches, especially the use of refined electrical stimulation using microelectrodes, have shown that there is a systematic motor map in cytoarchitectonic area 4 in the precentral gyrus (Fig. 15.12). This map is in register, in terms of somatotopic organization, with the somatosensory map in the postcentral gyrus. In addition to this area, called the motor cortex, there are other cortical areas known to play a role in voluntary movement control, in particular two areas in front of the motor cortex

– the premotor cortex and the supplementary motor area – and areas behind the somatosensory cortex – the posterior parietal cortices. Each of these areas is connected by cortico-cortical projections to each of the others and, in turn, receives cortico-cortical connexions from each of them.

The Motor Cortex

The motor cortex provides an important component of the direct connexions from cerebral cortex to spinal cord, the corticospinal tract. Other important contributions are made from the premotor cortex and the supplementary motor area, together with contributions from somatosensory areas. A subset of corticospinal

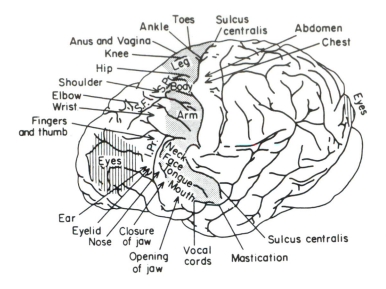

Fig. 15.12. The motor cortex of the chimpanzee. The motor area is indicated by *stippling*. Abbreviations: *I.Pr.*, inferior precentral sulcus; *S.F.*, superior frontal sulcus; *S.Pr.*, superior precentral sulcus. Note the somatotopic organization of the motor cortex. (Reproduced from Sherrington 1906.)

neurons makes important connexions with the spinal motor apparatus and, in primates, makes direct (monosynaptic) excitatory synapses with alpha-motoneurons. Many of the connexions made with the spinal motor apparatus, however, are made with the various interneurons that are intercalated between primary afferent fibres and the motor neurons (see Chap. 13), and thus the motor cortex can influence the working of the spinal mechanism. In addition to the direct connexions with the segmental motor apparatus, there are also indirect connexions via the brain stem motor nuclei, such as the red nucleus.

Individual corticospinal neurons in the motor cortex have been recorded in awake behaving primates. Many of these cells increase their firing just before the animal carries out a trained motor action (Fig. 15.13) and the firing of the cells appears to code for the force required to perform the movement rather than for the movement itself. Not only that, but individual corticospinal neurons appear to signal whether it is a dynamic change of force or a static level of force that is required. The motor cortex is itself informed of how well its instructions to the segmental motor apparatus have been carried out by feed-back from the spinal cord, and a similar role in comparing intended with actual performance is carried out by the cerebellum (see Chaps. 13 and 14).

Supramotor Areas of Cerebral Cortex

The motor cortex forms essentially an intermediate level of motor control. It executes motor plans specified from motor areas higher in the hierarchy of control. It is now believed that central motor programs are developed in the premotor areas and that motor acts may be initiated there.

Evidence for the role of the supplementary motor area in the self-initiation of motor acts came from work on squirrel monkeys. After bilateral removal of this area the frequency of vocalization decreased. Most interestingly, this was essentially due to the decreased frequency of a particular vocalization, the isolation peep, which is thought to be a learned, self-initiated long-distance call (Kirzinger and Jürgens 1982). The supplementary motor area also appears to be involved in thinking about motor acts in humans. Thus, when subjects were asked to think about carrying out a complex learned movement the regional cortical blood flow (rCBF) over this area increased, but thinking about a trivial repetitive task had little effect on rCBF. Thus it seems that the supplementary motor area is involved in translating a process from an idea to a movement, but only if the movement demands attention and not if the movement can be performed automatically.

In primates, including humans, the premotor cortex appears to be involved in guiding arm movements. Damage to the area leads to involuntary grasping in response to tactile stimulation of the palm. Some neurons in the area discharge as if they are responsible for preparing for arm movement. Finally, the posterior parietal areas seem to coordinate sensory information about the relationships of the body in space (again especially the limb positions) with movements aimed at particular targets. Some neurons in

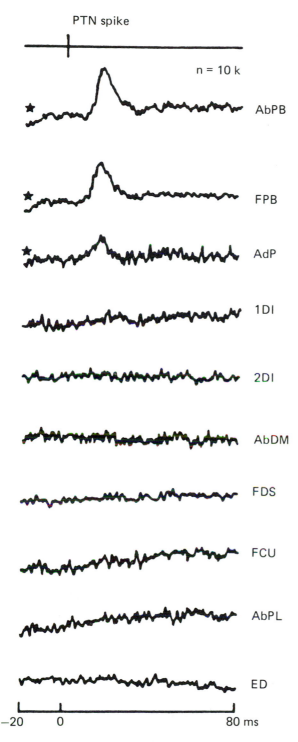

PTN spike

n = 10 k

AbPB

FPB

AdP

1DI

2DI

AbDM

FDS

FCU

AbPL

ED

−20   0   80 ms

Fig. 15.13. Correlation of a single impulse discharge in a corticospinal neuron and the EMG activity in muscles of the hand (monkey). The *top trace* shows the timing of the impulse in the neuron, and each of the other traces represents the averages of the EMG activity (averaged with respect to 1000 impulses in the neuron). Only three of the muscles (marked with an *asterisk*) show any facilitation. (Reproduced with permission from Lemon 1988.)

these areas only fire when the monkey manually explores an object, and others only fire when the monkey reaches for a particular object near to it.

Maps in the Brain

It should now be apparent to the reader from the present and the previous chapters that at all levels in the sensory and motor systems there are maps in the brain (and spinal cord). The presence of such maps imply a remarkable specificity in the way connexions are made between neurons. The following questions can be asked (following Cowey 1979): Why are there maps? Why is there usually more than one map (in a particular area)? What is it that is being mapped?

The answer to the first question – Why are there maps? – would seem to have to do with economy of neural material. It certainly would make for more economic use of neuronal cytoplasm to have neurons that carry out closely related operations situated near one another to keep the lengths of their axons to a minimum. Thus, in the visual system, analysis of the left and right eye inputs from the same part of the visual field and the orientation of stimuli at that part of the field are brought together in the hypercolumns of V1 and analysis of colour from similar parts of the visual field are brought together in the "blob" areas of V1; in the motor cortex, processing of motor commands to the spinal apparatus involved in particular movements is brought together in the motor cortex, and so on.

The second question – Why are there several maps at each level? – seems to need an answer in terms of function. Since the brain works in both a hierarchical and parallel fashion and also breaks down its processing into component parts (for example, in the visual system it appears to analyse form, movement, colour etc. by separate sets of neurons), multiple mapping again becomes an economical way to carry out this processing.

The third question – What is being mapped? – is more difficult. One often reads (or hears) that something "is represented in the maps". But surely the maps are *of* something rather than *representing* something. Sensory maps certainly do not represent the sensory receptors and motor maps certainly do not represent muscles. Surely, in agreement with Zeki (1981), the sensory maps are of transformations of and contrasts in the appropriate sensory data, and similarly the motor maps are maps of motor instructions coded in the way the nervous system operates.

Summary

1. Sensory systems show modality specificity, which is laid down by specific sensory receptors and maintained by the way they are connected through primary afferent fibres and the various ascending neuronal pathways to the cerebral cortex.

2. All specific sensory pathways are arranged in a topographical fashion so that the neighbourhood relations present on the receptor sheet are maintained at the various synaptic sites in the central sensory pathways.

3. The concept of receptive field is important for understanding neuronal operations in sensory (and motor) systems. In sensory systems receptive fields provide clues to how feature extraction is carried out.

4. Not all sensory neurons show complete modality specificity.

5. At all levels in sensory systems there are descending neuronal loops acting back from higher to lower levels and controlling the through-put of sensory impulses.

6. Motor systems operate with stimulus-triggered reactions (such as spinal reflexes) and centrally programmed movements. Stereotyped movements such as respiratory movements and locomotion are centrally programmed.

7. The isolated spinal cord is capable of generating sophisticated locomotor patterns in the output of motoneurons. Central pattern generators exist in the spinal cord.

8. Brain stem regions can access the spinal central pattern generators to initiate and influence locomotion, as can the cerebellum – via the brain stem or through the thalamus and motor cortex.

9. The motor cortex is responsible for controlling the segmental motor apparatus in the carrying out of voluntary (purposeful) movements. In turn, the motor cortex is instructed by premotor areas of the cerebral cortex. and there is a close working relationship between motor and sensory areas of the cortex to provide information of the relationship of the body parts in space.

10. There are many motor and sensory maps in the nervous system in which neurons of like function are brought close together in space. The sensory maps are maps of transformations of sensory data, and the motor maps (when revealed by recording rather than stimulating) are maps of neuronal operations responsible for controlling movement.

16 The Nervous System and Homeostasis – Interactions with the Internal and External Environments

A major function of the nervous system is to control the relative constancy of the internal environment of the organism. That is, to provide the right chemical environment for living processes to take place. This control of the internal environment is known as homeostasis. Any disturbances in the internal environment are monitored by sense organs: for example chemoreceptors sensitive to the partial pressure of oxygen in the arterial blood, mechanoreceptors sensitive to blood pressure, and chemoreceptors within the central nervous system itself sensitive to hydrogen ion concentration or to various hormones. The information from the sense organs is fed to the central nervous system, where it is processed and appropriate outputs sent to the effectors, muscle (striated, smooth and cardiac) and glands, to counteract the disturbance. Such a function is essentially the same as that carried out by a physical servosystem like a governor on a steam engine, or a central heating control system that measures room temperature and keeps it within certain limits by regulating the output of the heating unit (Fig. 16.1).

On the effector side, the nervous system provides direct control of muscle and glands by the somatic and autonomic motor systems. By far the greater control is exerted by the autonomic nervous system (see Fig. 1.7), which controls smooth muscle and cardiac muscle, exocrine glands and the adrenal medulla (endocrine gland). The somatic motor system has the important role of controlling the (striated) muscles of respiration. In addition, the brain controls the function of many organs and tissues by releasing hormones. This neuroendocrine function of the nervous system is extremely important. The hormones released by certain neurons may pass into the systemic circulation and directly affect target organs, in the same way as any hormone released from an endocrine gland, or may pass into a special portal circulation and control the release of hormones from the pituitary gland. Finally, the nervous system also provides appropriate outputs via the somatic motor system that lead to behavioural responses necessary to maintain the constancy of the internal environment (for example, feeding, drinking and thermoregulatory behaviour) and also to protect the individual animal and thus the species (aggression, emotional behaviour, reproductive behaviour). In this chapter neuroendocrine mechanisms will be discussed, and this will be followed by consideration of aspects of behavioural state control, motivational behaviour and control of nociception. Chapter 18 will consider some aspects of learning and memory which allow the organism to operate much more efficiently within the external environment.

The Neuroendocrine System

The neuroendocrine system provides a means of connecting the two major control systems in the

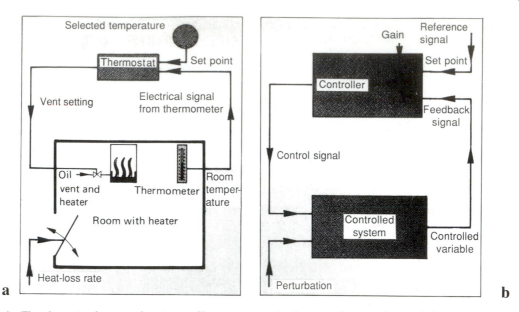

Fig.16.1a,b. The elements of a control system. **a** Shows an example of a control system for regulating room temperature. **b** Shows a block diagram of a generalized feed-back control system. (Reproduced from Schmidt 1978.)

body – the nervous system on the one hand with the endocrine system on the other. It allows both internal and external changes to be monitored by the sense organs of the nervous system, the neural signals to be processed by the nervous system (with the hypothalamus playing a major role) and converted to endocrine outputs. Furthermore, associated with the neuroendocrine system are special areas where the blood–brain barrier is breached. This is necessary both to allow hormones released from nerve fibres to enter the blood stream and also to allow hormones access to the brain, since many hormones circulating in the blood influence the brain, especially the neurosecretory system itself.

Several different sets of neurons in the hypothalamus release hormones into the blood. These hormones are all peptides; indeed, in other parts of the nervous system there are neurons that release the same peptides at synaptic junctions, where they act as neurotransmitters or neuromodulators. The several different sets of neuroendocrine neurons may be grouped into two categories: the magnocellular neurosecretory system and the parvocellular neurosecretory system. Both systems have ancient phylogenetic origins and are present in all vertebrates, indicating their importance.

The idea that neurons might secrete hormones was introduced by Speidel (1922), who observed large neurons that looked like secretory (gland) cells in the fish spinal cord. Later, Scharrer and Scharrer (1940) noted that hypothalamic neurons projecting into the posterior pituitary contained granules that stained selectively with a particular histological stain (Gomori's chrome alum haematoxylin). The granules were of a protein character and it was later shown (by du Vigneaud) that this material contained the hormones vasopressin and oxytocin (see du Vigneaud 1956).

Magnocellular Neurosecretory System

The magnocellular neurosecretory system consists of neurons which have their cell bodies in the supraoptic and paraventricular nuclei of the hypothalamus and which have axons that run through the pituitary stalk into the posterior part of the pituitary gland where they end in close relation to blood capillaries (Fig. 16.2). These neurons synthesise two main peptides, vasopressin (or antidiuretic hormone) and oxytocin. Each hormone is synthesized by separate sets of neurons and each is a nine amino acid peptide that is cleaved from a larger prohormone. The peptides are released from the nerves at their terminations in the posterior pituitary and enter the blood stream.

Oxytocin release controls two important reproductive functions, uterine contraction during labour (if the uterine smooth muscle is appropriately primed by oestrogens) and milk ejection from the mammary gland during lactation. Thus, in both cases oxytocin leads to contraction of smooth muscle. Vasopressin has important roles to play in the control of blood pressure and also in the control of body fluid composition (ionic

HYPOTHALAMIC-NEUROHYPOPHYSIAL SYSTEM	HYPOTHALAMIC-ADENOHYPOPHYSIAL SYSTEM

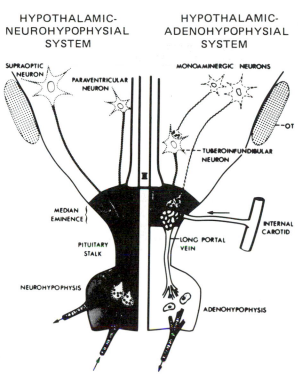

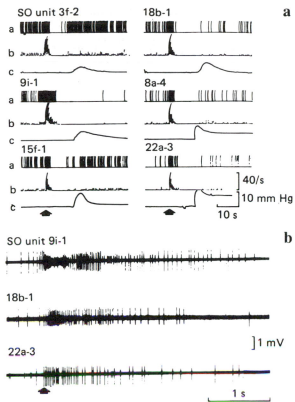

Fig. 16.2. Schematic representation of the hypothalamic regulation of the pituitary gland. On the *left* is the magnocellular system (hypothalamic-neurohypophysial system) and on the *right* is the tuberoinfundibular system (hypothalamic-adenohypophysial system). *OT*, optic tract. (Reproduced with permission from Martin et al. 1977.)

Fig. 16.3a,b. Activity of oxytocin-releasing neurons and the milk ejection reflex. **a** Polygraph records of activity in single supraoptic neurons in the lactating rat (*top*) and the integrated records of the unit activity (*middle*), together with a recording of intramammary pressure (*bottom*). **b** Expanded original traces of the discharges of three of the units. The *arrows* indicate the onset of the neurosecretory responses. (Reproduced with permission from Lincoln and Wakerley 1974.)

concentration) by acting on the kidney to prevent loss of body water in the urine. The release of these two hormones is controlled by separate systems.

Control of the oxytocin system has been studied by using the milk ejection reflex as the sign of hormone release. During suckling by rat pups the neurons fire bursts of impulses, and shortly afterwards there is contraction of the smooth muscle of the mammary gland ducts in the lactating female rat (Fig. 16.3). The suckling activates sensory receptors in the teats, and by means of a neural reflex (whose details have not yet been worked out) the oxytocin-releasing neurons are caused to fire. This relatively simple relex is influenced, however, by many other factors. Thus, many types of stress, in both animals and humans, can interfere with lactation, and in a lactating woman even the sound or sight of her infant can cause a reflex milk let-down.

Neurons that release vasopressin respond to both neural and humoral inputs. The neural inputs include those from the sensory receptors on the arterial side of the circulation that monitor blood pressure (the baroreceptors). The afferent im-

pulses travel via the ninth and tenth cranial nerves to the brain stem and then via noradrenergic neurons to the hypothalamus (see Fig. 7.8). The noradrenergic neurons exert a tonic inhibition on the magnocellular neurons, and lesions of the noradrenergic pathway (from the A1 group of catecholamine neurons) lead to increased plasma levels of vasopressin and increased blood pressure which may lead to death of the animal. Normally, increases in blood pressure lead to a reduction in vasopressin release and a lowering of blood pressure. The vasopressin-producing cells also respond to changes in the osmotic environment around them. If the osmotic pressure of the blood in the internal carotid artery, which supplies the hypothalamus, is increased then vasopressin release is increased, and this prevents water loss from the kidney. Vasopressin release is also increased if the concentration of the hormone angiotensin II in the blood increases. Angiotensin II is a peptide, and in order for it to affect vasopressin release it must cross the blood–brain barrier. Evidence suggests that it does so at the subfornical organ at the rostral end of the third ventricle, where there are angiotensin-sensitive neurons that are essentially outside of the blood–brain barrier. Connexions from the subfornical neurons to the supraoptic and paraventricular nuclei are responsible for controlling vasopressin release by this system. Angiotensin II is formed from precursors by the action of the hormone renin. Renin is secreted by the juxtaglomerular apparatus in the kidney in response to a fall in blood pressure at the renal arterioles and also to a decrease in the sodium content of the fluid in the renal tubule (in the distal nephron). Increased renin secretion in response to these stimuli leads to increased angiotensin II levels in the blood. Angiotensin II, in addition to its actions on the magnocellular neuroendocrine system, also causes aldosterone secretion from the adrenal cortex (leading to sodium retention by the kidney) and vasoconstriction in arterioles (leading to compensatory increases in blood pressure).

Parvocellular Neurosecretory System

The neurons of the parvocellular neurosecretory system (or the tuberoinfundibular system of the hypothalamus, as it is otherwise known) have their cell bodies in the medial basal hypothalamus (in the paraventricular, preoptic and arcuate nuclei and adjacent areas) and send their axons to the median eminence, where they release their hormones into the blood stream (see Fig. 16.2). Blood from capillaries in the median eminence passes to a second set of capillaries (this is therefore a portal system – the hypothalamohypophysial portal system) in the anterior pituitary gland, where the hormones act on hormone-secreting cells causing them either to release their hormones or to inhibit such release.

The parvocellular neuroendocrine system consists of five subsystems, each releasing a regulating hormone (a releasing or a release-inhibiting factor). The five factors are thyrotropin-releasing hormone (TRH), gonadotropin-releasing hormone (GnRH), somatostatin or growth hormone release-inhibiting hormone, growth hormone-releasing hormone (GRH) and corticotropin-releasing hormone (CRH). Each factor affects the release of one or more of the anterior pituitary hormones (Table 16.1).

It is beyond the scope of this book to present a discussion of the control of pituitary function by the brain and of the effects of the pituitary hormones on their various target hormones. Some generalizations are probably worth making:

1. The secretion of the various factors by the hypothalamic neurosecretory neurons occurs in a pulsatile fashion due to the neurons discharging in bursts. It has been shown that steady levels of the neurohormones in the blood are much less effective than if the same amounts are released in a pulsatile way, and this is thought to prevent so-called down regulation of receptors.

2. There is much evidence for feed-back regulation of anterior pituitary hormone release by blood levels of hormones released by the target cells. This feed-back appears to act at both the hypothalamus and the anterior pituitary. There are hormone-sensitive neurons in the hypothalamus and also in other parts of the brain (such as the limbic system), and changes in the circulating levels of various hormones can have remarkable effects on behaviour. The hormones must cross the blood–brain barrier, which they do at the median eminence, the subfornical organ and other places where the barrier is breached. Some examples of the effects of hormones on behaviour include the increased aggression seen when testosterone levels are high

Table 16.1. Hypothalamic releasing hormones

Pituitary hormone	Release-stimulating hormone	Release-inhibiting hormone
Growth hormone	Growth hormone-releasing factor	Somatostatin
Thyrotropin	Thyrotropin-releasing hormone	Somatostatin
Prolactin	Prolactin-releasing factor	Dopamine
Luteinizing hormone Follicle-stimulating hormone	Gonadotropin-releasing hormone	
Adrenocorticotropin Melanocyte-stimulating hormone	Corticotropin-releasing hormone	

and the increased female mating behaviour (e.g. lordosis in rats) when GnRH levels are high.

3. Release of neurohormones is under the control of other parts of the brain. Thus, inputs from various sensory systems, especially the olfactory, visual and auditory systems (e.g. during mating behaviour), strongly influence the release of GnRH. Copulation in rabbits leads to postcoital ovulation. Various stresses lead to adreno-corticotropin release via the action of CRH.

Behavioural State – Sleeping and Waking

The adaptive behaviour of an animal to its external environment (and to its internal environment) obviously depends on the function of many central nervous subsystems. It is convenient to distinguish between behavioural state and motivational state. In a behavioural state there appears to be no goal or termination point to the behaviour. Rather, the duration of the state is regulated autonomously. For a motivational state there are external goals (eating, drinking, mating) and achievement of the goals can terminate the particular behaviour.

Sleeping and Waking

Two behavioural states that are very different from each other are waking and sleeping. Only in the awake state does an animal react appropriately to its external environment. During sleeping an animal is, for the most part, cut off from the external environment or, at least, only reacts to large stimuli such as loud noises, pin-pricks etc. Waking and sleeping are so different that it might be expected that dramatic differences in brain function are responsible for them. Also, the two states alternate regularly in a cycle that appears to be governed by the alternation of night and day or by some internal clock that is in phase with the day–night cycle.

The outward appearances of animals and humans in these states are comparable. Thus, subjects are assessed as being in the waking state if they maintain an erect posture, have their eyes open and carry out apparently purposeful behaviour or respond reflexly in an appropriate manner. Animals or humans are judged to be asleep if they are recumbent with their eyes closed and with spontaneous and responsive movements greatly reduced. Within the sleeping state two major stages are recognizable: In one phase the muscles are relaxed and yet major postural adjustments take place; in the other phase most of the musculature is even further relaxed, although the eyes make rapid movements (REMs) and there are twitches of the extremities, but arousal is more difficult to evoke than in the first sleep phase. In humans dreaming occurs during REM sleep. At least, when wakened during REM sleep humans report they have been dreaming. Although other mammals in REM sleep also appear to be dreaming (e.g. they may vocalize or make various movements), it is not necessarily the case that they are dreaming. Indeed, it is probable that they are not, since dreaming in humans is a sensory-perceptual phenomenon with usually marked degrees of visual and linguistic components.

Neural Correlates of Sleeping and Waking

During waking the electrical activity of the brain as recorded from the surface of the scalp (the electroencephalogram; EEG) is characterized by low-voltage, fast activity. Most of the individual neurons in the forebrain are firing at a relatively fast rate (Fig. 16.4). With the transition to sleeping the EEG becomes progressively dominated by high-voltage, slow wave activity and most forebrain neurons decrease their firing rates (Fig. 16.4). This is non-REM or synchronized sleep, and in its deepest stage the EEG is characterized by synchronized waves of activity. During this synchronized sleep some neurons, in the paramedian pontine reticular formation, increase their firing. Synchronized sleep is punctuated by periods when the EEG suddenly becomes desynchronized and is characterized by low-voltage, fast activity similar to that of the awake state. In this state the electrical activity of the lateral geniculate nucleus shows distinctly clustered biphasic waves that are synchronous with the rapid eye movements that occur in this state of sleep. Most forebrain neurons increase their firing during REM sleep, and neurons of the paramedial pontine reticular formation are firing at their highest rates during REM sleep. In REM sleep, although the EEG appears similar to that of the awake state, the organism is much more difficult to arouse than when in the synchronized sleep state and there is also active inhibition of most sensory and motor systems. (For example, descending neuronal systems inhibit somatic sensory input by presynaptic inhibition at the primary

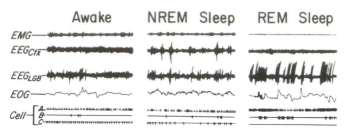

Fig. 16.4. Neural correlates of waking and sleeping in the cat. From the *top* down: *EMG*, electromyographic activity of skeletal muscle; *EEG*, electroencephalographic records from the cerebral cortex (*Ctx*) and the lateral geniculate body (*LGB*); *EOG*, electro-oculogram. At the *bottom* are records of different types of neuronal firing: *A*, typical of neurons in cerebral cortex and cerebellum; *B*, typical of motoneurons; *C*, aminergic neurons of the brain stem. (Reproduced with permission from Hobson and Steriade 1986.)

afferent fibre level in the spinal cord and also inhibit motoneurons by postsynaptic mechanisms.)

Circadian Rhythms and Behavioural State

The sleep–wake cycle in humans and other animals is synchronized with the 24-h day–night cycle. However, under experimental conditions of isolation when there are no light–dark clues, nor other indications of time, the sleep–wake cycle becomes decoupled from the 24-h cycle and tends to lengthen to one of 25 h. The sleep–wake cycle is normally also synchronized with the body's 24-hourly rhythm of temperature fluctuation, but under the above "free-wheeling" conditions these two cycles also become desynchronized. Thus both of these rhythms are endogenous and not simply a response to outside factors such as daylight.

The day–night cycle, however, does entrain the sleep–wake cycle as well as other circadian rhythms. The integrity of the suprachiasmatic nucleus of the hypothalamus is necessary for this entrainment, and lesions of the nucleus will lead to its loss. The monitoring of the day–night cycle is a function of the retina, and it is thought that a direct pathway from retina to the hypothalamus is responsible for carrying the afferent impulse traffic, since destruction of both the primary and accessory optic pathways does not affect entrainment. The suprachiasmatic nucleus is thought to be the site of origin of the circadian rhythms. But the sleep–wake cycle and the transition between synchronized and REM sleep are controlled by other brain systems.

Behavioural State Control

The transition from synchronized sleep to the awake state or to the REM sleep state seems to be controlled by the reticular formation and its related projection areas of the thalamus and cortex. Neurons in the midbrain reticular formation increase their firing before EEG and behavioural signs of both waking and REM sleep (Fig. 16.5) and, conversely, reduce and cease firing before the transition from waking to sleeping (Fig. 16.6). These reticular neurons excite neurons of the thalamus (intralaminar thalamic nucleus) which, in turn, excite neurons of the cerebral cortex.

The brain monoaminergic systems also play an important role in the sleep–wake cycle. Direct projections from the locus coeruleus (noradrenergic) and the raphe nuclei (serotoninergic) to the cortex as well as to the thalamic nuclei (see Figs. 7.7, 7.9) are involved in arousal, possibly by means of disinhibition, since their action on target neurons is to inhibit them. Destruction of the raphe nuclei produces complete insomnia in cats for several days. After this period some synchronized sleep reappears but REM sleep does not. However, the control system for REM sleep seems quite complex. There appears to be a REM sleep trigger and clock in the pons (the paramedian pontine reticular formation), since in a cat with its pons isolated by brain stem sections at its rostral and caudal ends REMs (and associated electrical activity) occur every 30 min or so. Neurons of the paramedian pontine reticular formation have the earliest and most prominent firing rate increase relative to REMs – 100–150 ms before the eye movement onset. This pontine generator is itself controlled by the aminergic (noradrenergic and serotoninergic) systems.

Function of Sleep

An animal must be awake in order to carry out its life-preserving functions such as the finding

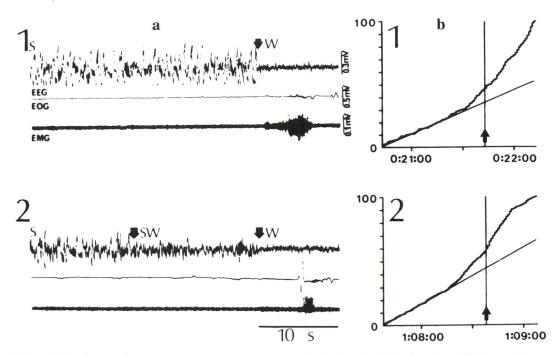

Fig. 16.5a,b. Midbrain reticular formation neurons increase their discharge before behavioural and EEG signs of activated states in the cat. **a** Shows (*1*) an abrupt change from sleep to wakefulness and (*2*) a more gradual change. **b** Shows the cumulative number of impulses of two neurons recorded from the midbrain reticular formation during the corresponding EEG and EMG traces. Note the increase in firing (deviation from the straight line) some 10–20 s before the EEG signs of waking (*arrows*). The graphs in **b** have been normalized for impulse discharge and show real time on the *abscissas*. (Reproduced with permission from Hobson and Steriade 1986.)

and ingesting of food and water, predator avoidance, mating etc. Sleep is an active process with complicated control systems. It is present in its fully developed form in mammals, birds and reptiles, and ambiguously present in fish and amphibia. It obviously has important functional roles, in both its synchronized and REM states.

Sleep provides rest, and an important function of sleep is to enable a genuine metabolic saving by the organism. During synchronized sleep the motoneurons, and therefore the muscles, are at rest. Furthermore, during sleep the nervous system is given a respite from processing sensory inputs. In

contrast, REM sleep is an active process which is internally driven. Its function is unknown, but it cannot be coincidence that REM sleep occupies much more of the total sleeping time in neonatal and immature animals than in adults. Thus, in humans, REM sleep occupies about 80% of the total sleep time in babies born 10 weeks prematurely and about 60% in babies born 2–4 weeks prematurely. At birth a full-term neonate has about 50% REM sleep, and by the age of 2 years this has fallen to about 33%. At 10 years of age the rate is about 25%, and this rate is maintained over the next five or six decades. Thus,

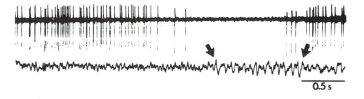

Fig. 16.6. Midbrain reticular neurons decrease their discharge rate before EEG signs of transition from waking to sleeping. The *upper trace* is the discharge of a midbrain reticular neuron in the cat. The neuronal discharge slows and stops before the first EEG spindle (*lower trace, first arrow*) and then starts again before the last spindle (*second arrow*). (Reproduced with permission from Hobson and Steriade 1986.)

the highest rates of REM sleep occur before birth, when sensory input is limited, and may have some important function during ontogenetic development of the nervous system. After birth the rates are high while the nervous system is still developing and at the time when the organism is learning the most rapidly. REM sleep occurs throughout life, and other functions, such as the active maintenance of brain circuitry, have been suggested for it.

Motivational Behaviour

During the behavioural state of waking there are two major components of motivational activity: non-specific activation and motivational behaviour. Non-specific activation includes such phenomena as arousal and drive (which are general components of motivational behaviour and which energize motivational behaviours), whereas motivational behaviour directs the animal's activities towards particular goals (eating, drinking, mating etc.). During the REM sleep state there is cortical arousal even though there is no motivational behaviour.

Non-specific Activation

Two major brain systems have been implicated in arousal. The earlier one to be recognized was the ascending reticular activating system described by Lindsley, Magoun and their colleagues, arising in the brain stem, receiving polysensory input onto individual neurons and projecting to all parts of the central nervous system. After extensive damage to this system the animal becomes somnolent and comatose and is incapable of arousal even when sensory input is extreme. More recently the central monoaminergic pathways have been recognized as playing an important role in arousal, and, since many reticular neurons contain biogenic amines, the emphasis nowadays is on these rather than the "ascending reticular activating system" concept.

Mesencephalic Dopaminergic System

The mesencephalic dopaminergic system arising in the substantia nigra and adjacent ventral tegmentum gives rise to the mesotelencephalic dopaminergic projection system to wide areas of the forebrain, including the striatum, limbic system and parts of the cerebral cortex. By means of its input to the striatum it can influence wide areas of the brain (Fig. 16.7).

Complete bilateral lesions of this system in rats leads to a severe state of behavioural unresponsiveness. The animals maintain a hunched-back posture, move little or not at all, pay little or no attention to sensory stimuli, do not eat and do not drink. They have an apparent inability to initiate coordinated movements or even orient towards a sensory stimulus. The lesions necessary to section the ascending dopaminergic nerve fibres involve the lateral hypothalamus, and it is interesting to note that early experiments in which the lateral hypothalamus was bilaterally destroyed were interpreted as destroying a "centre" responsible for eating, since the lesioned animals displayed aphagia. But the lateral hypothalamus contains fibres of passage rather than groups of cell bodies, and aphagia is only one of the behavioural deficits produced. In humans, damage to the dopaminergic connexions from the substantia nigra to the striatum lead to Parkinsonism, a disease characterized by a deficit in the initiation of voluntary movements.

Most of the effect of destruction of the dopaminergic mesotelencephalic system in animals may be reversed by drugs that activate dopamine receptors (such as apomorphine) and by grafts (or transplants) of dopamine-containing neurons into the striatum. If dopaminergic transmission is increased, by drugs such as L-dopa or amphetamine, then overactivity of the striatal output system occurs with hyperactivity and stereotyped movements in rats. Overactivity of the system in man (due to amphetamines) leads to similar hyperactivity, but also agitation, excitement and ultimately psychosis.

Thus, animals with damage to the dopaminergic mesotelencephalic system appear not to be arousable or at least not able to sustain arousal. The system sets the level of arousal that determines threshold for an appropriate behavioural response. It is worth noting that the dopamine-containing neurons of the substantia nigra do not modulate their firing rate during the sleep–wake cycle or during REM sleep, and therefore are presumably not involved in this aspect of behavioural state control. Finally, animals with extensive lesions of the dopamine system have marked similarities to animals with peripheral sympathectomy. Thus, such animals are unable to respond to acute challenges in their environment, although, if kept under controlled laboratory conditions, they will survive.

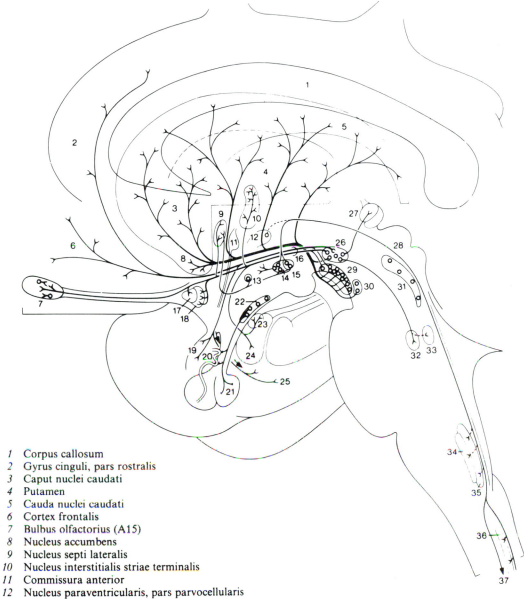

1   Corpus callosum
2   Gyrus cinguli, pars rostralis
3   Caput nuclei caudati
4   Putamen
5   Cauda nuclei caudati
6   Cortex frontalis
7   Bulbus olfactorius (A15)
8   Nucleus accumbens
9   Nucleus septi lateralis
10 Nucleus interstitialis striae terminalis
11 Commissura anterior
12 Nucleus paraventricularis, pars parvocellularis
13 Cell group A14
14 Cell group A13
15 Cell group A11
16 Fasciculus telencephalicus medialis
17 Nucleus olfactorius anterior
18 Substantia perforata anterior
19 Cortex praepiriformis
20 Eminentia mediana
21 Lobus posterior hypophyseos
22 Nucleus infundibularis (A12)
23 Nucleus centralis amygdalae
24 Nucleus basalis amygdalae
25 Cortex entorhinalis
26 Area tegmentalis ventralis (A10

27 Nucleus habenulae lateralis
28 Fasciculus longitudinalis dorsalis
29 Substantia nigra, pars compacta (A9)
30 Area tegmentalis lateralis (A8)
31 Nucleus raphes dorsalis
32 Locus coeruleus
33 Nucleus parabrachialis lateralis
34 Nucleus dorsalis nervi vagi
35 Nucleus solitarius
36 Substantia gelatinosa
37 Nucleus intermediolateralis

Fig. 16.7. Dopamine-containing cells and fibres in the brain. The mesencephalic dopaminergic system arises from the substatia nigra (29), the lateral tegmental area (30) and the ventral tegmental area (26) and projects to wide areas of the forebrain. (Reproduced from Nieuwenhuys 1985.)

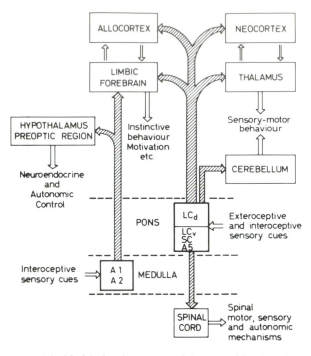

Fig. 16.8. Models for the neuromodulatory and level-setting actions of noradrenergic systems. (Reproduced with permission from Björklund and Lindvall 1986.)

Brain Stem Noradrenergic Systems

The brain stem noradrenergic systems (see Figs. 7.7, 7.8) arise from the locus coeruleus and sub-coeruleus, the lateral tegmentum and the dorsal medulla. They have widespread projections to the forebrain, cerebellum, brain stem and spinal cord. Functionally the systems are thought to have similarly widespread actions (Fig. 16.8) both on non-specific and motivational behaviour as well as on sensory-motor behaviour.

Neurons of the locus coeruleus discharge according to the level of arousal. Thus, their discharge is directly related to the animal's level of vigilance, decreasing during sleep and grooming and also during the drinking of sweet-water (that is, during internally generated repetitive behaviours), and increasing on awakening, in response to arousing stimuli and during orienting behaviour (that is, during externally generated behaviours).

Current ideas about the role of the central noradrenergic systems are that they are particularly involved in attention. The neurons of the locus coeruleus complex seem to signal that something important is going on. There is also evidence that activity in this system increases the signal-to-noise ratio in sensory systems and thus helps to filter out irrelevant signals. This atten-

tional function may also be an important role for the descending noradrenergic systems to the spinal cord. Activation of descending noradrenergic pathways can selectively depress the nociceptive component in the responses of dorsal horn cells, leaving the non-nociceptive component unaffected. Rather than being a function of pain control (a common interpretation of such observations), a role in attention may be more likely.

Homeostasis and Motivational Behaviour

The hypothalamus and the associated limbic system are important brain areas for the control of homeostatic mechanisms and their behavioural components. The hypothalamus exerts its influence in three major ways: through the endocrine system by its neurosecretory functions (see above), through the autonomic nervous system (over which it has control) and via other parts of the central nervous system, especially the limbic system, by controlling motivation.

The limbic system consists of the limbic lobe – the primitive cortical gyri that form a ring around the brain stem – and underlying structures. The limbic system (Fig. 16.9) includes the parahippocampal, the cingulate and subcallosal gyri and the hippocampal formation (the hippocampus, the dentate gyrus and the subiculum). In addition, the limbic system includes various other brain structures, such as parts of the hypothalamus, the septal area, part of the striatum, the amygdala and also some neocortical areas.

In the following sections two examples of homeostasis will be given, and emotional behaviour and motivation and reward will be discussed, to indicate some of the roles of the hypothalamus and limbic system.

Regulation of Body Temperature

Warm-blooded animals maintain a relatively constant body temperature in the face of considerable changes in the temperature of the external environment. The hypothalamus plays a pivotal role in the control of body temperature. Thermoreceptors in the periphery (cutaneous and visceral sense organs and also thermoreceptors in the spinal cord) and in the hypothalamus itself monitor the temperature in their surroundings and their activity is projected to and assessed in the hypothalamus. Electrical stimulation of the anterior hypothalamus leads to responses associated with heat loss, such as peripheral vasodilatation

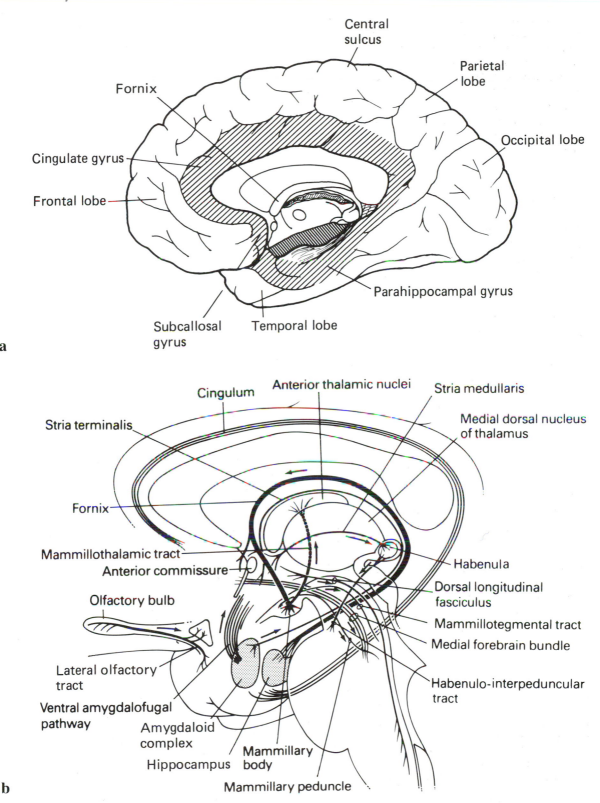

Fig. 16.9a,b. The limbic system. **a** A medial view of the human cerebrum with the limbic lobe (*dotted*) surrounding the upper brain stem. **b** Schematic representation of the inter-connexions of the deep-lying structures included in the limbic system. (Modified from Kandel and Schwartz 1985, after Nieuwenhuys et al. 1981.)

and sweating (these are mediated via the autonomic outflows), inhibition of thyroid hormone release (mediated via the neuroendocrine system) and behavioural responses appropriate to inducing heat loss such as panting and the seeking out of cool places in the environment. Stimulation in the posterior hypothalamus leads to responses associated with prevention of heat loss, such as peripheral vasoconstriction, increased output of thyroxine, shivering and the adoption of postures suitable for prevention of heat loss.

Regulation of Food and Water Intake

The regulation of food and water intake is also carried out, for the most part, via hypothalamic mechanisms. The control of water loss by the kidney through the vasopressin released from supraoptic and paraventricular hypothalamic neurons has been discussed in the first section of this chapter. Stimulation of the hypothalamus can lead to drinking behaviour; in animals such as goats, which are ruminants and can therefore store large volumes of fluid in their gastrointestinal tract, or in animals with oesophageal fistuli, which allow ingested water to drain away without entering the body fluid compartments, enormous volumes of water are drunk upon stimulation of the appropriate hypothalamic area. The control of food intake is largely a hypothalamic function, and, again, electrical stimulation of parts of the hypothalamus can lead to either feeding behaviour or to lack of it (aphagia). However, some non-specific systems, such as the dopaminergic pathways, ascend through the lateral hypothalamus, and it is difficult to dissect the roles of fibres of passage from those of intrinsic neuronal elements (see the section on the mesencephalic dopaminergic system, above). Nevertheless, the hypothalamus is important in the regulation of body weight, including feeding behaviour, and lesions to the hypothalamus may lead to obesity.

Emotional Behaviour

Early stimulation experiments indicated that the hypothalamus was involved in coordinating emotional responses. Thus stimulation of the lateral hypothalamus elicits responses of rage, whereas lesions of the same area results in placidity (but see the discussions above about the ascending dopaminergic pathways). If lesions are made in the medial hypothalamus the animal becomes over-excitable and has a much lowered threshold for aggression. Removal of parts of the neocortex produce a similar picture of so-called sham rage, in which the animal shows all the signs of rage and aggression, but also various autonomic phenomena such as micturition and defaecation as well as erection of the hairs along the back and tail (cats). These sham rage responses occur with very mild stimuli, and also apparently spontaneously, but soon subside in the absence of stimuli. These experiments imply that normally some part of the cortex suppresses the rage responses, and it has been shown that the parts of the neocortex responsible include some of the limbic system, especially the cingulate gyrus. Removal of other parts of the cortex (the temporal lobe) and limbic system (amygdala and hippocampal formation) leads to a syndrome characterized by a flattening of emotional responses and hypersexuality. Again, the implication is that these parts of the cortex and limbic system normally act to suppress such hypersexualty (and prevent the dulling of emotional responses). These cortical areas and the limbic system act on the hypothalamus, which integrates sensory (and endocrine) signals to produce outputs that control neuroendocrine, autonomic, and somatic motor functions.

Motivation and Reward

One of the most remarkable observations of relevance to understanding mechanisms of motivational behaviour was made by Olds and Milner in 1954. They showed that if electrodes were implanted in certain parts of the hypothalamus and limbic system, then the animals would behave as if electrical stimulation was itself a reward. The electrical stimulation could be used to initiate and sustain many types of operant behaviour and acted as a reinforcement, similar to food. However, food only acts as a reinforcement in hungry animals, whereas intracranial stimulation works irrespective of the particular drive state of the animal. The animals quickly learn to activate the stimulation themselves, and indeed will continue to do so until they are in danger of death from exhaustion.

This phenomenon is very complex. It does seem, however, that an important part is played by the ascending mesotelencephalic dopamine systems and also the endogenous opiate systems (enkephalinergic systems). There is evidence that these systems are not only involved in the phenomena of intracranial self-stimulation but also in the responses to certain addictive drugs such as amphetamine (which releases dopamine), cocaine and heroin.

Control of Nociception

As part of its requirements for successful control of its relationships with the environment, an animal must not only be aware of potential or actual damage to its body parts but it must to able to make the appropriate responses to such dangers. The monitoring of potential or actual damage is carried out by the nocireceptors, sense organs specifically responsive to nociceptive stimuli. These sense organs are innervated by primary afferent fibres of small calibre – either non-myelinated (C) fibres or fine myelinated (Aδ) fibres. The activity in these fibres from sense organs in skin, subcutaneous tissue, joints, periosteum, muscle and viscera enters the central nervous system via either spinal dorsal roots or various cranial nerves. In the central nervous system the activity in these fibres can influence very many different classes of central neurons, either directly or via other interneurons. Some neurons activated form part of ascending neural pathways to the thalamus and cortex and also to the brain stem reticular formation and form part of labelled lines specific for nociceptive information. Many neurons in the spinal cord, however, are excited by both nociceptive afferent fibres and others that respond to innocuous stimuli, that is, they are multireceptive. But some of the multireceptive neurons project to the brain too. Most spinal neurons, however, do not project out of the spinal cord but form part of various spinal cord neuronal circuits. Two major problems immediately present themselves:

1. If most spinal neurons respond to both innocuous and noxious stimuli, can the nervous system differentiate between the two sorts of stimuli on the basis of the discharges of these neurons or does it depend on the minority of neurons responding specifically?

2. If most spinal neurons have local functions in the cord is it sensible to consider them as part of a pain system, since pain is a conscious experience?

Unfortunately, these problems seem to be put aside by many workers in this area, who, for the most part, interpret their findings in terms of pain rather than in terms of how the central nervous system deals with input from nocireceptors.

The overriding importance of pain to humans, and especially the great difficulty of pain treatment and management in the clinical setting, is probably a major reason for the emphasis on pain rather than on nociception. Another reason stems from the classic studies of reflexes in spinal preparations. Under these conditions (a spinal cord free from influences from the brain and the absence of anaesthetics) responses to noxious stimuli, such as flexion reflexes, dominate all other reflexes. In intact animals, however, nociceptive inputs may not produce flexion reflexes. There are many documented cases of humans with severe injuries continuing with either sporting activities or with fighting in battle and having no pain sensation. Also, in many situations in which nocireceptors are excited, animals (and humans) are better protected from danger if their motor control remains intact and they are not disabled by flexion reflexes.

Segmental Control of Nociceptive Input

Nociceptive input is controlled at the first possible site in the central nervous system – at the terminals of the nocireceptive afferent fibres by means of presynaptic inhibition. Activation of large myelinated afferent fibres from low-threshold mechanoreceptors leads to presynaptic inhibition of small-diameter fibres from nocireceptors.

Activity in ascending tract neurons produced by C fibre inputs is also inhibited by previous activity in cutaneous A fibres. Some of this inhibition is due to the presynaptic effects described above, and there may be additional postsynaptic inhibitory components too. Figure 16.10 shows the C fibre (nocireceptive) component of a spinocervical tract neuron's discharge being completely inhibited by stimulation of low-threshold A fibres in the contralateral limb.

Descending Control of Nociception

A number of neuronal pathways descending from the brain act to inhibit nociceptive responses of spinal neurons, including both those spinal neurons giving rise to ascending projections and also those with local actions only. These descending pathways include serotoninergic fibres from the raphe nuclei of the brain stem, noradrenergic fibres from the locus coeruleus and dopaminergic fibres from the substantia nigra, hypothalamus and diencephalon. The actions of some of these systems on some spinal neurons are selective in inhibiting nociceptive responses, whereas in other neurons their action is non-selective and has rather a general damping-down effect. As descri-

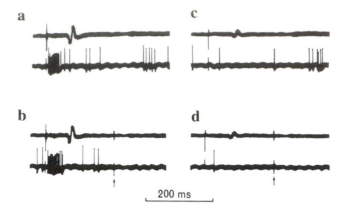

200 ms

Fig. 16.10a–d. Inhibition of C fibre-evoked discharges in a spinocervical tract cell by activity in A fibres of other cutaneous nerves. Each pair of records shows the compound action potential recorded from a cat's sural nerve (*upper trace*) and the corresponding discharge in the spinocervical tract neuron. In **a** and **b** both the A and C fibres in the sural nerve are conducting (the compound potential due to A fibre activity is largely off the trace due to the amplification needed to see the later C fibre volley). In **c** and **d** impulse conduction in the A fibres and a portion of the C fibres had been blocked. In **b** and **d** the contralateral sural A fibres were electrically stimulated at the *arrow*. Note the complete inhibition of the C fibre-evoked discharge in the spinocervical neuron (*right-hand end of trace* in **a** and **c**). (Reproduced with permission from Brown et al. 1975.)

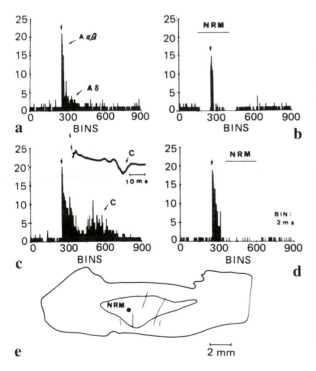

bed earlier in this chapter, these amine-containing neural pathways have important functions in sleep, arousal, attention, orienting behaviour etc. It seems important to keep these functions in mind in interpreting actions at the spinal level.

Stimulus-Produced Analgesia

Electrical stimulation of certain sites in the brain stem results in a profound analgesia, so strong that animals may be operated upon without anaesthetics. This stimulus-produced analgesia has been the subject of much investigation. A powerful site for the production of this effect is the periaqueductal grey matter (PAG). The PAG projects to the raphe nuclei (nucleus raphe magnus; NRM), the source of descending serotoninergic fibres. Stimulation of the NRM produces marked inhibition of spinal neuron responses to noxious inputs (Fig. 16.11).

Fig. 16.11a–e. Inhibition of the response of a primate spino-thalamic tract (STT) neuron by stimulation of the nucleus raphe magnus (*NRM*). **a–d** Peristimulus time histograms of the STT neuron's response. The STT cell was activated by stimulation of the sural nerve at strengths sufficient to excite A fibres (**a**) and A plus C fibres (**c**). These control responses were strongly inhibited by electrical stimulation of the NRM during the time shown by the *bars* (**b,d**). Note that most of the inhibitory effect is on the STT cell's response to the Aδ and C fibres, although the action is not completely selective. (Reproduced with permission from Gerhart et al. 1981.)

Opiate Analgesia

Opiates, such as morphine, have long been known to have powerful analgesic actions in addition to their addictive properties. Injection of morphine into the PAG produces powerful analgesia, and depletion of serotonin prior to morphine injection nullifies the analgesic effect of morphine. Opiates act also on the spinal cord directly and on various brain sites, including the locus coeruleus, the thalamus and the cerebral cortex. At these sites opioid receptors have been demonstrated. It is now known that the brain has its own opioid-like peptides – the enkephalins and endorphins – and neurons containing these peptides are present in many parts of the nervous system, including those parts thought to be concerned with nociception.

Summary

1.   Major functions of the nervous system are to control the internal environment of the animal, directly and by interaction with the external environment. Control of the internal environment is largely a function of the autonomic nervous system and the endocrine system, coordinated by the hypothalamus. Appropriate behavioural interactions with the external environment are also coordinated, in large part by the hypothalamus.

2.   The hypothalamus provides the link between the nervous system and the endocrine system through its magno- and parvocellular neuroendocrine outputs. The magnocellular division secretes the hormones vasopressin and oxytocin, which pass into the circulation. The parvocellular division secretes a variety of peptide hormones (regulating hormones) that control anterior pituitary function.

3.   Waking and sleeping are two behavioural states that are vastly different to each other. Only in the awake state does the animal respond appropriately to its external environment. The sleep–wake cycle is a circadian rhythm driven by internal clocks but strongly influenced by the day–night cycle. There are two states of sleep: slow wave sleep and REM or desynchronized sleep. REM sleep occupies a larger fraction of sleeping time in young animals and appears to be important during the development of the nervous system and in learning.

4.   During waking there are two major components of motivational activity: non-specific activation and motivational behaviour. Non-specific activation (which includes arousal and drive) appears to be controlled by central monoaminergic pathways, especially the dopaminergic mesotelencephalic projections and the noradrenergic systems. Motivational behaviour is controlled to a large extent by the hypothalamus and the associated limbic structures, which also are important in the control of emotional behaviour.

5.   An important aspect of an animals's interaction with the external environment is its response to harmful or potentially harmful stimuli. The neural input from specific nocireceptors is under a number of very powerful controls acting at several levels of the nervous system. Many pathways descending from the brain can inhibit nociceptive responses of central neurons, allowing motor function and other sensory functions to continue. The nervous system has its own morphine-like substances – the enkephalins and endorphins – which play important roles in analgesia.

17 Formation, Maintenance and Plasticity of Synapses

So far, the structure and function of the nervous systems of adult animals has been considered. Furthermore, very little attention has been paid to any dynamic functions over long time scales: neuromodulation and long-term potentiation are the only examples of such functions that have been mentioned. Likewise, no consideration has been given to any structural changes. But the nervous system, like all other systems, develops out of a single cell – the fertilized egg – and the formation of such a complex system that contains so many individual cells whose interconnexions are of paramount importance for its functioning must surely be controlled by a strict set of instructions. Also, during the course of the lifetime of an animal the nervous system may be exposed to numerous threats that might lead to damage (e.g. poisoning, wounds that result in loss of a limb or damage to parts of the central nervous system, infections etc.), and the question arises as to how the nervous system copes with such damage and indeed whether it can cope at all? A related question, even in the absence of externally imposed changes in neuronal structure, is: How are synaptic connexions, once formed during development, maintained during the rest of the animal's life? Is it necessary for a particular set of synaptic connexions to be used in order for their structural integrity to be maintained? These questions will be considered in this chapter. Finally, a prime function of nervous systems is to learn and to remember, and it would seem that in order to learn and remember there must be changes in the function and perhaps in the structure of synaptic connexions. Chapter 18 will address these problems.

Development of the Nervous System

The first step in the development of the nervous system is a process called determination, by which certain cells in the embryo are set off on the pathway to form the cells of the nervous system (the neurons and the glia). Neurons, in contrast to cells in most other tissues such as those of the skin, gastrointestinal tract, the immune system etc., once generated cannot in general be replaced (although there are some exceptions to this). Indeed, throughout life there is a continual loss of nerve cells due to cell death. The neurons must therefore be determined early in development. Following determination there is the process of differentiation, which consists of the proliferation of particular classes of nerve cells, their migration to specific positions and their maturation by the formation of dendritic trees, axons and specific connexions with other neurons (and with non-neuronal target cells – effectors). The three components of differentiation take place in parallel, that is, they overlap in time.

Determination of Nervous Tissue

The determination of nervous tissue is carried out by the process of gene expression. All neurons are nucleated and, like all other nucleated cells in the body (except the gametes), contain a full set of genetic instructions, the genome, in the DNA. The process of gene expression must be regulated so that cells destined to become part of the nervous system do so, and this regulation must differ in detail from that taking place in cells destined for other fates. An understanding of the control of gene expression is a central problem in molecular biology, but at present little is known of the process as it takes place in more advanced animal forms with nervous systems. In simpler forms such as bacteria (prokaryotes) gene expression is triggered by environmental influences which release genes from a normally repressed state. Information on how genes in higher organisms are expressed is, however, now being obtained. Certain genes (proto-oncogenes) are present in the genome and these control cell growth and proliferation and also probably cell differentiation. They appear to control "switches" that activate other genes responsible for growth and development. In neurons there appears to be a "switch" that turns off cell division and differentiation so that new neurons cannot be generated to replace those lost during the lifetime of the animal.

The cells of the nervous system in vertebrates arise from the ectoderm, the outer layer of the embryo, specifically from a part of the ectoderm known as the neural plate (Fig. 17.1). The neural

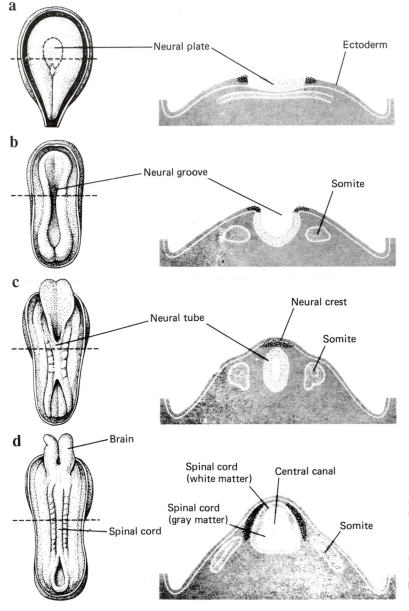

Fig. 17.1a–d. Stages in the development of the human nervous system at 3–4 weeks following conception. *Left:* dorsal views of the developing embryo. *Right:* cross-sections at the levels indicated by the *dashed lines* on the *left-hand figures.* **a** The neural plate arises from the ectoderm. **b** The plate folds to form the neural groove. **c** The groove closes to form the neural tube. **d** The brain forms from the anterior portion of the neural tube and the spinal cord from the posterior portion. (Reproduced with permission from Kandel and Schwartz 1985, after Cowan 1979.)

plate, originally a sheet of cells, folds into a tube-like structure – the neural tube. The rostral end of the neural tube ultimately forms the brain and the caudal part gives rise to the spinal cord. The tube-like structure remains throughout life, the central canal persisting as the ventricles in the brain and the central canal in the spinal cord. Determination of presumptive nervous tissue (the neuroectoderm) from the ectoderm is accomplished early in embryonic life and quickly fixes the fate of the cells. Once the embryo has formed its three germ layers (ectoderm, mesoderm and endoderm) by the process of gastrulation, transplantation of neurectoderm from its usual location to another place in the embryo leads to the development of nervous tissue at the transplanted site and ultimately to inappropriate sites in the fetus.

The determination of neuroectoderm is dependent on the presence of mesoderm underlying the ectoderm. By transplanting mesoderm from one early embryo (gastrula) to another it can be shown that the transplanted mesoderm can induce the formation of neuroectoderm from overlying mesoderm. Furthermore, this process of induction is caused by the passage of a substance or substances from the mesoderm to the ectoderm. Passage of inducing substances can be blocked by placing filters between the ectoderm and mesoderm. Filters with a pore size that prevents passage of substances with molecular weights below about 1000 prevents induction. This induction process not only specifies that ectoderm shall become neuroectoderm but also specifies which part of the nervous system the neuroectoderm will become. Thus mesoderm at the rostral end of the embryo specifies neuroectoderm to become forebrain, slightly more caudal mesoderm specifies mid-brain, and so on. Rostral neuroectoderm if transplanted to more caudal regions still develops into forebrain structures

Cell Differentiation

Once the neuraxis and the major regions of the central nervous system have been determined, the cells begin to differentiate. As mentioned above, there are three components to differentiation – cell proliferation, cell migration and cell maturation – that take place concurrently.

Once the neural tube has fused, cell proliferation begins. Initially the neural tube consists of a single layer of cells but soon becomes multilayered. Cell division takes place in germinal zones located at the surface of the neural tube next to the central canal (that is, the inner surface). The actively dividing cells (stem cells) have cytoplasm that stretches from the inner to the outer surface of the neural tube. The nuclei of the stem cells undergo movements in which the nucleus of the cell migrates from the inner to the outer surface of the neural tube, then back to the inner surface, where mitosis takes place followed by cell division (Fig. 17.2). The reasons for such strange behaviour of the nuclei are unknown: one suggestion is that the movement allows the nucleus to be exposed to different cytoplasmic substances in a necessary temporal sequence. The daughter cells then extend their cytoplasm to the outer surface of the neural tube and the migration of the nuclei starts over again. After several such cycles the daughter cells are incapable of further subdivision in the germinal zone and leave the germinal zone, migrating to some appropriate position, where they become either neurons (most of which are incapable of division) or glial cells (which can divide). The minority of neurons that can proliferate after migration includes those that ultimately form interneurons in the basal ganglia, granule cells in the cerebellar cortex and also cells derived from the neural crest, such as primary afferent neurons, postganglionic autonomic nerve cells and cells of the adrenal medulla (chromaffin cells), which secrete adrenaline and noradrenaline.

In invertebrate species, at least, stem cells are capable of giving rise to several different types of neurons, although many stem cells only generate a particular cell type. Furthermore, some cell types may only be differentiated from a particular stem cell, and removal of such a stem cell by experimental interference can result in the compete absence of a particular class of neurons.

Cell Migration

Since the vast majority of nerve cells are produced in the germinal zones of the neural tube it is necessary for them to migrate from their site of origin to take up their final places in the developing brain. This cell migration is a fundamental principle of development of the nervous system and applies to both glia as well as neurons.

The fact that neurons migrate during the development of the nervous system, and sometimes migrate over considerable distances relative to their size, poses many questions. How do the cells recognize their final positions? How do they make the correct journey to those positions?

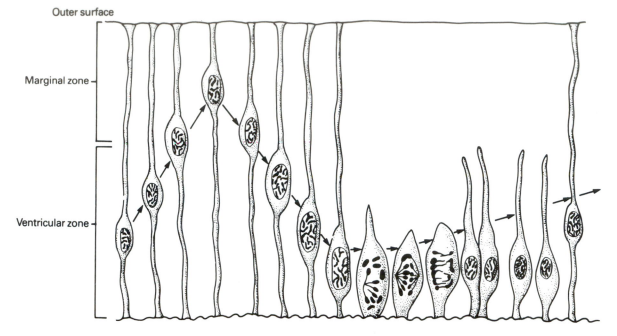

Fig. 17.2. Movements of the nuclei of actively dividing cells in the neural tube. DNA synthesis takes place in the S phase of the cell cycle and cell division in the M phase. (Modified from Kandel and Schwartz 1985, after Sauer 1935.)

What is the mechanism responsible for movement? What makes the cells stop moving when they have reached their appropriate positions? Can neurons move in adult animals? Answers to these questions are not available, but there is some information about aspects of cell migration.

Migration, and the Ultimate Fate, of Neurons Can Be Influenced By Their Original Location. As mentioned above, the neural crest gives rise to neurons of the autonomic ganglia. The parasympathetic ganglia arise from the rostral and caudal parts of the neural crest, whereas the sympathetic ganglia arise from the middle parts of the crest. There are histological differences between the cell nuclei of two species of birds – the domestic fowl and the quail – and if parts of the neural crest of one species are transplanted into the other the fate of the transplanted cells can be followed (Le Douarin et al. 1975). If presumptive sympathetic ganglion cells from the middle neural crest of a quail are transplanted into the rostral parts of the neural crest (tube) of a chick they migrate along paths appropriate for cells in the rostral crest and come to rest in the parasympathetic ganglia. Not only do these cells finish up in parasympathetic ganglia but they also behave as parasympathetic neurons: instead of producing noradrenaline (the sympathetic postganglionic transmitter) they produce acetyl-

choline (the parasympathetic transmitter). Transplantation of presumptive parasympathetic ganglion cells into neural crest regions that normally produce cells of the adrenal medulla also leads to migration and transmitter synthesis appropriate to the new location of the transplanted cells.

The transmitter synthesized by a neuron is not, however, completely specified by the cell's original location. If immature sympathetic neurons are grown in tissue culture they synthesize noradrenaline. But if they are cocultured with other cells (such as immature cardiac muscle cells) they may synthesize acetylcholine. Thus, the local environment can influence the expression of genes responsible for transmitter metabolism.

Glial Cells may be Responsible for Directing the Migration of Neurons. In the developing cerebellar cortex elongated glial cells radiate from the inner surface (near the ventricular canal) to the outer (pial) surface. The developing cerebellar granule cells migrate along the cytoplasmic extensions of the glial cells from their site of origin near the pial surface (the presumptive granule cells are one of the classes of neurons that proliferate after they have left the germinal zone of the neural tube) to their ultimate location near the ventricular surface. In a mutant mouse known as the "weaver", an autosomal recessive mutant, there is an extensive loss of granule cells. This loss of granule cells is found in regions of the cerebellar cortex where the glial cells have either degenerated or where they are arranged in a haphazard fashion. In other regions where the glia appear to have developed normally the granule cells also have a normal appearance. Thus, interactions between glia and neurons are important for neuronal migration.

Synapse Formation and the Maintenance of Connexions

In order for the nervous system to function properly and to produce appropriate behaviour, the connexions between neurons must also be appropriate. There is a high degree of specificity in the connexions made between neurons during development and also during regeneration after injury in those species (mainly non-mammalian) in which regeneration of central nervous tissue can occur. Both inherent (genetic) and environmental factors are involved in both the formation of connexions during development and during regeneration. Neurons behave as if they "know" which are their appropriate target cells and, not only that, they make connexions with particular parts of their target cells, for example with the soma and proximal dendrites rather than with distal dendrites. Neurons obviously receive connexions from other neurons as well as make them with other neurons and they behave as if they recognize when appropriate connexions have been made upon them. If neurons or other target cells such as muscle fibres are disconnected from their afferent nerve supply they undergo changes that include supersensitivity to transmitters, which are due to the appearance of new receptor molecules in their membranes. In this section the following will be considered: the formation of appropriate synaptic connexions in the visual system of non-mammalian vertebrates, nerve growth factor, the effects of denervation and reinnervation of skeletal muscle and neural transplantation in the mammalian brain.

Formation of Synaptic Connexions in the Visual System

Non-mammalian vertebrates such as frogs, toads, salamanders and goldfish have been used extensively in the study of how synaptic connexions are made, because of the remarkable ability of their central nervous tissue to show regeneration in adult animals. Furthermore, the development of microsurgical techniques has allowed remarkable studies of the developing visual system in these animals, since it is possible to make discrete lesions or perform rotations of the developing eye and transplantions of part of the eye in larval embryos.

In some now classic experiments, Sperry (see Sperry 1951) showed that if the optic nerve of an adult amphibian is sectioned apparently normal vision is reinstated after a few weeks, since appropriate behavioural responses to visual stimuli reappear. If, however, in addition to optic nerve section the eyes are rotated through 180°, then although visual reflexes reappear they are inappropriate, and the animal behaves as if its vision were upside-down and anterior-posterior reversed. The animals in Sperry's experiments never learned to make the correct visual responses. Electrophysiological experiments by Gaze and Jacobsen (see Gaze 1970) and their collaborators confirmed that under these conditions the optic nerve fibres had regenerated to their original locations in the optic tectum (analogous to the mammalian superior colliculus) where a normal retinotectal map was reformed. In other words, the retinal ganglion cells, the axons of which form the optic nerve, had regenerated to the optic tectum and made synaptic connexions at their previous locations, even though these connexions were now inappropriate for correct visual reflexes. The retinal ganglion cells can be said to be specified to make connexions with particular target cells in these adult amphibia.

In the goldfish, axons from the retina of one eye cross completely in the optic chiasm and terminate in the contralateral optic tectum. The axons enter the tectum along two tracts – a medial one from ganglion cells in the ventral retina and a lateral one from cells in the dorsal retina. Furthermore, axons from the anterior (nasal) parts of the retina terminate posteriorly in the tectum, whereas fibres from the posterior (temporal) retina terminate anteriorly in the tectum (Fig. 17.3). The pathway taken by an individual fibre from retina to tectum is, therefore, quite complex. Sperry performed experiments to determine whether regenerating optic nerve fibres showed particular preferences for their appropriate tracts. He cut the optic nerve, to allow degeneration of the central parts of the optic fibres and combined this with various ablations of the retina and then followed the regeneration of axons from the remaining retinal ganglion

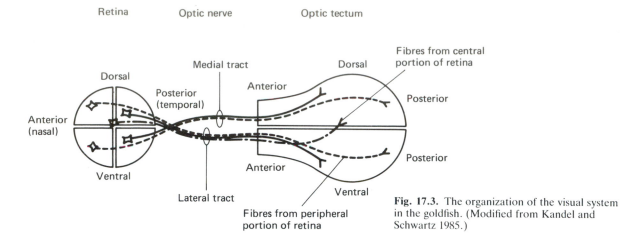

Fig. 17.3. The organization of the visual system in the goldfish. (Modified from Kandel and Schwartz 1985.)

cells. As shown in Fig. 17.4, such experiments demonstrated that the regenerating nerve fibres showed a preference for (1) their appropriate tract (medial or lateral), (2) their appropriate point of entry into the optic tectum at its circumference, and (3) their appropriate point of entry into the depths of the tactum. It is as if there were some guidance factors along the path of the regenerating fibres. Sperry's results, however, only show the final outcome of the regeneration process, and it is now known that during regeneration itself individual fibres may make apparently random growth over the tectal surface before finding their appropriate target.

In the above experiments and similar ones, the results showing specificity of regeneration of optic nerve fibres to the optic tectum indicate that not only are the optic nerve fibres specified in terms of the location of the retinal ganglion cells, but the tectal neurons must be specified in a matching fashion. However, the situation is more complex than such an explanation suggests. Thus, in the goldfish, if part of the tectum is removed and the optic nerve crushed, the regenerating fibres are capable of forming a complete map of the visual field in the tectum, but that field is compressed according to which parts of the tectum have been removed (Fig. 17.5). The optic fibres behave as if the tectum were intact.

Further clues to the mechanisms responsible for the formation of synaptic connexions come from work on amphibian larval embryos. Jacobson rotated the eye cups of early *Xenopus* embryos at times before the optic nerve fibres had begun to grow out from them. If the eye cup was rotated before embryonic stage 29 a normal projection to the optic tectum was formed (as tested electrophysiologically in the adult toad). Rotation of the eye cup at stage 30, only about 10 h later, led to a normal dorsoventral axis of the tectal retinotopic map but a reversed anteroposterior axis. Rotation at stage 31, a further 10 h later, produced a complete reversal of the map. Thus, the retinal ganglion cells are not specified in terms of position at stage 29, but within the next 20 h they become specified, and the specification in terms of the two axes (dorsoventral and anteroposterior) takes place separately. Because it seems highly unlikely that each single cell is uniquely specified genetically (due to the large number of retinal ganglion cells), the present hypotheses are that there are quantitative differences, rather than qualitative ones, between the cells: for example that gradients in the concentrations of a cell surface label (two gradients at right angles) determine the retinal coordinates, and similar gradients in the tectum also specify the location of tectal neurons. Another hypothesis, which does not invoke cell surface labels, is that each cell in the retina is uniquely specified as a result of a temporal sequence related to its birthdate and the time of its migration.

Matching of Neuronal Populations

Most neuronal proliferation during development seems to be genetically programmed. If the target cells of a particular neuronal population are absent, however, then the afferent population eventually degenerates and disappears. Thus, the postsynaptic target cells are of vital importance for the maintenance of an afferent neuronal populaton. Even during normal development, however, there is a remarkable amount of cell

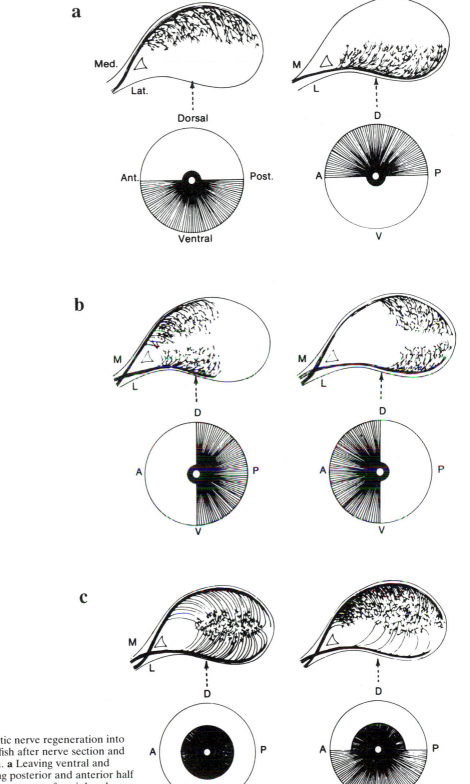

Fig. 17.4a–c. Patterns of optic nerve regeneration into the optic tectum of the goldfish after nerve section and partial ablation of the retina. **a** Leaving ventral and dorsal half retinae. **b** Leaving posterior and anterior half retinae. **c** Removing varying amounts of peripheral retina. (Reproduced with permission from Attardi and Sperry 1963.)

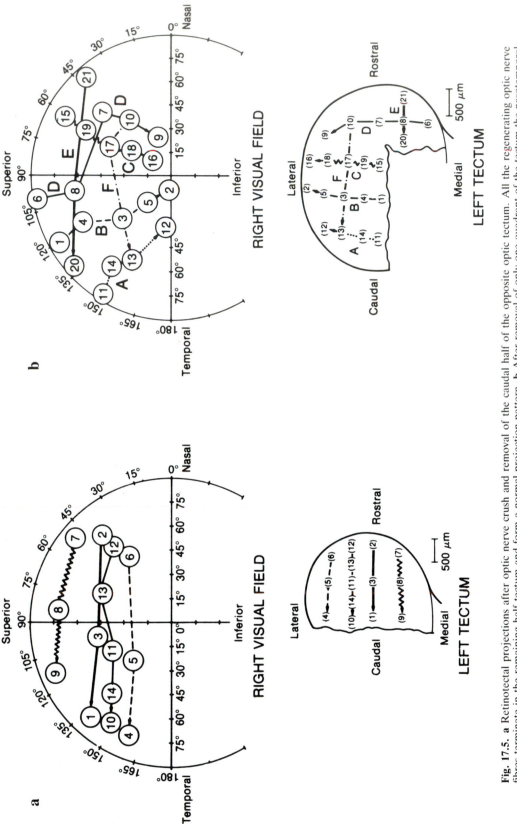

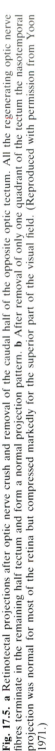

Fig. 17.5. a Retinotectal projections after optic nerve crush and removal of the caudal half of the opposite optic tectum. All the regenerating optic nerve fibres terminate in the remaining half tectum and form a normal projection pattern. **b** After removal of only one quadrant of the tectum the nasotemporal projection was normal for most of the retina but compressed markedly for the superior part of the visual field. (Reproduced with permission from Yoon 1971.)

death. Many more neurons are born than are required. In the developing amphibian spinal cord the number of motoneurons sending axons into the developing limb is considerably greater than the numbers that remain to innervate the skeletal muscle (Fig. 17.6). Ingrowing motor axons compete with each other for muscle fibres. Several axons may innervate a single muscle fibre initially, but eventually all but one are retracted. Motoneurons that do not succeed in innervating muscle die.

The size of the target population of neurons of effector cells also influences the size of the afferent population. As mentioned above, if the target cells are absent there is considerable cell death of the afferent population. Not only that, however, but if the target population is made greater than normal, for example by grafting additional limb buds onto an embryo, then fewer of the afferent neurons die than usual. Some signal, presumably chemical, is required by the afferent neuron that tells it that successful synaptic contacts have been formed.

Nerve Growth Factor

The identity of the trophic factor or factors responsible for the maintenance of neuronal populations is unknown. One substance of importance for the survival of sympathetic neurons (and dorsal root ganglion cells) is nerve growth factor – a protein with a molecular weight of about 130 000. Nerve growth factor (NGF) was discovered by Levi-Montalcini and Hamburger, who showed that implanting mouse sarcoma cells into a chick embryo led to the sarcoma being innervated by sympathetic ganglion cells. NGF is synthesized in and released from target cells of the sympathetic postganglionic neurons. It enhances the innervation of tissue by sympathetic axons and is necessary for the survival of the sympathetic neurons, being taken up by their axon terminals and transported, by retrograde transport, back to the nerve cell body, where it affects gene expression. It is likely that NGF is only one of many growth factors necessary for the outgrowth of neuronal processes and the maintenance of neuronal populations.

Effects of Nerve on Muscle

Nerve–muscle preparations have not only been important for our understanding of the mechanisms of synaptic transmission but have also been extremely useful in the study of the effects of neurons on their target cells. If, in an adult animal, the motor nerve to a muscle is cut, the axons distal to the nerve section undergo degeneration and several changes take place in the muscle. After a few days the individual fibres of the muscle begin to show spontaneous contractions. These contractions are not synchronized across the denervated muscle, which is said to show fibrillation. Fibrillation is associated with the appearance of a phenomenon of supersensitivity of the muscle fibres to a variety of stimuli, both chemical and mechanical.

Normally innervated skeletal muscle fibres are sensitive to their transmitter (acetylcholine; ACh) only at the end-plate region. After denervation they become sensitive throughout their length because of the appearance of ACh receptors in their membrane, as shown by the responses to ACh applied via an ionophoresis pipette. These extrajunctional ACh receptors do not originate from the position of the end-plate, because, if muscle fibres are cut in two, such that one part does not contain the end-plate region, then ACh receptors appear on parts of surviving muscle that did not previously receive innervation.

Nerve section with subsequent degeneration is not necessary for the appearance of extrajunctional ACh receptors. If impulse conduction in the motor nerve is blocked (by application of local anaesthetics or diphtheria toxin or α-bungarotoxin to the intact nerve) then extrajunctional ACh receptors appear, even though in this sort of preparation minitiature end-plate potentials still occur normally (Fig. 17.7). Thus, blockage of synaptic transmission is sufficient to elicit the appearance of extrajunctional receptors. Furthermore, in such nerve impulse-blocked preparations, direct electrical stimulation of the muscle can reverse the appearance of extrajunctional receptors (Fig. 17.8), and there is obviously an important effect of the muscle itself. Direct stimulation needs to be applied in bursts and carried out over several days and the efficaciousness of this direct stimulation of muscle depends on the frequency of stimulation and also on the periods between bursts of stimulation. Since denervated muscles undergo fibrillation, the question needs to be asked – Why does the fibrillation not prevent the appearance of extrajunctional ACh receptors? The answer is that although fibrillation is cyclical it does not produce enough muscle contractions.

Thus, in normally innervated muscle, ACh receptors are restricted to the end-plate, where they are in high concentration. If the muscle is

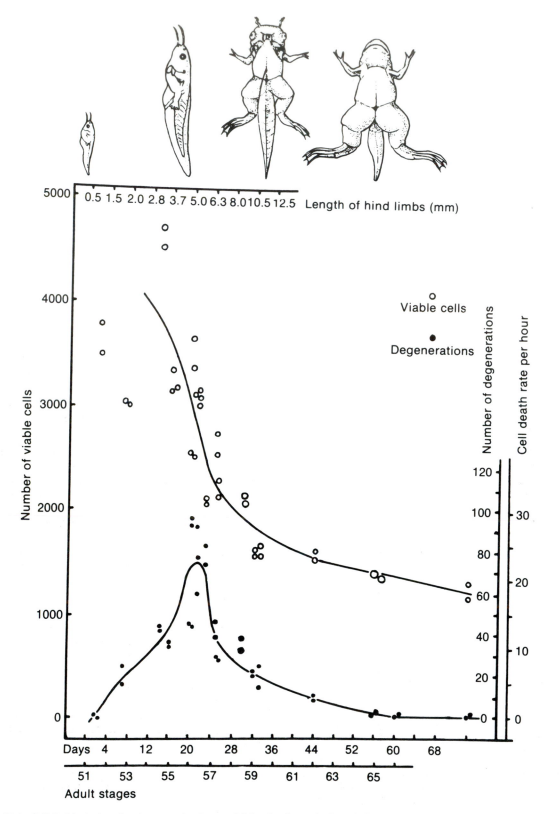

Fig. 17.6. Cell death during development in the amphibian lumbar spinal cord (Reproduced with permission from Hughes 1961.)

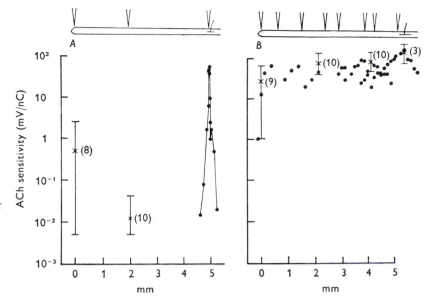

Fig. 17.7. Acetylcholine (ACh) sensitivity along a normal soleus muscle fibre in the rat (*A*) and after a 7-day local anaesthetic block of the motor nerve (*B*). *Crosses* and *bars* represent the mean and range of sensitivity of a number (in *brackets*) of adjacent fibres. (Reproduced with permission from Lømo and Rosenthal 1972.)

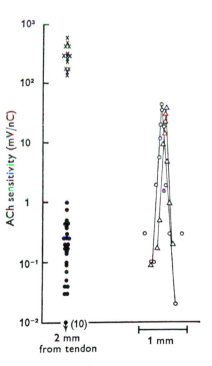

Fig. 17.8. Reversal of supersensitivity in denervated rat soleus muscle by direct electrical stimulation of the muscle fibres. *Crosses*, increased ACh sensitivity in a nerve-free portion of the muscle denervated for 14 days. *Filled circles*, sensitivity of a similar part of a soleus muscle denervated for 7 days and then, whilst still denervated, stimulated electrically intermittently for 7 days. *Open circles* and *triangles*, ACh sensitivity of the same muscle (denervated and directly stimulated) near their denervated end-plate regions. (Reproduced with permission from Lømo and Rosenthal 1972.)

denervated, or if muscle activity is prevented by blocking impulse conduction in the nerve, then ACh receptors appear all over the muscle surface, but at a lower density than they were previously at the end-plate. Reinnervation of denervated muscle or appropriate artificial stimulation of the muscle will lead to the disappearance of the extrajunctional ACh receptors. Furthermore, embryonic muscle, before innervation, is sensitive to ACh over all its surface, and once a muscle fibre has been innervated by one nerve it cannot receive innervation from an additional nerve. Obviously, there is considerable interaction between the nerve and muscle fibres, and it is generally considered that some chemical substance(s) may pass from nerve to muscle (in addition to ACh).

The ACh receptors that appear at extrajunctional sites under the above conditions are new receptors, manufactured by the muscle fibre and inserted into extrajunctional membrane. They are similar to but not identical with the junctional ACh receptors. Thus, although they open chemically gated channels for Na^+ and K^+, their open times are longer and also exhibit other differences, especially in their binding properties for various drugs such as curare and α-bungarotoxin.

Effects of Nerve on Muscle Contraction

There are other effects that motor nerves have on the muscle fibres they innervate. There are two basic types of muscle fibres in mammals: (1) fast (twitch) muscle, which is pale in appearance; and (2) slow (tonic) muscle, which is redder in appearance. Fast muscles are responsible for phasic movements and are dependent on glycolytic (anaerobic) metabolism, whereas slow muscles are responsible for tonic contractions of particular importance in maintenance of posture, are dependent on aerobic metabolism, and contain large amounts of myoglobin. Motoneurons and the muscle fibres they innervate are matched to one another. Thus, fast muscle is innervated by motoneurons whose axons conduct at high velocities and which are capable of relatively high frequencies of impulse firing because their action potential has only a brief after-hyperpolarization. Slow muscle, on the other hand, is innervated by motoneurons with more slowly conducting axons and which, because of longer after-hyperpolarizations, are incapable of generating impulses at frequencies as high as those in motoneurons innervating fast muscle.

At birth, the limb muscles of kittens are all slow muscles. Differentiation into the two main types, fast and slow, takes place over the first few weeks of extrauterine life. If the nerve to a slow muscle (soleus) is sectioned and sutured to the distal end of the nerve to gastrocnemius (a fast muscle), and vice versa, then the axons of slow motoneurons will innervate previously fast muscle and those of fast motoneurons will innervate previously slow muscle. Under these conditions the slow muscle becomes converted to a fast muscle and the fast muscle to a slow muscle. Thus, the nerve is capable of determining the function of the muscle by controlling its biochemistry, by affecting gene expression in the muscle fibre. Furthermore, since cross-innervation in adult life can produce these changes, it must be the case that throughout life the nerve is controlling the molecular biology of the muscle it innervates.

Effects of Denervation in the Central Nervous System

In the peripheral nervous system, as described above for the effects of nerve on muscle, denervation leads to changes in the target organ (and ultimately to degeneration in muscle if denervation is prolonged). If reinnervation is allowed, normal function can be restored and, furthermore, inappropriate reinnervation can take place and cause a switch in the properties of the muscle fibres. Similarly, sense organs are dependent

on innervation for the maintenance of their structure and function. In the mammalian central nervous system, on the other hand, little if any regeneration of nervous tissue can take place, at least in the specific sensory and motor systems. This is a serious problem, particularly in view of the relatively high incidence of central nervous system damage due to accidents etc. Even if central nerve fibres cannot regenerate after section it remains possible that the remaining neurons might be able to respond in some way to help restore function, for example by means of localized sprouting of normal fibres with the subsequent formation of new synapses at sites previously occupied by the damaged neurons. Alternatively, even though there may be no such formation of new connexions, it is possible that synaptic connexions that are already present but weak in their actions may become more effective. Study of such problems is bedevilled with technical difficulties, and there are many discrepancies in the original literature. A major problem is that it is often impossible to be sure that those neurons affected by a particular section of their afferent pathways are those neurons that are being studied weeks or months later.

Some of the most convincing evidence for reorganization after injury comes from studies of the somatosensory map in the cerebral cortex of primate species. As described in Chapter 15, there are detailed maps at all levels of the somaesthetic system, and in these maps the topographical relationships of the skin are maintained. What happens if a peripheral cutaneous nerve is sectioned? Figure 17.9 shows the normal somatotopic organization of the hand areas in cortical areas 3b and 1 in the squirrel monkey. After section of the median nerve, which supplies the medial side of the hand, initially no activity can be recorded from those areas of the cortex that responded to stimulation of the median nerve area. If the median nerve is prevented from regenerating, then, after several weeks, this previously unresponsive cortex becomes responsive – not to stimulation of the median nerve area but to skin innervated by the radial and ulnar nerves. These latter nerves had not grown into the median nerve in the hand and the reorganization must have occurred centrally.

Experiments, such as this have been interpreted in terms of the reorganization of the cortex. But there are several regions of synaptic interactions on the somatosensory pathways afferent to the cortex, and changes have been reported in some of these after peripheral nerve sections etc. Furthermore, even during block of impulse acti-

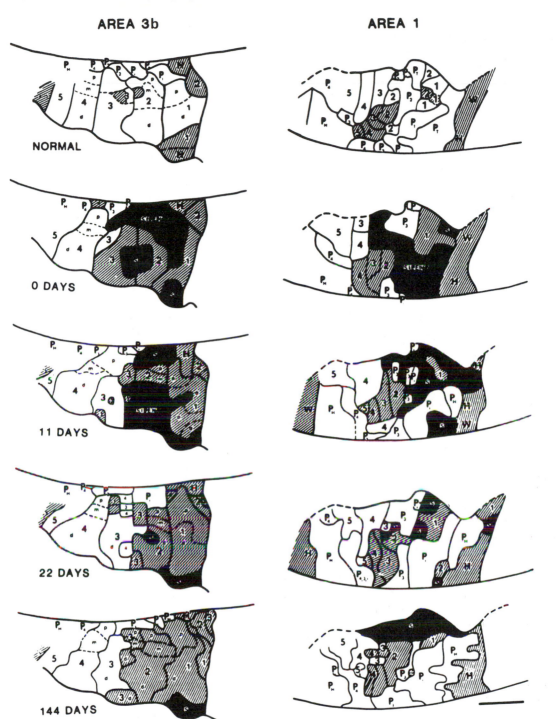

Fig. 17.9. Effects of median nerve section on the somatotopic representation of the hand in cortical areas 3b and 1 in the squirrel monkey. The normal somatotopic maps in these areas are shown in the *topmost figures*. The *lower figures* show the immediate loss of median nerve representation (0 days) and the subsequent changes over 144 days. Note the unresponsive areas (*black*) that are gradually taken over by representations from outside the median nerve area. Dorsal hand areas are *cross-hatched*. *1–5*, the number of the digits; *P*, palmar pads; P_H hypothenar eminence; *W*, wrist; *H*, dorsum of hand. (Reproduced with permission from Merzenich et al. 1983.)

vity in cutaneous nerves some central neurons show the appearance of receptive fields that were not obvious in the animal before nerve block. These latter observations are interpreted as due to the "unmasking" of previously ineffective connexions. It is obvious that the interpretation of such results is difficult, especially as it is not usually possible to know whether or not the same neurons are recorded in the two states; and where recordings are carried out on different occasions in the same animals or on different animals then the difficulties are compounded. If, in an area of the central nervous system a population of neurons falls silent, then other neurons, previously more difficult to record from, may now produce impulses visible above the noise level.

Abnormal Experience and the Formation of Synaptic Connexions

The visual systems of cats and primates have been used extensively in studies of how experience, particularly abnormal experience, influences development of synaptic connexions. The anatomy and physiology of the adult visual system has been described in Chapters 14 and 15. Neurons in the visual cortex (area 17) are highly specific for the type of stimulus to which they will respond: for example requiring the stimulus to be located in a particular part of the visual field, to have a particular orientation and to be presented preferentially to either the ipsilateral or contralateral eye. Newborn kittens and monkeys also show similar features in the responses of their visual cortical neurons. The distribution of ocular dominance among cortical neurons is similar in neonates to that in adults (Fig. 17.10). Obviously, in these animals, with little or no visual experience, the general features of visual cortical neuronal processing (and therefore the underlying anatomical organization) are genetically programmed. In Siamese cats a mutation which leads to the abnormal crossing of optic nerve fibres in the optic chiasm results in more contralateral fibres reaching the lateral geniculate nucleus than normal and terminating there in regions that would normally receive ipsilateral input. From the lateral geniculate in these animals there is a projection to the visual cortex which is anatomically correct but

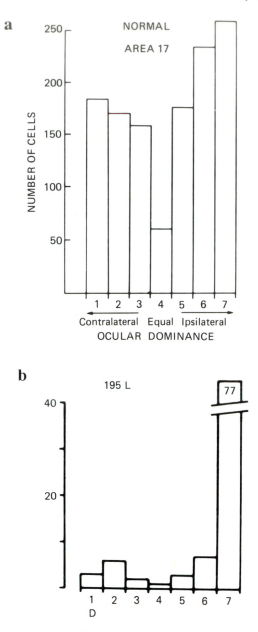

Fig. 17.10. Ocular dominance in normal monkey (**a**) and in a monkey in which the contralateral eye had been closed between 21 and 30 days of age and recordings made at 4 years (**b**). The cell groups 1–7 are classed according to whether the cell is influenced only from the contralateral eye (*1*) to only the ipsilateral eye (*7*); groups 3–5 show little preference for one particular eye. [Reproduced with permission from Wiesel and Hubel 1974 (**a**) and from LeVay et al. 1980 (**b**).]

functionally inappropriate, and an outward sign of this is the characteristic squint, or cross-eyed appearance, of Siamese cats.

Experience, however, does play an important role in the further development of the visual system. If the eyelids of one eye are sutured together at birth that eye never receives patterned visual input – only diffuse light. If the sutures are removed some months later and the properties of visual cortical cells examined electrophysiologically it is found that the vast majority of cells can now be driven only from the eye that had not been sutured. These functional effects are almost completely restricted to the cortical level of the visual system (Fig. 17.10), although there are anatomical changes in the geniculate. Striking anatomical changes occur in the cortex of these animals. The ocular dominance columns demonstrated by autoradiography show that the amount of cortex given over to the open eye is greatly enlarged at the expense of that given to the closed eye.

Eyelid closure in adult animals does not produce the above effects. It is necessary for the closure, and therefore the lack of visual experience, to occur within a certain critical time band – in the third and fourth week of life in kittens (which are born behaviourally blind with a very immature visual system) and during the first 6 weeks of life in monkeys. Animals which have suffered such lack of visual experience during the critical period never recover. The importance of these observations to human medicine is apparent. The critical visual period in babies occupies about the first year of life, and any visual problems at this time, for example congenital cataract or squint, can lead to serious problems if not corrected early. (It is known that the auditory system also has a critical period for correct development in early life.)

If both eyes are closed during the critical period it might be expected that even more serious effects would be observed, with cortical cells showing no or almost no responses to visual stimulation. Surprisingly this is not what happens. If both eyes are sutured in monkeys subsequent testing shows that visual cortical cells show ocular dominance, and that dominance is more obvious than in the normal animal. Very few cells can now be driven by both eyes (Fig. 17.11). Similar, but less dramatic, results are obtained in kittens. A reasonable conclusion from these experiments is that there is competition between the pathways from the two eyes for their target cells. A similar conclusion in support of competition comes from experiments in which one eye is sutured during the critical period and then, later in the critical period, the eye is opened and the other eye closed. These so-called reverse-sutured animals, when tested, show ocular dominance histograms in which most cortical cells respond

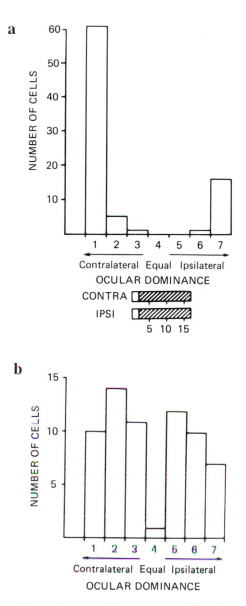

Fig. 17.11a,b. Effects of binocular eye closure in newborn monkey. **a** The monkey was delivered by Caesarian section and both eyes were sutured. Recordings were made at 30 days. **b** Ocular dominance columns in a normal 3-week-old monkey. (Reproduced with permission from Wiesel and Hubel 1974.)

to the newly opened eye, and the anatomically demonstrated ocular dominance columns also show expansion of the columns for the eye that was originally closed but later opened (Fig. 17.12). During the critical period, then, there is a remarkable amount of plasticity in the developing visual system, and the formation of synaptic connexions depends not only on genetic programmes but also on experience.

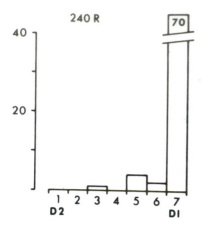

Fig. 17.12. Effects of reverse-suture on ocular dominance in the monkey. The ipsilateral eye was closed between days 2 and 21, and the contralateral eye was closed on day 21 and kept closed until the recordings were made at 9 months of age. Nearly all neurons respond only to the initially closed eye. (Reproduced with permission from LeVay et al. 1980.)

Summary

1.   The development of the nervous system consists of determination and differentiation of nervous tissue. In determination certain cells of the embryo are set off on the pathway to form the cells of the nervous system by the process of gene expression. Differentiation of nervous tissue consists of three processes – cell proliferation, cell migration and cell maturation – which take place concurrently.

2.   In order for the nervous system to function properly the connexions between neurons must be appropriate. There is a high degree of specificity in the connexions made between neurons. Both genetic and environmental factors are involved in the formation of connexions.

3.   Embryonic muscle fibres and adult muscle fibres that have been denervated are sensitive to acetylcholine (ACh) over their entire surface. Innervation leads to a restriction of ACh to the end-plate region. Furthermore, motoneurons are capable of determining the characteristics of muscle fibres by affecting gene expression in them.

4.   After central denervation in adult fish and amphibia regeneration of the lesioned axons can take place. In adult mammals there is no significant regeneration of sectioned central axons. There is some evidence for limited recovery in the latter species which is possibly due to strengthening of previously weak synaptic connexions.

5.   There are important critical periods in the development of mammalian nervous systems. If abnormal experience occurs during these periods, which are in early postnatal life, permanent effects on the anatomy and physiology of the brain will ensue.

18 Learning and Memory

The success of an animal species in its relationships with the external environment is dependent on how well it can adapt to changes in that environment. Part of this adaptation is, of course, evolutionary and leads to the emergence of new species over long periods of time. Within the lifetime of an individual animal success is strongly dependent on that animal's ability to adapt to the environment and, in particular, to alter its behaviour in appropriate ways. This capacity to alter behaviour is a result of changes in the nervous system; these changes constitute learning and memory.

Learning is the process, or set of processes, in which new knowledge about the environment is acquired. Remembering is the process, or set of processes, in which that new knowledge is recalled for use at a later date. The ability to remember obviously implies that there is a store of knowledge – memory – from which learnt knowledge can be recalled. Forgetting (amnesia) is the process, or set of processes, whereby previously acquired memory is lost. Amnesia can be particularly distressing in humans, both in old age, in premature senility (Alzheimer's disease) and as a result of other pathological states.

The study of learning, remembering and forgetting encompasses an enormous range of experimental, observational and clinical disciplines, with a correspondingly enormous literature. The range runs from the study of the molecular biology and cellular neuroscience of learning and memory at one end, through the study of neuronal networks and animal behaviour, to psychological and psychiatric studies in humans at the other end. In an introductory text such as this it is only possible to touch upon a few aspects of this large field. Some possible cellular mechanisms of learning in invertebrates and vertebrates will be considered, together with some attributes of memory and amnesia in humans. Although it is convenient to separate learning from memory it should be realized that in order to show that an animal has learnt something it is often that animal's memory that is tested. The two processes of learning and remembering are inextricably intertwined, at both the cellular and behavioural levels.

Forms of Learning and Memory

Learning may be non-associative or associative. In non-associative learning an organism is exposed to a stimulus, either at a single occasion or repeatedly, and learns about the properties of that stimulus. Non-associative learning is the most common form and includes the phenomena of habituation and sensitization. Habituation is the decrease in a response to a repeated stimulus, usually to an innocuous stimulus. Sensitization is the increase in a response to a repeated stimulus, usually to a noxious stimulus. A sensitized animal has an increased response to an innocuous stimulus after having received a noxious one. A sensitizing stimulus can override an habituating one to produce the phenomenon of dishabituation. For example, after a startle response to a loud noise has become habituated, a strong mechanical stimulus can restore the startle response to the noise. In associative learning the animal relates one stimulus to another (classical conditioning) or relates a stimulus to behaviour (operant conditioning). In classical conditioning an initially ineffective conditioned stimulus (CS) becomes effective in eliciting a response after it has been temporally paired with an unconditioned stimulus (US). This type of learning was originally described by Pavlov in famous experiments on gastric acid secretion in dogs: the CS was a bell rung just before the presentation of food (the US) and after conditioning had taken place the sound of the bell was sufficient to cause gastric secretion. The CS must be presented before the US and the time between the two presentations is critical – a few hundred milliseconds to a few seconds in different situations. In operant conditioning an animal's own behaviour is associated with a subsequent reinforcing event. For example, a hungry animal will be rewarded with food if it performs a certain task such as pressing a lever. Pressing the lever may be initially a random activity, but if it is followed in a short time by food presentation then the animal learns to press the lever to receive the food reward.

Learning and memory may also be non-declarative (reflexive) or declarative. In non-declarative learning there is no awareness of what has actually been learned, leading to a disposition to behave in a particular way with no memory of the events involved in learning. Examples of such learning are the acquisition of perceptual and motor skills. In declarative learning there is the ability to remember past experiences and to predict, by inference, a possible future outcome of behaviour. The distinction between declarative and non-declarative memory is not hard and fast. Declarative memory may be transformed into non-declarative memory. For example, learning to play a musical instrument, to drive a car or to speak a foreign language all initially require considerable conscious effort but gradually become more and more automatic (reflexive).

Memory has several stages and can be divided into short-term and long-term memory. These two stages can be dissociated from each other. Brain injury in both animals and humans, such as is caused by a blow to the head producing unconsciousness or by electroconvulsive shock, may lead to selective loss of memory for events that occurred just before the insult (retrograde amnesia) or for the period just after regaining consciousness (anterograde amnesia), whilst long-term memories may be unaffected. It takes time to transfer short-term memory into long-term stores, and, because the transfer is disrupted by blocking protein synthesis, it is believed that synthesis of new protein is required for the transfer.

Furthermore, in addition to the short- and long-term memory stores, a separate search and read-out system seems to be required that can access both stores, since after brain trauma there is often recovery from at least some of the original amnesia.

Cellular Mechanisms of Learning and Memory in Invertebrates

Invertebrate preparations have been especially useful in studying the cellular mechanisms of certain simple types of learning. This is partly due to the relative simplicity of their nervous systems and behavioural responses, and more particularly to the ease with which the same identified neurons may be recorded from in different individual animals.

Non-associative Learning: Habituation and Sensitization

The marine snail *Aplysia californica* has been used to excellent effect by Castellucci, Kandel and Kupfermann and their colleagues in studies of learning. They have used the reflex withdrawal of the animal's respiratory organ, the gill, and its siphon, which is used to expel sea water and waste materials. The gill and siphon withdrawal reflex is brought into play after a mild tactile stimulus to the siphon (Fig. 18.1). Repeated stimulation leads to habituation of the reflex.

The neuronal circuitry underlying the gill withdrawal reflex has been determined (Fig. 18.1) and consists of three sets of neurons only. There is a sensory neuron innervating the skin of the siphon and which makes monosynaptic excitatory synaptic connexions with motor neurons that innervate the muscles responsible for gill withdrawal; in addition, there is also a set of interneurons intercalated between the sensory and motor neurons. Tactile stimulation of the siphon skin leads to firing of the sensory neurons and large excitatory postsynaptic potentials (EPSPs) and impulses in the interneurons and motoneurons resulting in brisk gill withdrawal. Repeated presentation of the stimulus leads to progressively smaller and smaller excitatory responses in the interneurons and motoneurons (but not in the sensory neurons) until ultimately

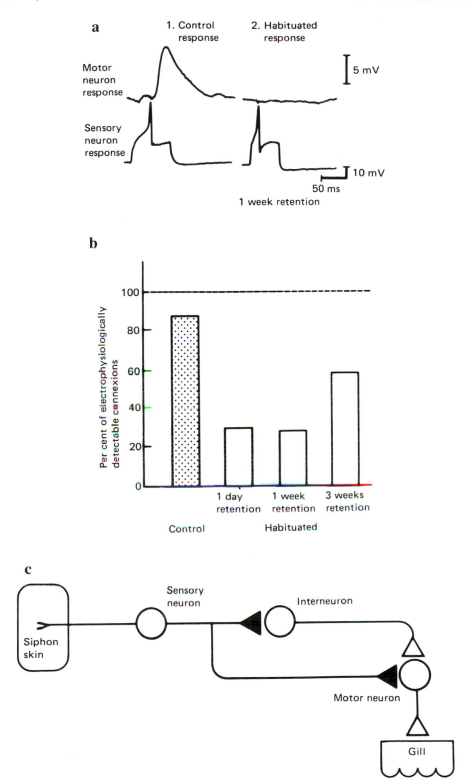

Fig. 18.1a–c. Habituation of the reflex withdrawal of the gill and siphon in *Aplysia*. **a** Shows the responses of the motor and sensory neurons in control animals and after habituation – the sensory neuron still responds but there is no response from the motoneuron. **b** Shows the duration of the habituation (more than 3 weeks). **c** Schematic diagram of the neuronal circuitry. (Modified from Kandel and Schwartz 1985.)

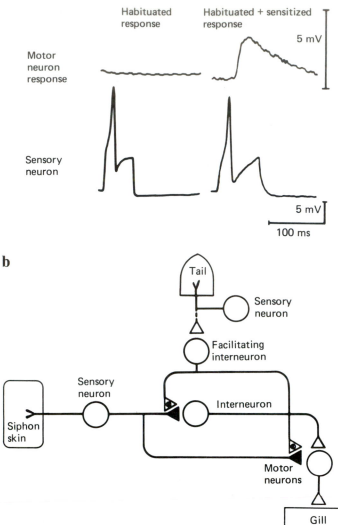

Fig. 18.2a,b. Sensitization of the habituated gill withdrawal reflex in *Aplysia*. **a** Restoration of synaptic transmission between the sensory neuron and motoneuron after a sensitizing, noxious, stimulus to the tail. **b** Schematic diagram of the neuronal pathways involved. (Modified from Kandel and Schwartz 1985.)

there is no gill withdrawal (Fig. 18.1). The habituation lasts for several hours after a single training session of ten repeated stimuli and can persist for several weeks after a series of repeated training sessions (Fig. 18.1).

As mentioned above, habituation does not affect the ability of the sensory neuron to respond to the mechanical stimulation of the siphon skin. Furthermore, there is no change in the properties of the motoneurons. The major mechanism of habituation in this preparation appears to be a partial inactivation of the Ca^{2+} channels in the presynaptic terminals. Such partial inactivation will lead to less transmitter being released (see Chap. 6). Habituation is therefore due to a change in the efficacy of synaptic transmission caused by a reduction in transmitter release.

Sensitization has also been studied by Kandel and his associates using the gill and siphon withdrawal reflex of *Aplysia*. Electrical stimulation of the tail (a noxious stimulus) leads to facilitation of the gill withdrawal reflex to mechanical stimulation of the siphon skin. The neuronal mechanism is one of presynaptic facilitation at axo-axonic synapses on the terminals of the sensory neurons (Fig. 18.2). The axo-axonic contacts are formed by the terminals of facilitory interneurons activated by noxious stimulation of the tail. These facilitatory interneurons are serotoninergic, releasing serotonin (5-HT) as their transmitter. Serotonin acts (see Chap. 8) via a G protein and adenylate cyclase, to increase the level of cyclic AMP in the sensory nerve terminals. The increased level of cyclic AMP in turn activates a protein kinase, which closes K^+ channels, leading to a prolongation of the action potentials in the sensory neuron. This prolongation of the action potential causes an increased opening time for Ca^{2+} channels with a subsequent increase of transmitter release from the sensory neurons. Sensitization is capable of reversing the effects of habituation (Fig. 18.2). Like habituation, sensitization in this preparation is due to a change in the efficacy of synaptic transmission, caused, in this case, by an increase in transmitter release.

Both habituation and sensitization change the effective number of synapses operating between the sensory neurons and the motoneurons in *Aplysia*. When tested electrophysiologically, habituation was shown to reduce the numbers of effective contacts between the sensory and motoneurons, whereas sensitization in long-term habituated animals was shown to increase the numbers of effective synapses back towards control values. In addition to these functional changes, there are corresponding anatomical changes in the terminals of the sensory neurons. Habituation reduces the number and size of active zones in the synapses and also reduces the number of synaptic vesicles associated with the active zones. Sensitization has the opposite effects to increase these numbers.

Associative Learning in Invertebrates: Classical Conditioning

Kandel and his associates have also used the gill and siphon withdrawal reflex of *Aplysia* to study cellular mechanisms of classical conditioning. Not only can noxious stimulation of the tail facilitate (sensitize) the gill withdrawal reflex to tactile stimulation of the siphon, but also, if the siphon stimulus (CS) precedes the tail stimulus (US) by 1–2 s, then the response enhancement is greater and lasts longer than that produced by sensitization. This conditioned response is temporally specific in that the CS must precede the US and the time between stimulus presentations is critical (up to 2 s for this conditioned reflex).

The crucial difference between sensitization (facilitation) and conditioning appears to be that if the CS and the US are timed to occur within 2 s of each other, the US following the CS, then even more Ca^{2+} is admitted to the terminals of the sensory neuron, by increased formation of cyclic AMP and closure of K^+ channels, leading to even greater transmitter release. Thus, the response of the terminals of the sensory neurons

to the facilitatory (US) input is much greater if those terminals have recently been active as a result of sensory input (CS). During training such pairing of the CS and US occurs.

In this invertebrate preparation, therefore, the site of conditioning is at the terminals of a presynaptic neuron – the postsynaptic neurons are not involved. Similar results have been obtained for the conditioning of phototactic behaviour by rotation in the marine snail *Hermissenda* by Crow and Alkon and their colleagues (see, for example, Crow 1988).

Cellular Mechanisms of Learning in Vertebrates

In 1949, Hebb suggested a mechanism for learning based on the coincidence of firing in presynaptic and postsynaptic neurons. The important point about this hypothesis was that learning (synaptic modification) would only take place when synapses were active in close temporal contiguity with strong postsynaptic activity. Work on mammalian preparations, in particular on the hippocampus, which is thought to be involved in learning and memory, has provided strong evidence supporting this hypothesis.

Mechanisms Underlying Long-term Potentiation in the Hippocampus

Long-term potentiation (LTP) in the mammalian hippocampus was first reported by Bliss and Lømo in 1973. It consists (Fig. 18.3) of an enduring increase in the EPSP amplitude of hippocampal pyramidal cells in response to a brief high-frequency activation of their afferent fibres. In the CA1 region of the hippocampus this potentiation takes a few seconds (about 3 s) before it starts to develop and then a further 15–20 s to reach its maximal value. After strong and repeated afferent stimulation LTP can last for days or even weeks, but there is no evidence that it becomes permanent.

In order for LTP to develop, a sufficient number of afferent fibres has to be active. Also, LTP shows the characteristics of an associative response – a weak input only leads to a potentiated response if it is preceded by a stronger tetanization of other afferent fibres, and more LTP is produced if two equally strong inputs are tetanized together. The role of the postsynaptic neuron

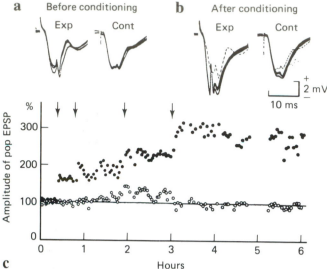

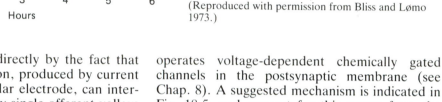

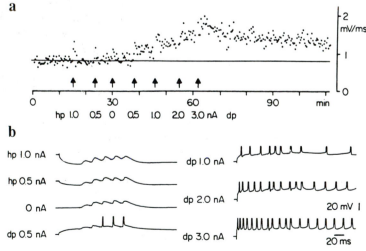

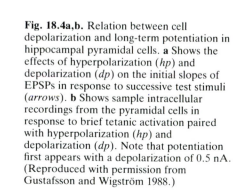

Fig. 18.3a–c. Long-term potentiation in the hippocampus of the rabbit. **a** Shows the population EPSP in the experimental and control pathways and **b** the potentials after conditioning. **c** The amplitudes of the conditioned and control responses plotted against time. The *arrows* indicate the timing of conditioning stimulation (15 Hz for 10 s) of the afferent fibres. (Reproduced with permission from Bliss and Lømo 1973.)

has been demonstrated directly by the fact that intracellular depolarization, produced by current pulses from an intracellular electrode, can interact with EPSPs evoked by single afferent volleys at low frequency to produce LTP, and LTP can be prevented by intracellular hyperpolarization (Fig. 18.4). These experiments also show that impulse firing in the postsynaptic neuron is not essential for the production of LTP – depolarization alone is sufficient.

A role for Ca^{2+} in the mechanism of LTP is indicated by the fact that injection of the Ca^{2+} chelating agent ethyleneglycol *bis* (β-aminoethylether)-N,N'-tetra-acetic acid (EGTA) into the cells will prevent its generation. Current hypotheses suggest an important role for the N-methyl-D-aspartate (NMDA) receptor that

operates voltage-dependent chemically gated channels in the postsynaptic membrane (see Chap. 8). A suggested mechanism is indicated in Fig. 18.5, and support for this comes from the observation that specific NMDA receptor antagonists will prevent the development of LTP. Furthermore, Morris et al. (1986) have shown that an NMDA receptor antagonist (AP5) selectively interferes with spatial learning in rats in a water maze test.

Long-term Depression in the Cerebellum

In the cerebellar cortex long-term depression (LTD) is thought to be an important mechanism

Fig. 18.4a,b. Relation between cell depolarization and long-term potentiation in hippocampal pyramidal cells. **a** Shows the effects of hyperpolarization (*hp*) and depolarization (*dp*) on the initial slopes of EPSPs in response to successive test stimuli (*arrows*). **b** Shows sample intracellular recordings from the pyramidal cells in response to brief tetanic activation paired with hyperpolarization (*hp*) and depolarization (*dp*). Note that potentiation first appears with a depolarization of 0.5 nA. (Reproduced with permission from Gustafsson and Wigström 1988.)

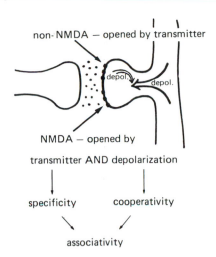

non-NMDA — opened by transmitter

depol.   depol.

NMDA — opened by

transmitter AND depolarization

specificity   cooperativity

associativity

Fig. 18.5. Suggested scheme for the mechanism of long-term potentiation. NMDA and non-NMDA receptors are located on each single dendritic spine of hippocampal pyramidal cells. Non-NMDA receptor channels are unconditionally opened by the transmitter. Opening of the NMDA receptor channels depends on concomitant depolarization of the post-synaptic cell. This depolarization is caused partly by ionic flux through non-NMDA (and NMDA) receptor channels and by spread of current from other active synapses. (Reproduced with permission from Gustafsson and Wigström 1988.)

underlying cerebellar motor learning (Ito 1989). If the two inputs to cerebellar Purkinje cells, from the parallel fibres and the climbing fibres, are caused to fire nearly synchronously then there follows a long-lasting depression of the transmission between parallel fibres and Purkinje cells – LTD. LTD only occurs when there is an excitation of parallel fibres from about 20 ms before to about 150 ms following climbing fibre activation.

LTD consists of an initial phase lasting about 10 min, followed by a later phase that has been followed for about 3 h. The depression of parallel fibre excitatory effects is intense and can be as much as 40% during the late phase, as tested by the ability of parallel fibres to cause Purkinje cells to fire. The underlying mechanism of LTD is thought to be a reduction of sensitivity of glutamate receptors, but unlike LTP the receptor is quisqualate-specific as opposed to NMDA-specific. The parallel fibres release glutamate at their synaptic terminals. The role of the climbing fibre input is to produce an inflow of Ca^{2+} ions (which underlies the dendritic action potential) in Purkinje cells. This influx of Ca^{2+} leads to desensitization of the quisqualate-specific glutamate receptors.

At present LTD is thought to work as follows. A region of cerebellar cortex forms a modifiable

side path into either a reflex arc or a command signal pathway for voluntary movement control through the connexions of mossy (parallel) fibres and Purkinje cells. This side path has signal transfer characteristics that are modified by activity in the climbing fibres. Climbing fibre signals represent feed-back control errors, and the LTD depresses the cerebellar network that was responsible for the error generation.

Learning and Memory in Humans

In the 1950s Scoville and Milner (see Scoville and Milner 1957) showed that damage to the hippocampal formation can lead to serious impairment of learning and memory in humans. Memory deficits may occur in humans with little other evidence of intellectual impairment, and not all cases have hippocampal damage. Thus, bilateral damage to the midline diencephalon can cause serious impairments in memory, and the parts of the brain most often implicated are the mammillary bodies of the hypothlamus and the mediodorsal nucleus of the thalamus.

Human memory may be subdivided into various components. As mentioned earlier in this chapter, memory may be divided into short-term and long-term memory. The study of amnesic patients supports this division. Korsakov's syndrome, the result of chronic alcohol abuse, is characterized by a loss of long-term memory with little, if any, impairment of short-term memory. A famous case study of a patient (H.M.) by Milner (1966) showed that memory may consist of several components. This patient underwent brain surgery for intractable epilepsy. The operation involved bilateral removal of the medial temporal lobe, including the anterior part (two-thirds) of the hippocampus and the hippocampal gyri: the lateral neocortex was spared. After the operation H.M. was densely amnesic and his ability to generate new long-term memory was grossly impaired, although he could remember his early life and also his immediate memory span was normal. Another patient, reported by Shallice and Warrington (1970) suffered damage to the perisylvian region of the left cerebral cortex. He had a very specific inability for the immediate recall of spoken verbal material in the short-term and yet could learn lists of words and remember them over the long-term.

A recent clinical case (patient R.B.) has provided important knowledge about the effects of hippocampal damage (Zola-Morgan et al. 1986). This patient suffered cerebral ischaemia during open heart surgery in 1978, when he was 52 years old. He was intensively investigated on a battery of psychological tests during the remaining 5 years of his life, and after his death in 1983 an extensive pathological examination of his brain was performed. There was a complete loss of pyramidal neurons in the CA1 region of the hippocampus bilaterally with minimal evidence of other neuronal damage (in particular, there were no signs of damage to the mammillary bodies or the mediodorsal nucleus of the thalamus). Between the time of the open heart surgery and his death he showed particular memory deficits. For example, he failed completely on a delayed prose recall test and poorly on several tests of both verbal and non-verbal learning ability. He repeated the same stories endlessly and also forgot events that had occurred earlier in the day. However, he appeared to have no deficits of his memory prior to the occurrence of cerebral ischaemia, that is, he had no retrograde amnesia as far as could be ascertained. It would appear from observations such as these that the hippocampus is involved in declarative learning in humans and in short-term memory, but that over a (short) period of time memory becomes independent of the hippocampus.

Summary

1. Learning and memory allow an animal to alter its behaviour in response to changes in the environment. Both learning and memory may be subdivided into various components.

2. Learning may be non-associative or associative. Non-associative learning includes the phenomena of habituation and sensitization. In invertebrate species habituation and sensitization have been shown to depend on presynaptic mechanisms that alter the effectiveness of synaptic transmission. Associative learning includes classical conditioning and operant conditioning. Classical conditioning in invertebrates has been shown to depend on mechanisms similar to sensitization and to alter the efficacy of synaptic transmission by presynaptic facilitation.

3. Long-term potentiation in the hippocampus of mammals has been extensively studied as a model for learning. It depends on concurrent pre- and postsynaptic activation and involves voltage-dependent chemically gated ion channels in the postsynaptic neuron, operated by the NMDA receptor.

4. Memory may be subdivided into several components, including short-term and long-term memory. Damage to different parts of the brain can disassociate these two components.

References

Armstrong CM, Bezanille R (1974) Charge movement associated with the opening and closing of the activation gates of Na channels. J Gen Physiol 63: 633–552

Armstrong CM, Bezanille R, Rojas E (1973) Destruction of sodium conductance inactivation in squid axons perfused with pronase. J Gen Physiol 62: 375–391

Armstrong DM (1988) The supraspinal control of mammalian locomotion. J Physiol (Lond) 405: 1–37

Attardi DG, Sperry RW (1963) Preferential selection of central pathways by regenerating optic fibers. Exp Neurol 7: 46–64

Baker PF, Hodgkin AL, Shaw TI (1961) Replacement of the protoplasm of a giant nerve fibre with artificial solutions. Nature 190: 885–887

Baker PF, Hodgkin AL, Shaw TI (1962) The effects of changes in internal ionic concentrations on the electrical properties of perfused giant axons. J Physiol (Lond) 164: 355–374

Barker D (1974) The morphology of muscle receptors. In: Hunt CC (ed) Muscle receptors. Springer, Berlin Heidelberg New York, pp 1–190 (Handbook of sensory physiology, vol III/2)

Baylor DA, Lamb TD, Yau K-W (1979) The membrane current of single rod outer segments. J Physiol (Lond) 288: 589–611

Björklund A, Lindvall O (1986) Catecholaminergic brain stem regulatory systems. In: Handbook of physiology, Section 1. The nervous system, vol IV. Intrinsic regulatory systems of the brain. American Physiological Society, Bethesda, Maryland. pp 155–235.

Bliss TVP, Lømo T (1973) Long-lasting potentiation of synaptic transmission in the dentate area of the anaesthetized rabbit following stimulation of the perforant path. J Physiol (Lond) 232: 331–356

Bodian D (1962) The generalized vertebrate neuron. Science 137: 323–326

Bodian D (1967) Neurons, circuits, and neuroglia. In: Quarton GC, Melnechuk T, Schmitt FO (eds) The neurosciences: a study program. Rockefeller University Press, New York, pp 6–31

Bretscher MS (1985) The molecules of the cell membrane. Sci Am 253: 86–90

Brodal A (1981) Neurological anatomy in relation to clinical medicine, 3rd edn. Oxford University Press, Oxford

Brown AG (1968) Cutaneous afferent fibre collaterals in the dorsal columns of the cat. Exp Brain Res 5: 293–305

Brown AG (1973) Ascending and long spinal pathways: dorsal columns, spinocervical tract and spinothalamic tract. In: Iggo A (ed) Somatosensory system. Springer, Berlin Heidelberg New York, pp 315–338 (Handbook of sensory physiology, vol II)

Brown AG (1981) Organization in the spinal cord: the anatomy and physiology of identified neurones. Springer, Berlin Heidelberg New York

Brown AG, Franz DN (1969) Responses of spinocervical tract neurones to natural stimulation of identified cutaneous receptors. Exp Brain Res 7: 231–249

Brown AG, Fyffe REW (1978) The morphology of Group Ia afferent fibre collaterals in the spinal cord of the cat. J Physiol (Lond) 274: 111–127

Brown AG, Fyffe REW (1981a) Direct observations on the contacts made between Ia afferent fibres and α-motoneurones in the cat's lumbosacral spinal cord. J Physiol (Lond) 313: 121–140

Brown AG, Fyffe REW (1981b) Form and function of dorsal horn neurones with axons ascending the dorsal columns in cat. J Physiol (Lond) 321: 31–47

Brown AG, Kirk EJ, Martin HF (1973) Descending and segmental inhibition of transmission through the spinocervical tract. J Physiol (Lond) 230: 689–705

Brown AG, Hamann WC, Martin HF (1975) Effects of activity in non-myelinated afferent fibres on the spinocervical tract. Brain Res 98: 243–259

Brown AG, Rose PK, Snow PJ (1977) The morphology of hair follicle afferent fibre collaterals in the spinal cord of the cat. J Physiol (Lond) 272: 779–797

Brown AG, Fyffe REW, Noble R, Rose PK, Snow PJ (1980) The density, distribution and topographical organization of spinocervical tract neurones in the cat. J Physiol (Lond) 300: 409–428

Brown AG, Koerber HR, Noble R (1987a) Excitatory actions of single impulses in single hair follicle afferent fibres on spinocervical tract neurones in the cat. J Physiol (Lond) 382: 291–312

Brown AG, Koerber HR, Noble R (1987b) An intracellular study of spinocervical tract cell responses to natural stimulation and single hair afferent fibres in cats. J Physiol (Lond) 382: 331–354

Brown HM, Ottoson D, Rydqvist B (1978) Crayfish stretch receptors: an investigation with voltage-clamp and ion-sensitive electrodes. J Physiol (Lond) 284: 155–179

Brown TG (1911) The intrinsic factor in the act of progression in the mammal. Proc R Soc Lond [Biol] 84: 308–319

Bullock TH (1959) Neuron doctrine and electrophysiology. Science 129: 997–1002

Bullock TH, Orkand R, Grinnell A (1977) Introduction to nervous systems. WH Freeman, San Francisco

Bunge RP (1968) Glial cells and the central myelin sheath. Physiol Rev 48: 197–251

Burke RE (1967) Composite nature of the monosynaptic excitatory postsynaptic potential. J Neurophysiol 30: 1114–1137

Burke RE, Rudomin P (1977) Spinal neurons and synapses. In: Kandel ER (ed) Handbook of physiology, Section 1. The nervous system, vol I. Cellular biology of neurons. American Physiological Society, Bethesda, Maryland. pp 877–944

Burkhardt D (1958) Die Sinnesorgane des Skeletmuskels und die nervöse Steuerung der Muskeltätigkeit. Ergeb Biol 20: 27–66

Cantley L (1986) Ion transport systems sequenced. Trends Neurosci 9: 1–3

Carter MC, Smith JL (1986) Simultaneous control of two rhythmical behaviors. II. Hindlimb walking with paw-shake responses in spinal cat. J Neurophysiol 56: 184–195

Chambers MR, Andres KH, Duering Mv, Iggo A (1972) The structure and function of the slowly adapting type II mechanoreceptor in hairy skin. Q J Exp Physiol 57: 417–445

Cole KS (1969) Membranes, ions and impulses. University of California Press, Berkeley

Conradi S (1969) On motoneuron synaptology in adult cats. Acta Physiol Scand 78 [Suppl 332]: 1–115

Coombs JS, Eccles JC, Fatt P (1955a) The electrical properties of the motoneurone membrane. J Physiol (Lond) 130: 291–325

Coombs JS, Eccles JC, Fatt P (1955b) The specific ion conductances and the ionic movements across the motoneuronal membrane that produce the inhibitory post-synaptic potential. J Physiol (Lond) 130: 326–373

Coombs JS, Eccles JC, Fatt P (1955c) Excitatory synaptic action in motoneurones. J Physiol (Lond) 130: 374–395

Coombs JC, Eccles JC, Fatt P (1955d) The inhibitory suppression of reflex discharges from motoneurones. J Physiol (Lond) 130: 396–413

Cowan WM (1979) The development of the brain. Sci Am 241: 112–133

Cowey A (1979) Cortical maps and visual perception. The Grindley Memorial Lecture. Q J Exp Psychol 31:1–17

Crow T (1988) Cellular and molecular analysis of associative learning and memory in *Hermissenda*. Trends Neurosci 11: 136–142

Crowe A, Matthews PBC (1964) The effects of stimulation of static and dynamic fusimotor fibres on the response to muscle stretching of the primary endings of muscle spindles. J Physiol (Lond) 174: 109–131

Curtis HJ, Cole KS (1940) Membrane action potentials from the squid giant axon. J Cell Comp Physiol 15: 147–157

del Castillo J, Katz B (1954a) Quantal components of the end-plate potential. J Physiol (Lond) 124: 560–573

del Castillo J, Katz B (1954b) The membrane change produced by the neuromuscular transmitter. J Physiol (Lond) 125: 546–565

Dowling JE, Boycott BB (1967) Organization of the primate retina: electron microscopy. Proc R Soc Lond [Biol] 166: 80–111

du Vigneaud V (1956) Hormones of the posterior pituitary gland, oxytocin and vasopressin. Harvey Lect 50: 1–26

Dykes RW, Rasmusson DD, Hoeltzell PB (1980) Organization of primary somatosensory cortex in the cat. J Neuro-

physiol 43: 1527–1546

Eccles JC (1964) The physiology of synapses. Springer, Berlin Göttingen Heidelberg New York

Eccles JC, Eccles RM, Lundberg A (1957) Synaptic actions on motoneurones in relation to the two components of the group I muscle afferent volley. J Physiol (Lond) 136: 527–546

Eccles JC, Eccles RM, Magni F (1961) Central inhibitory action attributable to presynaptic depolarization produced by muscle afferent volleys. J Physiol (Lond) 159: 147–166

Eccles JC, Schmidt RF, Willis WD (1963) Depolarization of the central terminals of cutaneous afferent fibers. J Neurophysiol 26: 646–661

Eccles JC, Ito M, Szentágothai J (1967) The cerebellum as a neuronal machine. Springer, Berlin Heidelberg New York

Eckert R, Randall D (1978) Animal physiology. WH Freeman, San Francisco

Eide E, Fedina L, Jansen J, Lundberg A, Vyklicky L (1969) Properties of Clarke's column neurones. Acta Physiol Scand 77: 125–144

Erlanger J, Gasser HS (1937) Electrical signs of nervous activity. University of Pennsylvania Press, Philadelphia

Evarts EV (1981) Role of motor cortex in voluntary movements in primates. In: Brooks VB (ed) Handbook of physiology, Section 1. The nervous system, vol II. Motor control, part 2. American Physiological Society, Bethesda, Maryland, pp 1082–1120

Eyzaguirre C, Kuffler SW (1955) Processes of excitation in the dendrites and in the soma of single isolated sensory nerve cells of the lobster and crayfish. J Gen Physiol 39: 87–119

Fatt P (1957) Sequence of events in synaptic activation of a motoneurone. J Neurophysiol 20: 61–80

Fatt P, Katz B (1952) Spontaneous subthreshold activity at motor nerve endings. J Physiol (Lond) 117: 109–128

Fesenko EE, Kolesnikor SS, Lynbarsky AL (1985) Induction by cyclic GMP of cationic conductance in plasma membrane of retinal rod outer segment. Nature 313: 310–313

Finkel AS, Redman SJ (1983) The synaptic current evoked in cat spinal motoneurones by impulses in single group Ia axons. J Physiol (Lond) 342: 615–632

Forssberg H, Grillner S, Halbertsma J (1980) The locomotion of the low spinal cat. I. Coordination within a hindlimb. Acta Physiol Scand 108: 269–281

Furshpan EJ, Potter DD (1959) Transmission at the giant synapse of the crayfish. J Physiol (Lond) 145: 289–325

Furukawa T, Furshpan EJ (1963) Two inhibitory mechanisms in the Mauthner neurons of goldfish. J Neurophysiol 26: 140–176

Gaze RM (1970) The formation of nerve connections. Academic Press, London

Gerhart KD, Wilcox TK, Chung JM, Willis WD (1981) Inhibition of nociceptive and nonnociceptive responses of primate spinothalamic cells by stimulation in medial brain stem. J Neurophysiol 45: 121–136

Gilbert PFC, Thach WT (1977) Purkinje cell activity during motor learning. Brain Res 128: 309–328

Gogan P, Gueritaud JP, Tyc-Dumont S (1983) Comparison of antidromic and orthodromic action potentials of identified motor axons in the cat's brain stem. J Physiol (Lond) 335: 205–220

Gorter E, Grendel F (1925) On bimolecular layers of lipoids on the chromatocytes. J Exp Med 41: 439–443

Granit R, Kernell D, Smith RS (1963a) Delayed depolarization and the repetitive response to intracellular stimulation of mammalian motoneurones. J Physiol (Lond) 168: 890–910

Granit R, Kernell D, Shortess GK (1963b) Quantitative aspects of repetitive firing of mammalian motoneurones caused by injected currents. J Physiol (Lond) 168: 911–931

Granit R, Kernell D, Lamarre Y (1966) Algebraic summation in synaptic activation of motoneurones firing within the primary range to injected currents. J Physiol (Lond) 187: 379–399

Grundfest H (1957) Electrical inexitability of synapses and some of its consequences in the central nervous system. Physiol Rev 37: 337–361

Gustafsson B, Wigström H (1988) Physiological mechanisms underlying long-term potentiation. Trends Neurosci 11: 156–162

Guy HR, Hucho F (1987) The ion channel of the nicotinic acetylcholine receptor. Trends Neurosci 10: 318–321

Hagiwara S, Morita H (1962) Electrotonic transmission between two nerve cells in leech ganglion. J Neurophysiol 25: 721–731

Hamill OP, Marty A, Neher F, Sakmann B, Sigsworth FJ (1981) Improved patch-clamp technique for high-resolution current recording from cells and from cell-free membrane patches. Pflugers Arch 391: 85–100

Hebb DO (1949) The organization of behaviour. Wiley, London

Heuser JE, Reese TS (1977) Structure of the synapse. In: Kandel ER (ed) Handbook of physiology, section 1. The nervous system, vol I. Cellular biology of neurons. American Physiological Society, Bethesda, Maryland, pp 262–294

Heuser JE, Reese TS, Landis DMD (1974) Functional changes on frog neuromuscular junctions studied with freeze-fracture. J Neurocytol 3: 109–131

Hille B (1970) Ionic channels in nerve membrane. Prog Biophys Mol Biol 21: 1–32

Hille B (1984) Channels of excitable membranes. Sinauer Associates Inc, Sunderland, Massachusetts

Hobson JA, Steriade M (1986) Neuronal basis of behavioral state control. In: Bloom FE (ed) Handbook of physiology, Section 1. The nervous system, vol IV. Intrinsic regulatory systems of the brain. American Physiological Society, Bethesda, Maryland, pp 701–823

Hodgkin AL (1937) Evidence for electrical transmission in nerve. J Physiol (Lond) 90: 183–210, 211–232

Hodgkin AL (1939) The relation between conduction velocity and the electrical resistance outside a nerve fibre. J Physiol (Lond) 94: 560–570

Hodgkin AL (1964) The conduction of the nervous impulse. Liverpool University Press, Liverpool

Hodgkin Al, Horowicz P (1959) The influence of potassium and chloride ions on the membrane potential of single muscle fibres. J Physiol (Lond) 148: 127–160

Hodgkin AL, Huxley AF (1939) Action potentials recorded from inside a nerve fibre. Nature (Lond) 144: 710–711

Hodgkin AL, Huxley AF (1952a) Currents carried by sodium and potassium ions through the membrane of the giant axon of Loligo. J Physiol (Lond) 116: 449–472

Hodgkin AL, Huxley AF (1952b) The components of membrane conductance in the giant axon of Loligo. J Physiol (Lond) 116: 473–496

Hodgkin AL, Huxley AF (1952c) The dual effect of membrane potential on sodium conductance in the giant axon of Loligo. J Physiol (Lond) 116: 497–506

Hodgkin AL, Huxley AF (1952d) A quantitative description of membrane current and its application to conduction and excitation in nerve. J Physiol (Lond) 117: 500–544

Hodgkin AL, Katz B (1949) The effect of sodium ions on the electrical activity of the giant axon of the squid. J Physiol (Lond) 108: 37–77

Hodgkin AL, Keynes RD (1955) Active transport of cations in giant axons from Sepia and Loligo. J Physiol (Lond) 128: 28–60

Hodgkin AL, Huxley AF, Katz B (1952) Measurement of current-voltage relations in the membrane of the giant axon of Loligo. J Physiol (Lond) 116: 424–448

Hökfelt T, Lundberg JM, Schultzberg M, Johansson O, Ljungdahl A, Rehfeld J (1980) Coexistence of peptides and putative transmitters in neurons. In: Costa E, Trabucchi M (eds) Neural peptides and neuronal communication. Raven Press, New York, pp 1–23

Hubel DH, Wiesel TN (1962) Receptive fields, binocular interaction and functional architecture in the cat's visual cortex. J Physiol (Lond) 160: 106–154

Hubel DH, Wiesel TN (1977) Functional architecture of macaque monkey visual cortex. Proc R Soc Lond [Biol] 198: 1–59

Hughes A (1961) Cell degeneration in the larval ventral horn of Xenopus laevis (Daudier). J Embryol Exp Morph 9: 269–284

Hunt CC, Kuffler SW (1951) Further study of efferent small nerve fibres to mammalian muscle spindles: multiple spindle innervation and activity during contraction. J Physiol (Lond) 113: 283–297

Huxley AF, Stämpfli R (1949) Evidence for saltatory conduction in peripheral myelinated nerve-fibres. J Physiol (Lond) 108: 315–339

Iggo A (1969) Cutaneous thermoreceptors in primates and sub-primates. J Physiol (Lond) 200: 403–430

Ito M (1989) Long-term depression. Annu Rev Neurosci 12: 85–102

Jack JJB, Miller S, Porter R, Redman SJ (1971) The time-course of minimal excitatory post-synaptic potentials evoked in spinal motoneurones by group Ia afferent fibres. J Physiol (Lond) 215: 353–380

Jones EG, Powell TPS (1969) Connexions of the somatic sensory cortex in the rhesus monkey. I. Ipsilateral cortical connexions. Brain 92: 477–502

Kandel ER, Schwartz JH (1985) Principles of neural science, 2nd edn. Elsevier, New York

Katz B (1966) Nerve, muscle, and synapse. McGraw-Hill, New York

Katz B, Miledi R (1967a) The timing of calcium action during neuromuscular transmission. J Physiol (Lond) 189: 535–544

Katz B, Miledi R (1967b) A study of synaptic transmission in the absence of nerve impulses. J Physiol (Lond) 192: 407–436

Kernell D (1965) High-frequency repetitive firing of cat lumbosacral motoneurones stimulated by long-lasting injected currents. Acta Physiol Scand 65: 74–86

Keynes RD (1958) The nerve impulse and the squid. Sci Am 199: 83–90

Kirsinger A, Jürgens V (1982) Cortical lesion effects and vocalization in the squirrel monkey. Brain Res 233: 299–315

Kuffler SW, Yoshikami D (1975a) The distribution of acetylcholine sensitivity at the post-synaptic membrane of vertebrate skeletal twitch muscles: iontophoretic mapping in the micron range. J Physiol (Lond) 244: 703–730

Kuffler SW, Yoshikami D (1975b) The number of transmitter molecules in a quantum: an estimate from iontophoretic application of acetylcholine at the neuromuscular junction. J Physiol (Lond) 251: 465–482

Kuffler SW, Nicholls JG, Orkand RK (1966) Physiological properties of glial cells in the central nervous system of amphibia. J Neurophysiol 29: 768–787

Kuffler SW, Nicholls JG, Martin AR (1984) From neuron to brain, 2nd edn. Sinauer Associates Inc, Sunderland,

Massachusetts

Kuno M, Miyahara JT (1969) Analysis of synaptic efficacy in spinal motoneurones from "quantum" aspects. J Physiol (Lond) 201: 479–493

Le Douarin NM, Renand D, Teillet MA, Le Douarin GH (1975) Cholinergic differentiation of presumptive adrenergic neuroblasts in interspecific chimeras after heterotopic transplantation. Proc Natl Acad Sci USA 72: 728–732

Lemon R (1988) The output map of the primate motor cortex. Trends Neurosci 11: 501–505

LeVay S, Hubel DH, Wiesel TH (1975) The patterns of ocular dominance columns in macaque visual cortex revealed by a reduced silver stain. J Comp Neurol 159: 559–576

LeVay S, Wiesel TN, Hubel DH (1980) The development of ocular dominance columns in normal and visually deprived monkeys. J Comp Neurol 191: 1–51

Lincoln DW, Wakerley JB (1974) Electrophysiological evidence for the activation of supraoptic neurones during the release of oxytocin. J Physiol (Lond) 242: 533–554

Livingstone MS, Hubel DH (1984) Anatomy and physiology of a color system in the primate visual cortex. J Neurosci 4: 309–356

Llínas R (1982) Calcium in synaptic transmission. Sci Am 247: 56–65

Llínas R, Heuser JE (1977) Depolarization-release coupling systems in neurons. Neurosci Res Prog Bull 15: 555–687

Llínas R, Nicholson C (1971) Electrophysological properties of dendrites and somata in alligator Purkinje cells. J Neurophysiol 34: 532–551

Llínas R, Sugimori M (1980a) Electrophysiological properties of in vitro Purkinje cell somata in mammalian cerebellar slices. J Physiol (Lond) 305: 171–195

Llínas R, Sugimori M (1980b) Electrophysiological properties of in vitro Purkinje cell dendrites in mammalian cerebellar slices. J Physiol (Lond) 305: 197–213

Loewenstein WR, Mendelson M (1965) Components of receptor adaptation in a Pacinian corpuscle. J Physiol (Lond) 177: 377–397

Lømo T, Rosenthal J (1972) Control of ACh sensitivity by muscle activity in the rat. J Physiol (Lond) 221: 493–513

Lorenté de Nó R (1934) Studies on the structure of the cerebral cortex. II. Continuation of the study of the Ammonic system. J Psychol Neurol 46: 113–177

MacDermott AB, Dale N (1987) Receptors, ion channels and synaptic potentials underlying the integrative actions of excitatory amino acids. Trends Neurosci 10: 280–284

Makowski L, Casper DLD, Phillips WC, Goodenough DA (1977) Gap junction structure. II. Analysis of the X-ray diffraction data. J Cell Biol 74: 629–645

Martin TFJ, Reichlin S, Brown GM (1977) Clinical neuroendocrinology. FA Davis, Philadelphia

Matthews PBC (1964) Muscle spindles and their motor control. Physiol Rev 44: 219–288

Maunsell JHR, Newsome WT (1987) Visual processing in the monkey extrastriate cortex. Ann Rev Neurosci 10: 363–401

Maxwell DJ, Fyffe REW, Réthélyi M (1983) Morphological properties of physiologically characterized lamina III neurones in the cat spinal cord. Neurosci 10: 1–22

McGeer PL, Eccles JC, McGeer EM (1978) Molecular neurobiology of the mammalian brain. Plenum Press, New York

Mendell LM, Henneman E (1971) Terminals of single Ia fibers: location, density and distribution within a pool of 300 homonymous motoneurons. J Neurophysiol 34: 171–187

Merzenich MM, Kaas JH, Wall JT, Sur M, Nelson RJ, Felleman DJ (1983) Progression of change following median nerve section in the cortical representation of the hand in areas 3b and 1 in adult owl and squirrel monkey. Neurosci 10: 639–665

Millar J, Basbaum AI (1975) Topography of the body surface of the cat to cuneate and gracile nuclei. Exp Neurol 49: 281–290

Milner B (1966) Amnesia following operation on the temporal lobes. In: Whitty CWM, Zangwill OL (eds) Amnesia. Butterworths, London

Morris RGM, Anderson E, Lynch GS, Baudry M (1986) Selective impairment of learning and blockade of long-term potentiation by an N-methyl-D-aspartate receptor antagonist, AP5. Nature 319: 774–776

Mountcastle VB, Darian-Smith I (1968) Neural mechanisms in somaesthesis. In: Mountcastle VB (ed) Medical physiology, 12th edn. CV Mosby, St Louis

Mountcastle VB, Talbot WH, Kornhuber HH (1966) The neural transformation of mechanical stimuli delivered to the monkey's hand. In: De Reuck EVS, Knight J (eds) Touch, heat and pain. Churchill, London; Little Brown, Boston

Mugnaini E (1970) Neurones as synaptic targets. In: Andersen P, Jansen JKS (eds) Excitatory synaptic mechanisms. Universitetsforlaget, Oslo

Nakajima S, Onodera K (1969) Membrane properties of the stretch receptor neurones of crayfish with particular reference to mechanisms of sensory adaptation. J Physiol (Lond) 200: 161–185

Nauta WJH, Fiertag M (1986) Fundamental neuroanatomy. WH Freeman, New York

Nieuwenhuys R (1985) Chemoarchitecture of the brain. Springer, Berlin Heidelberg New York Tokyo

Nieuwenhuys R, Voogd J, Van Huijzen C (1981) The human nervous system: a synopsis and atlas, 2nd edn. Springer, Berlin Heidelberg New York Tokyo

Noda M, Ikeda T, Kayano T et al. (1986) Existence of distinct sodium channel messenger RNAs in rat brain. Nature 320: 188–192

O'Brien DF (1982) The chemistry of vision. Science 218: 961–966

Ochs S, Ranish N (1969) Characteristics of the fast transport system in mammalian nerve fibers. J Neurobiol 1: 247–261

Olds J, Milner P (1954) Positive reinforcement produced by electrical stimulation of septal area and other regions of rat brain. J Comp Physiol Psychol 47: 419–427

Ottoson D, Shepherd GM (1971) Transducer properties and integrative mechanisms in the frog's muscle spindle. In: Loewenstein WR (ed) Principles of receptor physiology. Springer, Berlin Heidelberg New York, pp 442–499 (Handbook of sensory physiology, vol I)

Peters A, Palay SL, Webster H de F (1976) The fine structure of the nervous system: the neurons and supporting cells. WB Saunders, Philadelphia

Powell TPS, Mountcastle VB (1959) Some aspects of the functional organization of the cortex of the precentral gyrus of the monkey: a correlation of findings obtained in single unit analysis with cytoarchitectonics. Bull Johns Hopkins Hosp 105: 135–162

Rexed B (1952) The cytoarchitectonic organization of the spinal cord in the cat. J Comp Neurol 96: 415–495

Robertson JD (1960) The molecular structure and contact relationships of cell membranes. Prog Biophys 10: 343–418

Romanes GJ (1951) The motor cell columns of the lumbosacral cord of the cat. J Comp Neurol 94: 313–364

Ruch TC, Fulton JF (eds) (1960) Medical physiology and biophysics, 18th edn. WB Saunders, Philadelphia

Sauer FC (1935) Mitosis in the neural crest. J Comp Neurol 62: 377–405

Scharrer E, Scharrer B (1940) Secretory cells within the hypothalamus. Res Publ Assoc Res Nerv Ment Dis 20: 170–194

Schmidt RF (1971) Presynaptic inhibition in the vertebrate central nervous system. Ergeb Physiol 63: 20–101

Schmidt RF (1973) Control of the access of afferent activity to somatosensory pathways. In: Iggo A (ed) Somatosensory system. Springer, Berlin Heidelberg New York, pp 151–206 (Handbook of sensory physiology, vol II)

Schmidt RF (1978) Fundamentals of neurophysiology, 2nd edn. Springer, Berlin Heidelberg New York

Schmidt RF, Thews G (eds) (1983) Human physiology. Springer, Berlin Heidelberg New York

Scoville WB, Milner B (1957) Loss of recent memory after bilateral hippocampal lesion. J Neurol Neurosurg Psychiatry 20: 11–21

Shallice T, Warrington EK (1970) Independent functioning of verbal memory stores: a neuropsychological study. Q J Exp Psychol 22: 261–273

Shepherd GM (1972) The neuron doctrine: a revision of functional concepts. Yale J Biol Med 45: 584–599

Shepherd GM (1972) Synaptic organization of the mammalian olfactory bulb. Physiol Rev 52: 864–917

Shepherd GM (1988) Neurobiology, 2nd edn. Oxford University Press, Oxford

Sherrington CS (1906) The integrative action of the nervous system. Yale University Press, New Haven, Connecticut

Sigworth FJ, Neher E (1980) Single Na$^+$ channel currents observed in cultured rat muscle cells. Nature 287: 447–449

Singer SJ, Nicolson GL (1972) The fluid mosaic model of the structure of cell membranes. Science 175: 720–731

Speidel CC (1922) Further comparative studies in other fishes of cells that are homologous to the large irregular glandular cells in the spinal cord of the skates. J Comp Neurol 34: 303–317

Sperry RW (1951) Mechanisms of neural maturation. In: Stevens SS (ed) Handbook of experimental psychology. Wiley, New York, pp 236–280

Stevens SS (1961) The psychophysics of sensory function. In: Rosenblith WA (ed) Sensory communication. MIT Press, Cambridge, Massachusetts

Strausfeld NJ (1976) Atlas of an insect brain. Springer, Berlin Heidelberg New York

Szentágothai J (1975) The "module concept" in cerebral cortex architecture. Brain Res 95: 475–496

Takeuchi A, Takeuchi N (1959) Active-phase of frog's end-plate potential. J Neurophysiol 22: 395–411

Talbot WH, Darian-Smith I, Kornhuber HH, Mountcastle VB (1968) The sense of flutter-vibration: comparison of the human capacity with response patterns of mechanoreceptive afferents from the monkey hand. J Neurophysiol 31: 301–334

Tasaki I (1939) The electrosaltatory transmission of the nerve impulse and the effect of narcosis upon the nerve fibre. Am J Physiol 127: 211–227

Van Essen DC (1979) Visual areas of the mammalian cerebral cortex. Annu Rev Neurosci 2: 227–263

Whittaker VB, Essman WB, Dowe GHC (1972) The isolation of pure cholinergic synaptic vesicles from the electric organs of elasmobranch fish of the family Tarpedinida. Biochem J 128: 833–846

Wiesel TN, Hubel DH (1974) Ordered arrangement of orientation columns in monkeys lacking visual experience. J Comp Neurol 158: 307–318

Willis WD, Grossman RG (1973) Medical neurobiology. CV Mosby, ST Louis

Yoon M (1971) Reorganization of retinotectal projection following surgical operation on the optic tectum in goldfish. Exp Neurol 33: 395–411

Zeki SM (1975) The functional organization of projections from striate to pre-striate visual cortex in the rhesus monkey. Cold Spring Harbor Symp Quant Biol 40: 591–600

Zola-Morgan S, Squire LR, Amoral DG (1986) Human amnesia and the medial temporal region: enduring memory impairment following a bilateral lesion limited to field CA1 of the hippocampus. J Neurosci 6: 2950–2967

Further Reading

Chapter 1

Brodal A (1981) Neurological anatomy in relation to clinical medicine, 3rd edn. Oxford University Press, Oxford

Bullock TH, Orkand R, Grinnell A (1977) Introduction to nervous systems. Chap 10: Survey of animal groups. WH Freeman, San Francisco

Nauta WJH, Fiertag M (1986) Fundamental neuroanatomy. WH Freeman, New York

Peters A, Palay SL, Webster H deF (1976) The fine structure of the nervous system: the neurons and supporting cells. WB Saunders, Philadelphia

Chapters 2, 3, 4

Cole KS (1968) Membranes, ions and impulses. University of California Press, Berkeley

Hille B (1977) Ionic basis of resting and action potentials. In: Kandel ER (ed) Handbook of physiology, section 1. The nervous system, vol. I. Cellular biology of neurons. American Physiological Society, Bethesda, Maryland, pp 99– 136

Hille B (1984) Ionic channels of excitable membranes. Sinauer Associates Inc, Sunderland, Massachusetts

Hodgkin AL (1964) The conduction of the nervous impulse. Liverpool University Press, Liverpool

Hubbard JI, Llínas R, Quastel DM (1969) Electrophysiological analysis of synaptic transmission. Edward Arnold, London

Katz B (1966) Nerve, muscle, and synapse. McGraw-Hill, New York

Sakmann B, Neher E (eds) Single channel recording. Plenum Press, New York

Chapters 5, 6, 7, 8

Eccles JC (1964) The physiology of synapses. Springer, Berlin Heidelberg New York

Heuser JE, Reese TS (1977) Structure of the synapse. In: Kandel ER (ed) Handbook of physiology, section 1. The nervous system, vol I. Cellular biology of neurons. American Physiological Society, Bethesda, Maryland, pp 261–294

Hökfelt T, Johansson O, Ljungdahl A, Lundberg JM, Schultzberg M (1980) Peptidergic neurones. Nature 284: 515–521

Hubbard JI, Llínas R, Quastel DM (1969) Electrophysiological analysis of synaptic transmission. Edward Arnold, London

Katz B (1966) Nerve, muscle, and synapse. McGraw-Hill, New York

Katz B (1969) The release of neural transmitter substances. Liverpool University Press, Liverpool

Llínas R (1982) Calcium in synaptic transmission. Sci Am 247: 56–65

Martin AR (1977) Junctional transmission. II: Presynaptic mechanisms. In: Kandel ER (ed) Handbook of physiology, section 1. The nervous system, vol I. Cellular biology of neurons. American Physiological Society, Bethesda, Maryland, pp 329–355

Nicoll RA (1982) Neurotransmitters can say more than just "yes" and "no". Trends Neurosci 5: 369–373

Nieuwenhuys R (1985) Chemoarchitecture of the brain. Springer, Berlin Heidelberg New York Tokyo

Ochs S (1972) Fast transport of material in mammalian nerve fibers. Science 176: 252–260

Schmidt RF (1971) Presynaptic inhibition in the vertebrate central nervous system. Ergeb Physiol 63: 20–101

Schwartz JH (1980) The transport of substances in nerve cells. Sci Am 242: 122–135

Takeuchi A (1977) Junctional transmission. I: Postsynaptic mechanisms. In: Kandel ER (ed) Handbook of physiology, section 1. The nervous system, vol I. Cellular biology of neurons. American Physiological Society, Bethesda, Maryland, pp 295–327

Chapters 9, 10, 11

Bodian D (1962) The generalized vertebrate neuron. Science 137: 323–326

Bullock, TH (1959) Neuron doctrine and electrophysiology. Science 129: 997–1002

Brown AG (1981) Organization in the spinal cord: the anatomy and physiology of identified neurones. Springer, Berlin Heidelberg New York

Burke RE, Rudomin P (1977) Spinal neurons and synapses. In: Kandel ER (ed) Handbook of physiology, section 1. The nervous system, vol I. Cellular biology of neurons. American Physiological Society, Bethesda, Maryland, pp 877–944

Eccles JC (1964) The physiology of synapses. Springer, Berlin Heidelberg New York

Shepherd, GM (1972) The neuron doctrine: a revision of functional concepts. Yale J Biol Med 45: 584–599

Chapter 12

Dowling JE, Boycott BB (1967) Organization of the primate retina: electron microscopy. Proc R Soc Lond [Biol] 166: 80–111

Dowling JE (1979) Information processing by local circuits: the vertebrate retina as a model system. In: Schmitt FO, Worden FG (eds) The neurosciences, fourth study program. MIT Press, Cambridge, Massachusetts, pp 163–181

Matthews PBC (1972) Mammalian muscle receptors and their central actions. Edward Arnold, London

Matthews PBC (1981) Evolving views on the internal operation and functional role of the muscle spindle. J Physiol (Lond) 320: 1–30

O'Brien DF (1982) The chemistry of vision. Science 218: 961–966

Stevens SS (1961) The psychophysics of sensory function. In: Rosenblith WA (ed) Sensory communication. MIT Press, Cambridge, Massachusetts, pp 1–33

Chapters 13, 14, 15

Armstrong DM (1988) The supraspinal control of locomotion. J Physiol (Lond) 405: 1–37

Barlow HB, Mollon JD (eds) (1982) The senses. Cambridge University Press, Cambridge

Brodal A (1981) Neurological anatomy in relation to clinical medicine, 3rd edn. Oxford University Press, Oxford

Brown AG (1981) Organization in the spinal cord: the anatomy and physiology of identified neurones. Springer, Berlin Heidelberg New York

Burke RE, Rudomin P (1977) Spinal neurons and synapses. In: Kandel ER (ed) Handbook of physiology, section I. The nervous system, vol 1. Cellular biology of neurons American Physiological Society, Bethesda, Maryland, pp 877–944

Cowey A (1979) Cortical maps and visual perception. The Grindley Memorial Lecture. Q J Exp Psychol 31: 1–17

Eccles JC, Ito M, Szentágothai J (1967) The cerebellum as a neuronal machine. Springer, Berlin Heidelberg New York

Evarts EV (1981) Role of motor cortex in voluntary movements in primates. In: Brooks VB (ed) Handbook of physiology, section 1. The nervous system, vol II. Motor control, part 2. American Physiological Society, Bethesda, Maryland, pp 1082–1120

Gordon G (1973) The concept of relay nuclei. In: Iggo A (ed) Somatosensory system. (Handbook of sensory physiology, vol II) Springer, Berlin Heidelberg New York, pp 137–150

Grillner S (1981) Control of locomotion in bipeds, tetrapods and fish. In: Brooks VB (ed) Handbook of physiology, section 1. The nervous system, vol II. Motor control, part 2. American Physiological Society, Bethesda, Maryland, pp 1179–1236

Hubel DH, Wiesel TN (1977) Functional architecture of macaque monkey visual cortex. Proc R Soc Lond [Biol] 198: 1–59

Ito M (1984) The cerebellum and neural control. Raven Press, New York

Lemon R (1988) The output map of the primate motor cortex. Trends Neurosci 11: 501–506

Maunsell JHR, Newsome WT (1987) Visual processing in the monkey extrastriate cortex. Annu Rev Neurosci 10: 363–401

Merzenich MM, Kaas JH (1980) Principles of organization of sensory-perceptual systems in mammals. Prog Psychobiol Physiol Psychol 9: 1–42

Mountcastle VB (1978) An organizing principle for cerebral function: the unit module and the distributed system. In: Edelman GM, Mountcastle VB (eds) The mindful brain: cortical organization and the group-selection theory of higher brain function. MIT Press, Cambridge, Massachusetts

Phillips CG, Porter R (1977) Corticospinal neurones: their role in movement. Academic Press, London

Wiesendanger M (1981) Organization of secondary motor areas of cerebral cortex. In: Brooks VB (ed) Handbook of physiology, section 1. The nervous system, vol II. Motor control, part 2. American Physiological Society, Bethesda Maryland, pp 1121–1147

Zeki S (1981) The mapping of visual functions in the cerebral cortex. In: Katsuki Y, Norgren R, Sato M (eds) Brain mechanisms of sensation. Wiley, Chichester, pp 105–128

Chapter 16

Björklund A, Lindvall O (1986) Catecholaminergic brain stem regulatory systems. In: Bloom FE (ed) Handbook of physiology, section 1. The nervous system, vol IV. Intrinsic regulatory systems of the brain. American Physiological Society, Bethesda, Maryland, pp 155–235

Foote SL, Bloom FE, Aston-Jones G (1983) Nucleus locus ceruleus: new evidence of anatomical and physiological specificity. Physiol Rev 63: 844–914

Hobson JA, Steriade M (1986) Neuronal basis of behavioural state control. In: Bloom FE (ed) Handbook of physiology, section 1. The nervous system, vol IV. Intrinsic regulatory systems of the brain. American Physiological Society, Bethesda, Maryland, pp 701–823

Sagar SM, Martin JB (1986) Hypothalamo-hypophysiotropic peptide systems. In: Bloom FE (ed) Handbook of physiology, section 1. The nervous system, vol IV. Intrinsic regulatory systems of the brain. American Physiological Society, Bethesda, Maryland, pp 413–462

Willis WD (1982) Control of nociceptive transmission in the spinal cord. Progress in sensory Physiology, vol 3. Springer, Berlin Heidelberg New York

Chapters 17, 18

Hopkins W, Brown MC (1984) Development of nerve cells and their connections. Cambridge University Press, Cambridge

Learning, Memory (1988) Trends Neurosci 11, No 4

Movshon JA, Van Sluyters RC (1981) Visual neural development. Annu Rev Psychol 32: 477–522

Purves D, Lichtman J (1985) Principles of neural development. Sinauer Associates Inc, Sunderland, Massachusetts

Ribchester RR (1986) Molecule, nerve and embryo. Blackie, London

Teyler TJ, DiScenna P (1987) Long-term potentiation. Annu Rev Neurosci 10: 131–161

Wiesel TN (1982) The postnatal development of the visual cortex and the influence of environment. Nature 299: 583–592

Subject Index

Acetylcholine (ACh) 57, 64–5, 67, 68, 71, 73–6, 83, 91, 93–5, 102, 237–9
Action potential 45
  antidromic 108
  changes in internal ion concentrations due to 42
  events taking place 37
  ionic basis of 29–37
  prediction of 37
Adaptive behaviour 217
Adenosine triphosphate (ATP) 22, 103, 104
Adenylate cyclase 103, 104
Adrenaline 76
Afferent fibres. *See* Group Ia; Group Ib; Group II; Hair follicle afferent fibres; Nociceptive afferent fibres; Pacinian corpuscle afferent fibres
After-hyperpolarization (AHP) 111–12
Alpha-adrenergic receptor 92
Alpha helix proteins 16
Alpha-motoneurons 96, 107, 118, 157, 210
Alzheimer's disease 245
Amacrine cells 146
Amino acids 58, 76
Amnesia 245
Amphibian lumbar spinal cord 238
Analgesia
  opiate 226–7
  stimulus-produced 226
Angiotensin II 216
Antidromic action potential 108
Antidromic excitation 107
Aplysia 248, 249
Arousal 220
Ascending reticular activating system 220
Ascending sensory messages 191
Aspartate 76, 83
Astrocytes 9
Auditory pathways 181
  anatomical organization of 181

Avogadro's Law 19
Axo-axonic synapse 99
Axon hillock region of motoneuron 108, 119
  see also Initial Segment of axon
Axonal transport 89–90
Axons
  effect on conduction velocity of nerve impulses 46–7
  extracellular recording from single 49–50
  in nerve impulses 49
  myelinated 49
  potential recorded externally from 50

Basal ganglia 195
Basket cells 171
Behavioural state control 218
Behavioural states 217–20
Beta-adrenergic receptor 105
Biogenic amines 76
Blood-CSF barrier 11
Body temperature regulation 222–4
Boyle's Law 19
Brain maps 211–12
Brain stem 191
  electrical stimulation 226
  noradrenergic system 222

Cat lumbosacral spinal cord 129
Cat somatosensory system 200
Cat spinal cord motoneurons 119
Catecholamines 76
Caudate nucleus 195
Cell death 238
Cell differentiation 231–3
Cell division 231
Cell membrane
  distribution of major ions across 15
  electrically excitable 37–41

passive electrical properties 45–9
  proteins of 16
  structure of 15–18
Cell migration 231–3
Cell proliferation 231, 234–7
Central excitatory synapses 95–7
Central nervous system 7
  denervation 240–2
Central pattern generators (CPGs) 208
Centrally programmed movements 207–8
Centrifugal control
  sense organs 155–7
  sensory systems 207
Cerebellar cortex 169, 170
  afferent nerve supply to 170
  circuitry operation 171
  module of 170–3
Cerebellar folium 171, 173
Cerebellum
  in control of spinal locomotor apparatus 208
  long-term depression in 251–2
  modular design 169–73
  structure of 169
  zones of 194
Cerebral cortex 240
  afferent motor pathways 183–6
  columnar organization of 174
  major divisions of 184
  modular organization in 170–5
  supramotor areas of 210–11
  see also Motor cortex; Somatosensory cortex; Visual cortex
Cerebrocerebellum 194
Cerebrospinal fluid (CSF) 10–11
Cerebrum, structure of 169
Charles's Law 19
Chemically gated channels, voltage-dependent 101–2
Chemically gated ion channels 93–103
Chloride ions, distribution across membrane 24
Cholecystokinin 84